Physical
Therapist's
Clinical
Companion

Physical Therapist's Clinical Companion

Springhouse Corporation ■ Springhouse, Pennsylvania

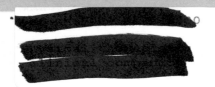

STAFF

Vice President
Matthew Cahill

Publisher
Judith A. Schilling McCann, RN, MSN

Clinical Manager
Joan M. Robinson, RN, MSN, CCRN

Creative Director
Jake Smith

Design Director
John Hubbard

Executive Editor
H. Nancy Holmes

Clinical Editors
Joanne Bartelmo, RN, MSN; Jill M. Curry, RN, BSN, CCRN; Maryann Foley, RN, BSN

Editor
Peter H. Johnson

Copy Editors
Brenna H. Mayer (manager), Priscilla DeWitt, Jaime Stockslager, Pamela Wingrod

Designers
Arlene Putterman (associate design director), Kate Nichols (book designer), Linda Franklin (project manager), Joseph John Clark, Donna S. Morris, Jeff Sklarow

Electronic Production Services
Diane Paluba (manager), Joy Rossi Biletz (technician)

Manufacturing
Deborah Meiris (director), Patricia K. Dorshaw (manager), Otto Mezei (book production manager)

Editorial and Design Assistants
Tom Hasenmayer, Beverly Lane, Liz Schaeffer

Indexer
Ellen Brennan

Printed in the United States of America.

PTCC- D N O S A J J M A M
03 02 01 00   10 9 8 7 6 5 4 3 2 1

A member of the Reed Elsevier plc group

Library of Congress Cataloging-in-Publication Data

Phywical therapist's clinical companion
   p.; cm.
   Includes bibliographical references and index.
   1. Physical therapy — Handbooks, manuals, etc.
   I. Springhouse Corporation.
   [DNLM: 1. Physical therapy — Handbooks. 2. Movement Disorders — rehabilitation — Handbooks. WB 39 P5774 2000]
RM701 .P475 2000
615.8′2 — dc21   99-052570
ISBN 1-58255-004-2 (alk, paper)

Contents

15 Medications

Appendices

Contributors and consultants

Elaine L. Bukowski, PT, MS, (D) ABDA
Associate Professor of Physical Therapy
Richard Stockton College of New Jersey
Pomona

Susan Christie, PT, BS, ATP
Supervisor, Assistive Technology Center
Bryn Mawr Rehab
Malvern, Pa.

Christine Conroy, PT, BS, MHS
Assistant Professor of Physical Therapy
Midwestern University
Downers Grove, Ill.

Gary Corso, PT, MS, OCS
Physical Therapist
Corso Physical Therapy, P.C.
Corso Rehabilitation and P.T. Associates, P.C.
Hauppauge, N.Y.
Adjunct Professor of Physical Therapy
Touro College
Bay Shore, N.Y.

Matthew Durst, PT, MA
Physical Therapist
Rehabilitation Hospital of Connecticut
Hartford

Lisa L. Dutton, PT, MS
Physical Therapy Program Director
University of Findlay (Ohio)

Jane M. Eason, PT, PhD
Assistant Professor of Physical Therapy
Louisiana State University Medical Center
New Orleans

Cathy Ellis, PT, BS, NDT
Director, Inpatient Physical Therapy,
Occupational Therapy, Training and
Vocational Rehabilitation
National Rehabilitation Hospital
Washington, D.C.

Christian Evans, PT, PhD
Physical Therapist
Westlake Community Hospital
Melrose Park, Ill.
Lecturer
Midwestern University
Downers Grove, Ill.

Erica Fletcher, PT, BS
Physical Therapist
Body Rebuilders Physical Therapy
Graduate Hospital
Bala Cynwyd, Pa.

Sharon Gallagher, PT, BS
Home Health Physical Therapist
Deaconess Home Health
St. Louis

Noel M. Goodstadt, MPT
Physical Therapist
Nova Care, Inc.
Huntingdon Valley, Pa.

Charles J. Gulas, PT, BAGCS, CWS
Clinical Director of Physical Therapy
Rehab Choice Inc.
St. Charles, Mo.

JoAnne L. Kanas, PT, BS, CPO
Administrator and Director of Clinical
Services
Atlantic Prosthetic & Orthotic Services,
Inc.
Smithville, N.J.

Marcia A. Kiernan, PT, BS
Physical Therapist
Rhode Island Hospital
Providence

Pamela C. Martin, MSPT, MPH
Assistant Professor of Physical Therapy
University of South Alabama
Mobile

Kathleen Nusbickel, PT, BS
Home Care Physical Therapist
Ostrow and Turner Physical Therapy
  Associates, P.C.
Exton, Pa.

E. Anne Rura, PT, MEd, CCI
Instructor of Physical Therapy
Howard University
Washington, D.C.

Sheila Sage, MPT
Physical Therapy Clinical Supervisor
National Rehabilitation Hospital
Washington, D.C.

Constance L. Seymour, RN, BSN
Nurse Epidemiologist
Consultant
Hatboro, Pa.

Mary Swagler, PT, BS
Physical Therapist
Hamilton (Ohio) City Schools

Pamela Unger, PT, CWS
Clinical Director and Partner
The Center for Advanced Wound Care
Wyomissing, Pa.

Susan Wainwright, PT, MS
Assistant Professor of Physical Therapy
University of the Sciences in Philadelphia

Jennifer L. Werdell, PT, MS
Physical Therapist
Laurel, Md.

Foreword

With the constant changes in health care legislation, practicing physical therapists and physical therapy students are more than ever aware of the limited time they have to treat their patients. The variety of environments in which physical therapists practice and the broad spectrum of patients' disabilities presents clinician and student with intellectual and clinical challenges. Today's practitioners must be prepared for skilled assessments and swift decision making in order to provide the most beneficial patient interventions in a cost-effective manner.

The *Physical Therapist's Clinical Companion* provides PTs with information of essential clinical relevance so that the therapist has a thorough understanding of a patient's condition and can formulate the most appropriate treatment plan. Its unique feature is its broad-based clinical approach that meets the needs of therapists in diversified clinical settings, such as acute care, hospital rehabilitation centers, and outpatient clinics.

This handy guide is an up-to-date and comprehensive resource for delivering quality physical therapy. Its easy-to-follow approach presents chapters in a logical order. The first three chapters give the reader an overview of current assessment methods geared to orthopedic, cardiovascular, and neurologic evaluations; the causes and further interpretation of assessment findings; and the use of important functional outcome measurement tools. The next two chapters impart an understanding of the value of various diagnostic tests, including the interpretation of ECG readings.

The therapist working in an outpatient setting will be especially interested in the musculoskeletal disorders section of chapter 6; chapter 7 on traumatic injuries; chapter 9 on therapeutic exercise; and chapter 13, which covers the various modalities utilized by the physical therapist.

In addition to the chapter on traumatic injuries, the acute-care physical therapist will find the following chapters invaluable: chapter 8, which deals with cardiac rehabilitation, and chapter 14 on wound care.

Chapters 10, 11, and 12, which discuss gait, selection of prosthetics and orthotics, and the intricacies of wheelchair fit, are extremely important to the therapist in a rehabilitation center.

The text has been enhanced by the addition of chapter 15 on medications, which includes the generic and trade names, indications, adverse reactions, and special considerations for the physical therapist. The therapist usually has to seek out another source for this important information.

The book's unique features are called to the reader's attention by graphic logos. These features include important points for teaching patients, alerts that offer tips and advice for handling unusual clinical situations, and women's health highlights for managing care and promoting health in this special population. Appendices include a guide to skeletal muscles, a review of the Americans with Disabilities Act, the very helpful section of English and Spanish words and phrases, and a list of common abbreviations and acronyms.

Readers will surely find the *Physical Therapist's Clinical Companion* to be an outstanding personal reference that is wide-ranging in content, readily accessible, and easily carried.

H.H. Merrifield, PhD, PT, FACSM
Associate Dean
Chair, Department of Rehabilitation Science
Texas Tech University Health Science Center
Lubbock

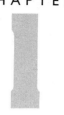

CHAPTER

General assessment

Reviewing the techniques

History

Initial interview

Assessment is done to elicit information about the patient's health status at specific times. A thorough initial assessment can yield baseline information about the physical and psychological aspects of the symptoms that cause the patient to complain. This information helps you determine the current level of function, including how the chief complaint affects the patient's personal and social life. Based on this assessment, the treatment plan you develop will help you analyze the patient's strengths and weaknesses, prioritize problems, and set treatment goals.

Ongoing assessments evaluate the results of the treatment plan and guide needed modifications. This chapter discusses interviewing techniques, assessment of activities of daily living, overall patient health, and a variety of techniques used to evaluate pain and body system function in detail.

A quick initial screening of the patient is the first step in the evaluation process. Developing an effective interviewing technique will help you collect pertinent health history information efficiently. Use the following guidelines to enhance your interviewing skills.

Be prepared

• Before the interview, review all available information, including current clinical records and previous records, if applicable.
• If possible, ask the patient to fill out a screening profile, providing details about his health history, his current problem, and how the problem impacts his work and personal life.

Provide a pleasant interviewing atmosphere

• Select a quiet, relaxed setting with good lighting, comfortable seating, and privacy to help to lessen anxiety and promote open dialogue, which is important in the assessment process.
• Sit with the patient as you review your present information, including the profile that the patient has provided.
• Make both subjective and objective assessments. Listen to the patient's description of the problem and then determine what specific assessments need to be made. Keep the interview informal but professional.

Set the tone and focus

• Encourage the patient to talk about his chief complaint. Allow him enough time to answer questions fully and add his own perceptions.
• Speak clearly and avoid medical jargon.

ALERT Be sure the patient understands you, especially if he's elderly. If you think he doesn't, ask him to restate the information. If the patient is a child, direct as many questions to him as appropriate. You should rely on the parents for information, though, if the child is very young.

• Pay close attention to the patient's words and actions, interpreting not only what he says but also what he doesn't say.

Choose your words carefully

• Ask open-ended questions to encourage the patient to provide complete and pertinent information. Avoid "yes-or-no" and leading questions.
• Listen carefully to the patient's answers. Use his words in your subsequent questions to encourage him to

elaborate on his signs, symptoms, and other problems.

Take notes

• Avoid documenting everything during the interview but be sure to jot down important information, such as dates, times, and key words or phrases. Use these later to help you recall the complete history for the medical record.

Assessing overall health

For a quick look at your patient's overall health, ask these questions:
• How has your health been during this past year?
• Has your weight changed? Do your clothes, rings, and shoes fit?
• Do you have any nonspecific symptoms, such as weakness, fatigue, night sweats, or fever?
• Can you keep up with normal daily activities?
• Can you perform your occupational or job-related activities?
• Have you had any unusual symptoms or problems recently?
• What prescription and over-the-counter drugs do you take?

Assessing activities of daily living

For a comprehensive look at your patient's functional status, determine the level of his daily living skills. (See *Assessing ADLs quickly*, page 4.) The information you gather will help you judge the patient's independence level, the level of assistance required, and whether adaptive devices will increase his independence level in a reasonable amount of time. Start by asking general questions and

progress to more specific questions, such as the following, as appropriate.

Feeding

• Can you feed yourself from a table or tray with eating utensils? Can you cut food such as meat? Are you able to pour liquid from an open container?
• Does using a spork or other feeding aid help you to feed yourself in a reasonable amount of time?
• Can you feed yourself if assisted by another person, for example, if you're helped to raise a cup to your mouth or to cut food?
• Can you feed yourself without help from another person?

Dressing the upper body

• Can you get your clothes out of drawers and closets and robe and disrobe your upper body unassisted? Can you handle items such as pullovers, bras, slips, and front-opening shirts and blouses with fasteners, such as buttons, hooks, snaps, and zippers?
• If your clothes are laid out or handed to you, can you dress and undress your upper body without help even if it takes a little more time, or do you need some help with fasteners, such as buttons, hooks, snaps, and zippers? Have you tried using aids, such as button hooks, dressing hooks, reachers, and zipper pulls?
• Do you need help putting on your blouse, shirt, or sweater because you are hampered by weakness, pain, or limited range of motion?
• Can you only dress your upper body with help from another person?

Dressing the lower body

• Can you put on undergarments, slacks, socks, stockings, and shoes by yourself? Can you tie your shoelaces?
• Can you put on undergarments, slacks, socks, stockings, and shoes by

---

ASSESSING A.D.L.S QUICKLY

Asking these questions will give you a quick overview of your patient's mobility and how current problems have affected his ability to perform activities of daily living (ADLs).

At work
• How has your problem affected your ability to work?
• What do you normally do that you can't do now?

At home
• What difficulties are you having at home since the problem began?
• Can you get up from a chair independently? When you're lying in bed, can you sit up and then stand up without any help?
• What problems are you having with dressing? Are fasteners a problem?
• What area of personal care is a problem? Can you bathe and take care of your toileting needs independently? Is eating a problem?
• Can you handle homemaking jobs, such as cooking, cleaning, doing laundry, and yard work independently?
• Are there other things you find difficult to do at home?

On the move
• What is your usual way of getting around? Independent walking? Assisted walking? Wheelchair? Powered wheelchair? Has this changed in the past year?
• How far can you walk or wheel before having to stop? Has this changed recently?
• Are stairs, curbs, or uneven surfaces a problem?
• Do you have other problems in moving about?

At leisure
• Are you able to enjoy your free time despite this problem?
• What is this problem preventing you from doing that you really enjoy?

---

yourself if they are laid out for you or handed to you? Do you use dressing aids such as long-handled reachers? Do you avoid shoes that have laces or buckles? Do you use elastic laces or Velcro shoe closures by yourself?
• Does someone help you to put on undergarments, slacks, socks, stockings, or shoes?
• Do you depend on another person to dress your lower body?

Grooming

• Can you comb, brush, and shampoo your hair; shave; apply makeup; clean your teeth or dentures; and care for your nails unassisted and without any special effort?

• Do you use special methods or devices to help with grooming? (These may include long-handled combs or brushes, suction brushes for cleaning nails or dentures, adapted shaving equipment, or keys for rolling toothpaste tubes.) Can you complete your grooming alone if someone places what you need within reach?
• Does someone help you to brush or shampoo your hair, shave, apply makeup, clean your teeth or dentures, or perform nail care?
• Do you depend on someone else entirely for your grooming needs?

Care of perineum and clothing at the toilet

• Can you go to the bathroom by yourself, including managing your clothes, wiping yourself, and placing sanitary napkins or tampons (if applicable)?
• Can you manage your clothing at the toilet and wipe yourself independently (but with difficulty), or do you use aids such as an extended reacher for wiping yourself?
• Does someone help you with your clothing at the toilet or assist you with wiping yourself or placing sanitary napkins or tampons (if applicable)?
• Do you require someone else to manage your clothes at the toilet for you, wipe you, or place sanitary napkins or tampons (if applicable)?

Washing and bathing

• Are you able to wash and dry your entire body by yourself, including your back and feet? Are you able to turn water faucets?
• Do you use bathing aids such as long-handled bath brushes or sponges? Do you have trouble reaching some parts of your body while bathing or drying but can still do it without help?
• Do you bathe and dry most parts of your body by yourself and then have someone help you with the rest?
• Does someone else bathe you?

Exercise and sleep

• Do you have a special exercise program? What is it? How long have you been following it? How do you feel after exercising?
• How many hours do you sleep each day? When? Do you feel rested afterward?
• Do you fall asleep easily?
• Do you take any drugs or do anything special to help you fall asleep?

• Do you have sleepy spells during the day? When?
• Do you take naps routinely?
• Have you ever been diagnosed with any sleep disorders, such as narcolepsy and sleep apnea?

Vocation

• Do you work full-time in your usual occupation? Are you a full-time homemaker who requires no assistance? Are you retired for a reason that isn't medical?
• Are you unable to work full-time either inside or outside the home?

Recreation

• What do you do when you aren't working?
• What kind of unpaid work do you do for enjoyment?
• How much leisure time do you have?
• Are you satisfied with what you can do in your leisure time?
• How do your weekends differ from your weekdays?

Tobacco, alcohol, and drug use

• Do you use tobacco? If so, what kind? How much do you use each day? Each week? For how long have you used it? Have you ever tried to stop?
• Do you drink any alcoholic beverages? If so, what kind?
• How much alcohol do you drink each day? Each week? What time of day do you usually drink?
• Do you feel dependent on coffee, tea, or soft drinks? How much of these beverages do you drink in an average day?
• Do you use any drugs not prescribed by a primary care provider, such as marijuana, sleeping pills, and tranquilizers?

Mobility

Supine to sitting

• When lying on your back, can you sit up without having to use your arms or rolling to one side? Can you sit up easily?

• Do you use your arms to help you sit up, or do you roll to the side before sitting up? Do you have to try several times before sitting up?

• Do you need someone to help you to sit up?

• Are you able to sit up?

Sitting to standing

• Can you stand up from sitting in a chair without using your arms?

• Do you need to use your arms to help you stand up, or do you need to try several times?

• Does someone need to help you stand up out of a chair?

• Do you depend on someone else entirely to get you out of a chair?

Toilet transfers

• Can you get on and off the toilet easily and without using your arms?

• Do you need to use your arms to help you get on and off the toilet, or do you use helps such as elevated toilet seats or grab bars?

• Do you need someone to help you get on and off the toilet?

• Are you unable to use the toilet?

Tub and shower transfers

• Can you get in and out of a tub or shower easily and safely?

• Can you get in and out of a tub or shower with the help of grab bars or a special seat or lift?

• Does someone need to help you get in and out of the tub or shower?

• Are you unable to get in and out of the tub or shower?

Automobile transfers

• Can you get in and out of a car easily, and can you open and close the door by yourself?

• Can you get in and out of a car by yourself if you use aids such as grab bars?

• Do you need someone to help you get in and out of a car?

• Are you unable to get in and out of a car even with assistance?

Walking on level ground

• Can you walk two blocks without using the help of a cane, crutches, modified shoes, or a walker?

• Do you need a cane, crutches, modified shoes, or walker to walk two blocks?

• Can you walk one block with assistance?

• Are you unable to walk one block even with assistance?

Walking outdoors

• Can you walk outdoors for at least two blocks without having to avoid uneven terrain, such as grass, sand, gravel, curbs, ramps, or hills?

• Do you try to avoid uneven ground? Do you use a crutch or cane for safety or balancing only when outdoors?

• Do you have to use crutches or a cane to walk at least two blocks on uneven ground?

• Are you unable to walk on any kind of uneven surface?

Climbing up and down stairs

• Can you go up and down at least five steps safely without using a handrail or other support?

• Can you go up and down at least five steps if you use a handrail, a cane, or crutches, or if you go one step at a time?

• Do you need someone to help you climb at least five steps?

• Are you unable to climb at least five steps even with help?

Wheelchair

• Can you push your wheelchair without help for 10 yards? Can you turn corners and get close to a bed, table, and toilet?
• Do you use a motorized wheelchair?
• Do you need someone to help you steer your wheelchair around corners or to help you position it?
• Are you unable to push your wheelchair 10 yards?

Cardiovascular examination

Counting respirations

To determine a patient's respiratory rate, you should count the number of respirations in 60 seconds. A rate of 14 to 20 breaths/minute is normal for an adult. (If the patient knows you're counting how often he breathes, he may subconsciously alter the rate. To avoid this, take his respirations while you are taking his pulse.)

You should observe the depth of the patient's respirations by watching his chest rise and fall. Is his breathing shallow, moderate, or deep? You should also observe the rhythm and symmetry of his chest wall as it expands during inspiration and relaxes during expiration. Be aware that skeletal deformity, broken ribs, and collapsed lung tissue can cause unequal chest expansion.

The use of accessory muscles can enhance lung expansion when oxygenation drops. Patients with chronic obstructive pulmonary disease or respiratory distress may use abdominal muscles and neck muscles, including the sternocleidomastoid, for breathing. Normal respirations are regular, quiet, and easy.

Measuring blood pressure

When you assess your patient's blood pressure, you're measuring the fluctuating force that blood exerts against arterial walls as the heart contracts and relaxes. To measure accurately, perform the following steps.

Applying the cuff and stethoscope

• To obtain a reading in an arm (the most common measurement site), wrap the sphygmomanometer cuff snugly around the upper arm above the antecubital area (the inner aspect of the elbow), with the cuff bladder centered over the brachial artery.

ALERT Avoid wrapping the cuff too loosely; this can result in a false high reading. Avoid wrapping the cuff too tightly as well; this can result in a false low reading.
• Most cuffs have arrow marks that should be placed over the brachial artery. Be sure to use the proper size cuff for the patient.

ALERT When taking an infant's or child's blood pressure, be sure to use the appropriate size cuff. Because blood pressure may be inaudible in children under age 2, consider using an electronic stethoscope to get a more accurate measurement.
• You should keep the mercury manometer at eye level; if the sphygmomanometer has an aneroid gauge, place it level with the patient's arm. You can keep the patient's arm level with the heart by placing it on a table or chair arm or by supporting it with your hand. Rest a recumbent patient's arm at his side. You shouldn't use the patient's muscle strength to hold up the arm because tension from the muscle contraction can ele-

vate systolic pressure and distort your results.

• Next, palpate the brachial pulse just below and slightly medial to the antecubital area. Then you should place the earpieces of the stethoscope in your ears and position the stethoscope head over the brachial artery just distal to the cuff or slightly beneath it, as shown below.

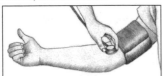

Generally, you'll use the easy-to-handle, flat diaphragm to auscultate the pulse. However, you may need to use the bell of the stethoscope if the patient has a diminished or hard-to-locate pulse because the bell detects the low-pitched sound of arterial blood flow more effectively.

Obtaining the blood pressure reading

• Watching the manometer, pump the bulb until the mercury column or aneroid gauge reaches approximately 20 mm Hg above the point at which the pulse disappeared. Then slowly open the air valve and watch the mercury drop or the gauge needle descend. Release the pressure at a rate of about 3 mm Hg per second, and listen for pulse sounds (Korotkoff's sounds). These sounds, which determine the blood pressure measurement, are classified as follows:

Phase I
Onset of clear, faint tapping, with intensity that increases to a louder tap

Phase II
Tapping that changes to a soft, swishing sound

Phase III
Return of clear, crisp tapping sound

Phase IV (first diastolic sound)
Sound that becomes muffled and takes on a blowing quality

Phase V (second diastolic sound)
Sound that disappears

As soon as you hear blood begin to pulse through the brachial artery, note the reading on the aneroid dial or the mercury column. Reflecting phase I (the first Korotkoff's sound), this sound coincides with the patient's systolic pressure. Continue deflating the cuff, noting the point at which pulsations diminish or become muffled — phase IV (the fourth Korotkoff's sound) — and then disappear — phase V (the fifth Korotkoff's sound). For children and highly active adults, many authorities consider phase IV the most accurate reflection of blood pressure.

The American Heart Association and the World Health Organization recommend documenting phases I, IV, and V. To avoid confusion and make your measurements more useful, follow this format for recording blood pressure: systolic/muffling/disappearance (for example, 120/80/76).

Measuring heart rate

Heart rate reflects the rhythmic expansion of the arteries as the heart ejects blood with each beat. To assess the patient's pulse, you'll note the rhythm, rate, and amplitude (strength) of the beat as you palpate or auscultate over a pulse point. A normal pulse for an adult is between 60 and 100 beats/minute.

Palpate the most accessible site — the radial pulse — with the pads of your index and middle fingers. In a cardiovascular crisis, you may palpate pulses over the femoral and carotid arteries. Because these arteries are larger and closer to the heart, they more directly reflect the heart's activity.

After you locate the pulse, check for a regular rhythm. Next, count the beats over 15 seconds and multiply that sum by 4 to calculate the pulse rate per minute. If the rhythm is irregular, count the pulsations over 60 seconds to determine the rate. When you note an irregular pulse that wasn't present before, notify the patient's primary care provider.

Next, assess the amplitude (or force) of the pulse. Document your findings with a numerical rating from + 3 (for a bounding pulse) to 0 (for an unpalpable pulse). Alternatively, simply describe the force of the pulse as strong, medium, or weak.

Whenever you encounter an irregularity, auscultate the apical pulse and palpate the radial pulse at the same time. Remember, every time you hear a heartbeat you should be able to palpate it. If you can't, document the difference between the apical pulse rate and the radial pulse rate. This difference, known as the pulse deficit, indirectly evaluates the heart's ability to pump blood to peripheral vessels.

Palpating arterial pulses

To palpate arterial pulses, you'll apply gentle pressure with your index and middle fingers.

Carotid pulse

Lightly place your fingers just medial to the trachea and below the jaw angle, as shown at top of next column.

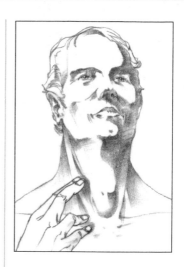

Brachial pulse

Position your fingers medial to the biceps tendon, as shown below.

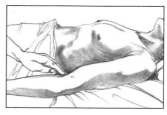

Radial pulse

Apply gentle pressure to the lateral and ventral side of the wrist just below the thumb, as shown below.

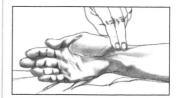

Femoral pulse

Press relatively hard at a point inferior to the inguinal ligament, as shown below. For an obese patient, palpate in the crease of the groin halfway between the pubic bone and the hip bone.

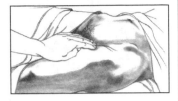

Popliteal pulse

Press firmly against the popliteal fossa at the back of the knee, as shown below.

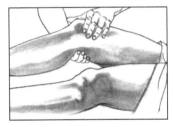

Posterior tibial pulse

Apply pressure behind and slightly below the malleolus of the ankle, as shown below.

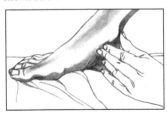

Dorsalis pedis pulse

Place your fingers on the medial dorsum of the foot while the patient points the toes down, as shown at top of next column. In this site the pulse

is difficult to palpate and may seem to be absent in some healthy patients.

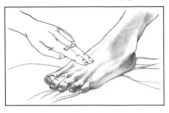

Assessing for edema

Examination of the skin is best performed in a room with good lighting. Start by observing the skin's overall appearance. Inspect and palpate the skin area by focusing on color, texture, turgor, moisture, and temperature. Look for localized areas of bruising, cyanosis, pallor, and erythema. Check for uniformity of color and hypopigmented or hyperpigmented areas.

Inspect and palpate the skin's texture, noting its thickness and mobility. It should be smooth and intact. Skin that isn't intact may indicate local irritation and trauma.

Palpation will also help you evaluate the patient's state of hydration. Dehydration and edema cause poor skin turgor. Overhydration causes skin to appear edematous and spongy. Localized edema can also result from trauma or systemic disease.

Look for edema in dependent parts of the body. For ambulatory patients, this involves inspecting the arms, hands, legs, feet, and ankles. However, if the patient is on bed rest, check for signs in the buttocks and sacral area.

Palpate the suspected area against a bony prominence and record your findings. Describe characteristics of the patient's edema, such as extent and location; type (pitting or nonpitting); degree of pitting (when present); and symmetry (unilateral or symmetrical). The degree of pitting is determined by depth. When recording

edema use the following scale:
0 = none present
+ 1 = 0″ to ¼″ = mild edema as shown below; indentation disappearing rapidly

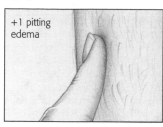

+1 pitting edema

+ 2 = ¼″ to ½″ = moderate pitting; indentation disappearing in 10 to 15 seconds
+ 3 = ½″ to 1″ = severe pitting; indentation disappearing in 1 to 2 minutes
+ 4 = > 1″ = very severe pitting, as shown below; indentation present after 5 minutes

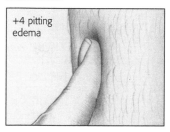

+4 pitting edema

When the skin swells so much that the fluid can't be displaced, it's called brawny edema. This condition, as shown below, resists pitting but makes the skin appear distended.

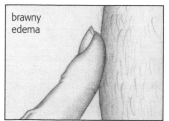

brawny edema

ALERT Keep in mind that poor skin turgor also occurs as a normal result of aging, so pitting edema may not be a reliable indicator of hydration in the elderly.

Palpate the skin for temperature, which can range from warm to cool. Warm skin suggests normal circulation. Be sure to distinguish between generalized and localized coolness and warmth.

Localized skin coolness can result from vasoconstriction associated with cool environments or impaired arterial circulation to a limb. General coolness can result from conditions such as shock or hypothyroidism.

Localized warmth can occur in an area of infection, inflammation, or burn. Generalized warmth occurs with fever or systemic diseases such as hyperthyroidism.

During inspection, you may see variations in the skin's texture and pigmentation. Evaluate all lesions for size, color, shape, and borders. Variations in color within the borders of the lesion, an irregular border, a raised and irregular surface, asymmetrical shape, a firm to hard consistency, and ulceration or crusting of the lesion are all reasons for concern. Question the patient about any changes in size, shape, or color and find out if his primary care provider is aware. It would be appropriate to suggest that the patient visit his primary care provider or for you to telephone the referring primary care provider.

Orthopedic examination

Examination guidelines

• Perform a visual screening of general posture and ease of mobility.

• Perform a range-of-motion screening to determine if a specific goniometric assessment is indicated.
• Test the unaffected side first, unless bilateral movement is necessary.
• Perform active movement before passive movement.
• Test resisted isometric movement.
• Perform painful movements last and, if joint range isn't full, provide support.
• Apply overpressure to joints to determine the end feel of joints when the patient is doing active motion and if the range is normal.
• Repeat movements several times to determine if symptoms increase or decrease or if substitute patterns emerge.
• Determine the quality of movement.
• Perform a muscle screening test to quickly determine a level of strength. If weakness is exhibited, perform a specific manual muscle test to focus on factors such as resistance, positions, grades, and substitutions.
• If testing myotomes (a group of muscles supplied by a single nerve root), each contraction should be held for a minimum of five seconds because myotomal weakness takes time to develop.
• Let the patient know that the examination may initially increase symptoms.

Assessing posture

Posture often reflects the state of muscles and joints. Strong flexible muscles of the trunk, hip, and legs are essential for good posture. The back has three natural curves: the cervical curve, the thoracic curve, and the lumbar curve. Hip, knee, and ankle joints balance the back curves as a person moves, making it possible to maintain good posture in any position.

A systematic approach to postural analysis involves viewing the body's anatomic alignment from different perspectives:
• Perform the assessment with the patient minimally clothed to provide a clear view of the physical contours and landmarks used for reference.
• Instruct the patient to assume a comfortable and relaxed posture.
• Perform a lateral posture assessment with the patient standing. An imaginary vertical line should run from the ear to the shoulder, hip, knee, and ankle, and the three curves of the back should be visible, as shown below.

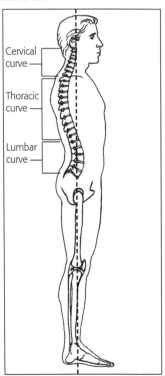

Cervical curve

Thoracic curve

Lumbar curve

 ALERT Be sure to perform the lateral assessment from both sides to detect any rotational abnormalities that might go undetected if observed from only one side.
• Perform a posterior view examination with the patient standing. An imaginary vertical line from the cen-

ter of the head should run down the center of the body to the floor. The head should be centered, not tilted or turned. Shoulders and hips should be level, as shown below.

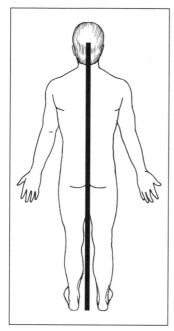

• Perform an anterior view examination with the patient standing. An imaginary vertical line should run from nose to sternum to navel. Shoulders and hips should be level, as shown at top of next column.

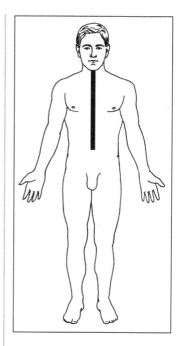

• Perform an examination of posture with the patient seated. Sitting posture should show an erect trunk and head, with the three curves of the back visible. The patient's feet should be flat on the floor, and hips and knees flexed at about 90 degrees, as shown below.

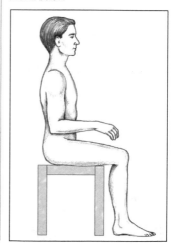

Assessing joint and muscle function

Two techniques most commonly used to evaluate joint and muscle function are goniometry and manual muscle testing. Goniometry uses a light metal or plastic goniometer to measure (in degrees) the amount of motion available at any given joint. Active and passive range of motion (ROM) can be measured. Active motion is produced by the contraction of a muscle or group of muscles moving the joint; passive motion is produced by an outside force such as when you move the joint through its range. Comparing the active and passive ROM, and also comparing that ROM with the comparable ROM seen on the unaffected side, elicits information about the nature of the patient's problem.

Using a goniometer

To ensure accuracy, the center of the goniometer must be placed at the joint line with one arm stabilized along the shaft of the proximal long bone and the other arm along the shaft of the distal bone. After the proximal bone is stabilized, the joint is actively or passively moved through its ROM. The resulting measurement is the joint's ROM.

To measure hip or shoulder range, the stable arm of the goniometer is placed on the trunk's longitudinal plane parallel to the body midline or on the horizontal plane of the shoulder or pelvis. The mobile arm is placed on the femur or humerus as appropriate.

The American Academy of Orthopedic Surgeons supports the system of measurement based on 0 to 180 degrees, with 0 representing the starting, or anatomical, position of the joint.

Measuring joint ROM

• Place the patient in a position of stability — supine, prone, sitting, or standing.
• Expose the joint you are measuring.
• Explain and demonstrate the desired motion.
• Passively perform the motion to relax and eliminate substitute motions.
• Find the joint line. Place the goniometer with its fulcrum on the joint line, keeping the stationary arm parallel to the longitudinal midline of the fixed segment and in line with the appropriate landmark and the moving arm parallel to the longitudinal bone of the moving segment and in line with the appropriate landmark.
• Take readings at the beginning and at the completion of each motion. It's assumed that the beginning measurement is 0. If it's different, record both beginning and end measurements.

Assessing ROM

Assessment of ROM tests the joint's function. To assess joint ROM, ask the patient to move specific joints through the normal ROM. If he can't do so, move the joints through passive ROM.

For a complete summary of ROM testing, see *Joint range of motion*.

Manual muscle testing

Manual muscle testing is a method of assessing the strength of a given muscle or group of muscles. The information obtained can establish a basis for treatment or reeducation. It can determine how functional a person can be, help provide a diagnosis, and define a patient's prognosis. To

(Text continues on page 21.)

JOINT RANGE OF MOTION

The chart below summarizes specific degrees of range of motion and preferred patient testing positions.

Joint motion being tested	Range in degrees	Preferred patient position	Goniometer alignment
Shoulder			
Flexion	0 to 180	Supine with hips and knees flexed	• Fulcrum centered close to the acromion
Extension	180 to 0	Prone with head comfortably positioned	• Stationary arm aligned with the midaxillary line of the thorax
Hyperextension	0 to 45	Prone with head comfortably positioned	• Moving arm aligned with the lateral humerus in line with the lateral epicondyle
Abduction	0 to 180	Supine with hips and knees flexed	• Fulcrum centered close to the anterior aspect of the acromion
Adduction	180 to 0	Supine with hips and knees flexed	• Stationary arm aligned with the midline of the anterior aspect of the sternum • Moving arm aligned with the medial midline of the humerus
Medial rotation	0 to 65	Supine with hips and knees flexed	• Fulcrum centered over the olecranon process
Lateral rotation	0 to 90	Supine with hips and knees flexed	• Stationary arm aligned either parallel to or perpendicular to the floor • Moving arm aligned with the ulna in line with the ulnar styloid
Horizontal adduction	0 to 120	Sitting	• Fulcrum of the goniometer superiority centered on the acromion process through the head of the humerus
Horizontal abduction	0 to 30	Sitting	• Stationary arm aligned on the midline of the shoulder toward the neck • Moving arm aligned with the lateral epicondyle of the humerus
Elbow			
Flexion	0 to 145	Supine with upper limb parallel to the lateral midline of the trunk and forearm in anatomic position	• Fulcrum centered over the lateral epicondyle • Stationary arm aligned with the lateral midline of the humerus in line with the center of the acromial process
Extension	145 to 0	Supine with arm parallel to the lateral midline of the trunk and forearm supinated	• Moving arm aligned with the radius in line with the radial styloid

(continued)

JOINT RANGE OF MOTION (continued)

Joint motion being tested	Range in degrees	Preferred patient position	Goniometer alignment
Radioulnar			
Supination	0 to 90	Sitting	• Fulcrum centered lateral to the ulnar styloid process • Stationary arm aligned parallel to the anterior midline of the humerus • Moving arm aligned across the ventral aspect of the forearm just proximal to the radial and ulnar styloid processes
Pronation	0 to 90	Sitting	• Fulcrum centered lateral to the ulnar styloid process • Stationary arm aligned parallel to the anterior midline of the humerus • Moving arm aligned across the dorsal aspect of the forearm just proximal to the radial and ulnar styloid processes
Wrist			
Flexion	0 to 90	Sitting with forearm supported on the table in pronation	• Fulcrum centered over the triquetrum of the lateral wrist • Stationary arm aligned with the lateral midline of the ulna in line with the olecranon • Moving arm aligned with the lateral midline of the fifth metacarpal
Extension	90 to 0	Sitting with forearm supported on the table in pronation	
Hyperextension	0 to 70	Sitting with forearm supported on the table in pronation	
Abduction	0 to 25	Sitting with elbow flexed and forearm pronated on the table	• Fulcrum centered over the capitate • Stationary arm aligned with the dorsal midline of the forearm in line with the lateral epicondyle • Moving arm aligned with the dorsal midline of the third metacarpal
Adduction	0 to 35	Sitting with elbow flexed to 90 degrees, forearm pronated on the table, and hand supported	
Fingers *Metacarpophalangeal (MCP) joint* Flexion	0 to 90	Sitting with elbow flexed to 90 degrees and forearm supported	• Fulcrum centered over MCP joint's dorsal aspect • Stationary arm over the dorsal midline of the metacarpal • Moving arm over the dorsal midline of the proximal phalanx

JOINT RANGE OF MOTION *(continued)*

Joint motion being tested	Range in degrees	Preferred patient position	Goniometer alignment
Fingers *MCP joint (continued)*			
Extension	90 to 0	Sitting with elbow and shoulder flexed and forearm in midposition between supination and pronation	• Fulcrum centered over the palmar aspect of the MCP joint • Stationary arm over the palmar midline of the metacarpal • Moving arm over the palmar midline of the proximal phalanx
Hyperextension	0 to 30		
Abduction	0 to 20	Sitting with elbow flexed and wrist in a neutral position	• Fulcrum centered over the dorsal aspect of the MCP joint • Stationary arm over the dorsal midline of the metacarpal • Moving arm over the dorsal midline of the proximal phalanx
Adduction	0 to 20	Sitting with elbow flexed, forearm pronated, and wrist in a neutral position	
Proximal interphalangeal (PIP) joints			
Flexion	0 to 120	Sitting with elbow flexed, forearm supported on the table in midposition between supination and pronation, and wrist slightly hyperextended	• Fulcrum centered over the dorsal aspect of the PIP joint • Stationary arm over the dorsal midline of the proximal phalanx • Moving arm over the dorsal midline of the middle phalanx
Extension	120 to 0	Sitting with elbow flexed, forearm supported on the table in midposition between supination and pronation, wrist in anatomic position, and fingers relaxed in flexion	• Fulcrum centered over the palmar aspect of the PIP joint • Stationary arm over the palmar midline of the proximal phalanx • Moving arm over the dorsal midline of the middle phalanx
Hyperextension	0 to 10		
Distal interphalangeal (DIP) joints			
Flexion	0 to 80	Sitting with elbow flexed and forearm in midposition between supination and pronation	• Fulcrum centered over the dorsal aspect of the DIP joint • Stationary arm over the dorsal midline of the middle phalanx • Moving arm over the dorsal midline of the distal phalanx *(continued)*
Extension	80 to 0		
Hyperextension	0 to 10		

JOINT RANGE OF MOTION (continued)

Joint motion being tested	Range in degrees	Preferred patient position	Goniometer alignment
Thumb			
Carpometacarpal (CMC) joint			
Flexion	0 to 15	Sitting with elbow flexed and forearm supinated and supported	• Fulcrum centered over the palmar aspect of the first CMC joint • Stationary arm aligned with ventral midline of the radius aligned with the radial styloid • Moving arm aligned with ventral midline of the first metacarpal
Extension	0 to 70	Sitting with elbow flexed and forearm pronated and supported	• Fulcrum centered over the dorsal aspect of the first CMC joint • Stationary arm aligned with dorsal midline of the radius aligned with the radial styloid • Moving arm aligned with dorsal midline of the first metacarpal
Abduction	0 to 60	Sitting with elbow flexed and forearm pronated and supported	• Fulcrum centered over the lateral aspect of the radial styloid process • Stationary arm aligned with lateral midline of second metacarpal in line with second MCP joint • Moving arm aligned with the lateral midline of the first metacarpal in line with the first MCP joint
Adduction	60 to 0	Sitting with elbow flexed and forearm pronated and supported	
MCP joint			
Flexion	0 to 50	Sitting with elbow flexed and hand supinated and supported	• Fulcrum centered over the dorsal aspect of the MCP joint • Stationary arm over the dorsal midline of the metacarpal • Moving arm aligned with the dorsal midline of the proximal phalanx
Extension	50 to 0		
Hyperextension	0 to 10		
Interphalangeal (IP) joint			
Flexion	0 to 90	Sitting with elbow flexed and forearm supinated and supported	• Fulcrum centered over dorsal surface of IP joint • Stationary arm aligned with the dorsal aspect of the proximal phalanx • Moving arm aligned with the dorsal aspect of the distal phalanx
Extension	90 to 0		
Hyperextension	0 to 90		

JOINT RANGE OF MOTION *(continued)*

Joint motion being tested	Range in degrees	Preferred patient position	Goniometer alignment
Hip			
Flexion	0 to 125	Supine	• Fulcrum centered over the greater trochanter
Extension	125 to 0	Side-lying on the non-test hip with the same hip flexed to 90 degrees	• Stationary arm aligned with the lateral midline of the pelvis • Moving arm aligned with the lateral midline of the femur in line with the lateral epicondyle
Hyperextension	0 to 10	Prone	
Abduction	0 to 45	Supine	• Fulcrum centered over the anterior superior iliac spine (ASIS) • Stationary arm aligned with the opposite ASIS • Moving arm aligned with midline of the patella
Adduction	0 to 20	Supine	
Medial rotation	0 to 45	Supine with knee flexed to 90 degrees over the table edge	• Fulcrum centered over the anterior aspect of the patella • Stationary arm perpendicular or parallel to the floor • Moving arm aligned with the tibial crest at a point midway between the malleoli
Lateral rotation	0 to 45	Supine with knee flexed to 90 degrees over the table edge	
Knee			
Flexion	0 to 130	Supine with hip flexed 90 degrees	• Fulcrum centered over the lateral epicondyle • Stationary arm aligned with the lateral femur in line with the greater trochanter • Moving arm aligned with the lateral fibula in line with the lateral malleolus
Extension	130 to 0	Supine with hip joint extended	
Ankle			
Dorsiflexion	0 to 20	Supine with knee joint flexed 20 to 30 degrees and supported by a pillow	• Fulcrum centered over the lateral malleolus • Stationary arm aligned with the lateral fibula in line with the head of the fibula • Moving arm aligned with the lateral aspect of the base of the fifth metatarsal
Plantar flexion	0 to 45	Supine with hip and knee joints extended and ankle in anatomic position	

(continued)

JOINT RANGE OF MOTION (continued)

Joint motion being tested	Range in degrees	Preferred patient position	Goniometer alignment
Ankle			
(continued)			
Inversion	0 to 30	Supine with hip in anatomic position and ankle relaxed	• Fulcrum centered over the anterior aspect of the ankle midway between malleoli
Eversion	0 to 25	Supine	• Stationary arm aligned with the tibial tuberosity • Moving arm aligned with the anterior midline of the second metatarsal
Toes			
Metatarsophalan-geal (MTP) joint			
Flexion	0 to 40	Any comfortable position with ankle in anatomic position	• Fulcrum centered over the dorsal aspect of the MTP joint • Stationary arm aligned with the dorsal midline of the metatarsal • Moving arm aligned with the proximal phalanx
Extension	40 to 0	Any comfortable position with ankle in anatomic position	• Fulcrum centered over the plantar aspect of the MTP joint • Stationary arm aligned with the plantar midline of the metatarsal • Moving arm aligned with the plantar phalanx
Hyperextension	45 to 0	Any comfortable position with ankle in anatomic position	
PIP joint			
Flexion	0 to 90 (great toe) 0 to 35	Any comfortable position with ankle in anatomic position	• Fulcrum centered over the dorsal aspect of the PIP joint • Stationary arm aligned with the dorsal midline of the proximal phalanx • Moving arm aligned with the phalanx distal to the joint line
Extension	90 to 0 (great toe) 35 to 0	Any comfortable position with ankle in anatomic position	• Fulcrum centered over the plantar aspect of the PIP joint • Stationary arm aligned with the plantar midline of the proximal phalanx • Moving arm aligned with the plantar midline shaft of the distal phalanx of the great toe or over the middle phalanges of the other toes
Hyperextension	Minimal	Any comfortable position with ankle in anatomic position	

JOINT RANGE OF MOTION (continued)

Joint motion being tested	Range in degrees	Preferred patient position	Goniometer alignment
Toes *(continued)* *DIP joint*			
Flexion	0 to 60	Any comfortable position with ankle in anatomic position	• Fulcrum centered over the dorsal aspect of the DIP joint
Extension	60 to 0	Any comfortable position with ankle in anatomic position	• Stationary arm aligned with the dorsal midline of the middle phalanx • Moving arm aligned with the dorsal midline of the distal phalanx
Hyperextension	minimal	Any comfortable position with ankle in anatomic position	
Cervical Spine			
Flexion	0 to 45	Sitting with trunk well supported and neck in anatomic position	• Fulcrum centered over the external auditory meatus
Extension	45 to 0	Sitting with trunk well supported and neck in anatomic position	• Stationary arm aligned perpendicular or parallel to the floor • Moving arm aligned with the base of the nares
Lateral flexion	0 to 60	Sitting with trunk well supported and neck in anatomic position	• Fulcrum centered over the C7 spinous process • Stationary arm aligned perpendicular to the ground • Moving arm aligned with the midline of the occipital protuberance
Rotation	0 to 75	Sitting with trunk well supported and neck in anatomic position	• Fulcrum centered over the center of the cranial aspect of the head • Stationary arm aligned parallel to an imaginary line running through both acromions • Moving arm aligned with the tip of the nose (with tongue depressor placed in the mouth to extend the reference point)

perform a muscle test or screening, follow these steps:

• Explain to the patient the purpose of the test and give directions in understandable terms.

• Place the patient in a comfortable, stable position.

• Ensure that the room is free of distractions so the patient can be fully attentive and provide full effort in contracting the muscles being tested.

• Expose the area to be examined so that it can be accurately palpated and viewed during testing.

MUSCLE TEST GRADING

Grade	Value	Movement
5	Normal	Complete range of motion (ROM) against gravity with maximal resistance
4	Good	Complete ROM against gravity with moderate resistance
3+	Fair +	Complete ROM against gravity with minimal resistance
3	Fair	Complete ROM against gravity
3 –	Fair –	Some but not complete ROM against gravity
2+	Poor +	Initiates motion against gravity
2	Poor	Complete ROM with gravity eliminated
2–	Poor –	Initiates motion if gravity is eliminated
1	Trace	Evidence of slight contractility but no joint motion
0	Zero	No contraction palpated

• Test the muscles on the unaffected side first to give the patient an awareness of the motion desired and the therapist an indication of "normal" strength or tone for comparison.

The ability of the muscle or muscle group to move a joint through a complete test ROM is a measure of muscle strength. The weight of the limb and gravity are factors in the ability to move. Muscle grades are based on the effects of gravity and manual resistance. (See *Muscle test grading*.)

ALERT In grading a muscle it's important to consider the patient's age. A normal rating will feel different in a 5-year-old child, a 20-year-old football player, and a 70-year-old woman. This is a reason to test both affected and unaffected limbs.

• Test muscles first, if possible, in a position where gravity and maximal resistance are factors. If the muscles can't move the joint through the full ROM, then the position should be changed so that the muscle can move the joint with gravity eliminated.

• Palpate the muscle as it's contracting to evaluate its strength and to determine if the substitution of other muscles is involved.

• When providing manual resistance in muscle testing, be consistent in how you apply the resistance. Manual resistance is applied at right angles to the long axis of the limb and at the distal end of the bone without crossing another joint. For example, in testing the biceps of the arm, stabilize the shoulder and place the resisting hand above the wrist to provide resistance as the patient bends his elbow and attempts to touch his shoulder.

• Resistance can be given throughout a motion or can be provided at the end point of contraction with the patient performing an isometric contraction. Isometric contractions are generally stronger than moving contractions.

• In either method, resistance is provided and decreased gradually allowing the patient time to fully contract and then relax the muscle. The resistance to the muscle is provided in a plane opposite to the muscle's rotational pull.

• As weakness is detected, palpate the muscle during contraction to evaluate the quality of contraction. When weakness of one muscle or group of muscles occurs, commonly other muscles are called upon to perform wanted movement. This can be minimized by careful and appropriate positioning, stabilizing the joint, and observation by the therapist.

The following is a sampling of various manual muscle tests.

Deltoid

With your patient's arm fully extended, place one of your hands over his deltoid muscle and the other on his wrist or proximal to the elbow. Ask him to abduct his arm to a horizontal position against your resistance; palpate for deltoid contraction, as shown below.

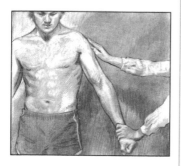

Biceps

With your hand on the patient's wrist, ask him to flex his forearm against your resistance, as shown below. Observe for biceps contraction.

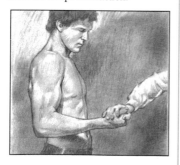

Triceps

Ask the patient to hold his arm midway between flexion and extension. Hold and support his arm at the wrist, as shown below, and then ask him to extend it against your resistance. Observe for triceps contraction.

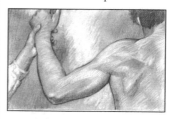

Dorsal interossei

Ask the patient to spread his fingers apart, as shown below, and then resist your attempt to squeeze them together.

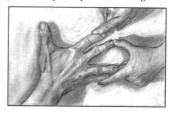

Forearm and hand

Ask the patient to grasp your middle and index fingers and squeeze them as hard as he can, as shown below.

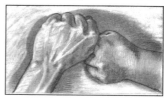

Psoas

While you support his leg, ask the patient to raise his knee by flexing his hip against your resistance, as shown at top of next page. Observe for psoas contraction.

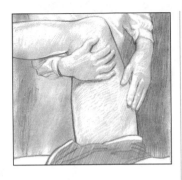

Quadriceps
Ask the patient to bend his knee slightly. Then ask him to extend his knee against your resistance, as shown below. Palpate for quadriceps contraction.

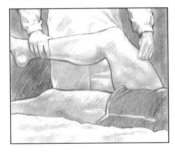

Gastrocnemius
With the patient in the prone position, support his foot and ask him to plantarflex his ankle against your resistance, as shown below. Palpate for gastrocnemius contraction.

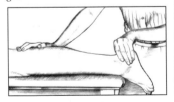

Anterior tibial
With the patient sitting on the side of the exam table with his legs dangling, place your hand on his foot, as shown at top of next column. Ask him to dorsiflex his ankle against your resistance.

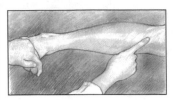

Extensor hallucis longus
With your finger on his great toe, ask the patient to dorsiflex the toe against your resistance, as shown below. Palpate for extensor hallucis contraction.

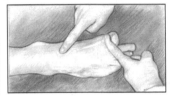

Resisted isometric movements
• Place the joint in a neutral or resting position.
• Ask the patient to contract the muscle strongly while you apply resistance to prevent movement of the joint and to ensure maximum effort by the patient.

If present, muscle weakness may be due to an upper neuron lesion, injury to a peripheral nerve, injury at the neuromuscular junction, or the muscles themselves. This test provides information about the muscle, tendons, and their attachments.
• Strong, pain-free contractions indicate no lesion of the muscles being tested.
• Strong but painful movement indicates a minor lesion of the muscle or tendon. This could be a strain or muscle tendinitis.
• Weak and painful movement indicates a severe lesion such as a fracture or incomplete tear. The weakness often results from reflex inhibition of the muscles around the joint.
• Weak and pain-free movement indicates the complete rupture of a

muscle or involvement of the nerve supplying that muscle.

When assessing a joint for pain, it's often necessary to look at the synovial joint itself. This can be done during the course of the joint examination.

• With the joint exposed, look for gross deformities, which may be congenital or traumatic in nature.

• Compare the soft tissue on both the affected and unaffected joint. Note areas of atrophy or swelling. Compare color, texture, and temperature. Heat often indicates inflammation, whereas coldness can indicate vascular compromise. Shiny skin can indicate diabetes, vascular problems, or peripheral nerve lesions.

• Look for scars that might indicate past trauma or surgery.

• Examine around the affected area for swelling.

• Palpate for pulses and compare to those on the unaffected limb.

• Palpate for any muscle spasm, which might indicate an attempt to immobilize a traumatized joint.

You should move the joint passively throughout its ROM noting when pain begins as well as the "feel" of the joint throughout the available range. Then assess the uninvolved side to obtain a baseline against which the involved joint can be compared. The sequence of pain and resistance during the passive ROM provides information about whether the joint pathology is acute or chronic.

Stage 1
The patient experiences pain before you feel any resistance. This indicates an acute joint injury.

Stage 2
The patient feels pain at the same time you feel resistance. This is a subacute joint injury, so treatment should be slightly more aggressive than in Stage 1.

Stage 3
You feel resistance before the patient feels pain. This indicates a lack of active inflammation and a chronic problem. Therapy in stage 3 should be aggressive.

Note if the patient demonstrates joint hypomobility or hypermobility on the unaffected side in comparison with possible hypermobility or hypomobility on the involved side. Hypomobile joints, those which show decreased ROM, may be more susceptible to muscular strains, overuse tendinitis, and nerve entrapment syndromes. Hypermobile joints, those which show increased ROM, are more susceptible to recurrent injury, sprains, early degenerative joint changes, and tendinitis resulting from muscular imbalance. Determining joint laxity can be achieved by performing appropriate testing. (See *Orthopedic tests*, pages 26 to 36.)

Neurologic examination

Pain assessment

Pain is often what brings the patient to your door. Standardized tools, such as the McGill pain questionnaire, simple figure (pain) drawings, and the visual analog scale, can elicit useful information from the patient about his complaint.

The McGill pain questionnaire includes 20 categories of words used to describe pain. The patient chooses one word from each category. The word columns are divided into four categories. Entries 1 to 10 describe sensory qualities of the pain experience; entries 11 to 15 describe affective, or emotional, qualities of the pain experience; entry 16 consists of words to describe the intensity of the

(Text continues on page 36.)

ORTHOPEDIC TESTS

The chart below lists common tests performed by physical therapists (PTs) to help identify orthopedic abnormalities. A positive result on one test doesn't make a diagnosis; rather, combined with results of the entire assessment process, it helps lead the PT toward a diagnosis.

Test and purpose	Procedure	Positive result
Cervical spine Brachial tension test To detect nerve root compression	With the patient supine, slowly abduct and externally rotate the arm just to the point of pain. Then have the patient supinate and flex the forearm while you support it at the shoulder.	Symptoms are reproduced or increased.
Distraction test To identify nerve root compression	Place one hand under the patient's chin, place the other hand under the occiput, and slowly lift the head (distraction).	Radiating pain decreases.
Spurling test (Foraminal compression test) To identify nerve root compression	Ask the patient to laterally flex the head. Carefully press down on the head (compression).	Pain radiates in the arm toward the flexed side.
Vertebral artery test To detect vertebral artery compression	With the patient supine, place the head into a position of extension, lateral flexion, and rotation and hold that position for 30 seconds. Test each side separately.	The patient feels dizzy or nauseous, or you observe nystagmus.
Pelvis Supine iliac compression test To identify sacroiliac (SI) joint dysfunction	With the patient supine, cross your arms and place your palms on his anterior SI spines. Press down and laterally to strain the SI ligaments.	Pain occurs in the gluteal or posterior crural areas. Repeat the test using more support if pain occurs in the lumbar region.
Supine-sit test To evaluate SI torsion by comparing functional leg lengths	With the patient supine, hold both of his ankles and give a slight, even traction force to make sure he's lying straight. With your thumbs placed just distal to the medial malleoli of the ankles, compare leg lengths. Ask the patient to rise into the straight-leg sitting position, then compare leg lengths again. Note whether the relationships remain the same or change with the change of position.	Change in length between the two positions indicates SI torsion. No change in relationship suggests no torsion. Posterior torsion is identified when the shorter leg in the supine position becomes the longer leg in the sitting position. Anterior torsion is identified when the longer leg in the supine position becomes the shorter leg in the sitting position. Posterior torsional dysfunctions are more common than anterior torsional dysfunctions.

ORTHOPEDIC TESTS (continued)

Test and purpose	Procedure	Positive result
Lumbar spine Straight leg raise test (Laseque's test) To identify sciatic nerve root compression	With the patient supine, extend one of his legs and raise it while watching his reaction. Stop when he complains of back or leg pain (not hamstring tightness). Also, dorsiflex the ankle to further increase the traction on the sciatic nerve. Repeat with the opposite leg.	Back pain suggests a central herniation, and leg pain suggests a lateral disc protrusion.
Slump test (Sitting root test) To identify sciatic nerve compression	With the patient seated and his neck flexed, actively extend his knee while the hip remains flexed.	Pain increases.
Quadrant test (Scouring test) To assess nonspecific hip joint pathology	With the patient supine, flex the hip and knee of the test leg toward the patient's opposite shoulder. Enough hip flexion and adduction should occur to take up the tissue slack. Then move the hip through an arc of abduction while maintaining the hip flexion.	You feel any movement irregularities, such as crepitus, glitches, and bumps, or the patient looks apprehensive or reports pain.
Hoover's test To discriminate lower limb weakness from possible malingering	With the patient supine, place one hand under each of his heels and ask him to do a straight-leg raise (knee extended).	The patient can't lift the leg, and you feel no downward pressure from the opposite leg.
Shoulder Sulcus sign To detect inferior instability	With the patient standing, his arm by his side and his shoulder muscles relaxed, grasp his forearm and pull distally.	A space larger than one thumb width appears between the acromion and the humeral head.
Anterior apprehension test To determine whether a patient has a history of anterior dislocations	With the patient supine, slowly abduct and externally rotate his arm.	The patient becomes apprehensive and resists further motion.
Posterior apprehension test To determine whether a patient has a history of posterior dislocations	With the patient supine, slowly flex his arm to 90 degrees, internally rotate the arm, and apply a posterior force to the patient's elbow.	The patient becomes apprehensive and resists further motion.
Clunk test To detect a tear of the glenoid labrum	With the patient supine, place one hand on the posterior aspect of his shoulder over the humeral head. Fully abduct the arm over the patient's head and push anteriorly with your hand over the humeral head.	You palpate a "clunk" or grinding. Also, patient apprehension may indicate anterior instability.

(continued)

ORTHOPEDIC TESTS (continued)

Test and purpose	Procedure	Positive result
Shoulder (continued) Jerk test To detect posterior shoulder instability	With the patient seated, flex his shoulder 90 degrees and internally rotate it until the elbow is flexed approximately 90 degrees. Then apply one hand to the elbow and produce an axial load through the humerus to the glenohumeral joint. Next, move the shoulder into horizontal adduction while maintaining the axial load.	The shoulder suddenly jerks during horizontal adduction.
Adson's test To detect thoracic outlet syndrome	Turn the patient's head toward his shoulder on the side being tested, then externally rotate and extend the shoulder while the patient extends his head.	The radial pulse disappears while the patient holds a deep breath.
Roos test Used in the assessment of thoracic outlet syndrome	With the patient standing and both shoulders abducted to 90 degrees, ask him to slowly open and close his hands for 3 minutes.	An inability to maintain upper arm position and presence of ischemic pain, numbness or paresthesia of the limb, or heaviness of the arm indicates thoracic outlet syndrome.
Speed's test (Biceps test) To detect bicipital tendinitis	With his forearm supinated and elbow fully extended, ask the patient to try to flex the arm against your resistance.	There is increased pain in the area of the bicipital groove.
Yergason's test To identify tendinitis of the long head of the biceps	With the patient's arm at his side and the elbow flexed to 90 degrees, have him supinate his forearm against your resistance.	Pain occurs in the biceps tendon in the area of the bicipital groove.
Supraspinatur test To detect a tear in the supraspinatus tendon	With the patient seated, position his arms horizontally at 30 degrees anterior to the frontal plane and internally rotated. Then apply a downward force on the arms.	Pain and weakness occur on the involved side.
Neer's impingement test To assess impingement of the shoulder involving either the supraspinatus or long head of the biceps	With the patient seated and his shoulder at 90 degrees of flexion, passively and forcibly abduct the shoulder horizontally.	Pain occurs at the extreme of horizontal adduction, indicating impingement of the supraspinatus, the long head of the biceps, or both.
Hawkins-Kennedy impingement test To identify supraspinatus tendinitis	With the patient standing, flex his arm to 90 degrees and then forcibly internally rotate the shoulder.	Pain occurs during the maneuver.

ORTHOPEDIC TESTS (continued)

Test and purpose	Procedure	Positive result
Shoulder *(continued)* Acromioclavicular (AC) shear test To assess pathology of the AC joint	With the patient seated or standing, cup your hands and place the base of one hand over the spine of the scapula and the other anteriorly over the clavicle. Then squeeze the heels of your hands together.	Pain or abnormal movement in the AC joint occurs.
Elbow Varus stress test To assesses stability of the lateral (radial) collateral ligament	With the patient's elbow slightly flexed and his forearm supinated, place one of your hands on the medial aspect of the elbow joint and the other along the radial forearm, either midshaft or distally. Then apply a varus force by adducting the forearm relative to the arm, using the elbow as a fulcrum. (Externally rotating the arm's soft-tissue mass helps maintain position during testing and allows easier application of a varus force by not allowing any shoulder rotation.) Also test the uninvolved side for comparison.	Pain occurs, or you see or feel excessive gapping along the lateral aspect of the joint.
Valgus stress test To assess stability of the medial (ulnar) collateral ligament	With the patient's elbow slightly flexed and his forearm supinated, places one of your hands on the lateral aspect of the elbow joint and the other medially on the midportion or distal forearm. Then apply a valgus force to the elbow by pulling the forearm away from the body, using the elbow as a fulcrum. (Internally rotating the arm's soft-tissue mass helps maintain position during testing and allows easier application of valgus force by not allowing any shoulder rotation.) Also test the uninvolved side for comparison.	Pain occurs, or you see or feel excessive gapping along the medial aspect of the joint.

(continued)

Test and purpose	Procedure	Positive result
Lateral epicondylitis test (Tennis elbow) Method 1 To detect muscle inflammation originating on and around the lateral epicondyle by imposing contradictory stress	With the patient's forearm pronated and the elbow slightly flexed, apply force to resist wrist extension and finger extension. The following testing positions are used: • wrist extension and radial deviation to assess the extensor carpi radialis longus and brevis • wrist extension and ulnar deviation to assess the extensor carpi ulnaris • finger extension to assess the extensor digitorum.	Sudden pain occurs in the origin of the muscles being contracted. Because the extensor carpi radialis brevis is often involved in pathology, it's important to differentiate this structure from the extensor carpi radialis longus by palpating and recognizing the specific site of pain. With involvement of the extensor carpi radialis longus, pain occurs above the lateral epicondyle, where it originates on the supracondylar ride. Conversely, the extensor carpi radialis brevis responds with localization of pain at its origin on the lateral epicondyle.
Lateral epicondylitis test (Tennis elbow) Method 2 To detect inflammation of the extensor muscles of the wrist and hand originating on and about the lateral epicondyle by elongating or stretching the muscle	Extend the patient's elbow, causing his forearm to pronate, while simultaneously flexing and deviating the wrist toward the ulna. *Important:* Perform these motions to the end ranges of motion to ensure complete stretching of the extensor musculature.	Pain occurs at or near the lateral epicondyle. (The method described in the previous test can locate the specific tendon. The patient's position for this test may also be used in treatment as flexibility conditioning.)
Medial epicondylitis test (Golfer's elbow) Method 1 To assess inflammation of the common flexor tendons of the wrist by contracting the muscle	With the patient's elbow slightly flexed and forearm supinated, resist flexion of the wrist.	Pain occurs in the region of the medial epicondyle. (Identifying the specific flexor muscle involved is clinically impossible because of the common origin of flexor muscles.)
Medial epicondylitis test (Golfer's elbow) Method 2 To detect inflammation of the common flexor tendons around the elbow by stretching the muscle	With the patient's forearm fully supinated, place the elbow and wrist in maximal extension.	Pain occurs over the medial epicondyle. (As in method 1, localization of the specific flexor tendon involved isn't possible. This position may also be used in flexibility training of the affected structures.)

ORTHOPEDIC TESTS (continued)

Test and purpose	Procedure	Positive result
Tinel's sign To assess the integrity of the ulnar nerve where it lies in the ulnar groove between the olecranon process and the medial epicondyle	With the patient's elbow flexed at 90 degrees, tap the ulnar nerve where it lies in the ulnar groove.	Tingling sensation within the distribution of the ulnar nerve in the forearm and hand indicates neuroma or neuritis of the ulnar nerve.
Hip Faber test (Patrick test) To detect arthritis of the hip	With patient supine, flex his knee and flex, abduct, and externally rotate the hip until the lateral malleolus rests on the opposite knee just above the patella. Then gently force downward the knee on the side being tested.	Pain occurs, indicating osteoarthritis of the hip.
Ortolani's sign To identify a congenital hip dislocation in infants	With the infant positioned supine, his hips flexed 90 degrees, and his knees fully flexed, grasp his legs so that your thumbs are on his medial thighs and your fingers are on his lateral thighs. Then gently abduct the thighs and apply a gentle force to the greater trochanters with the fingers of each hand.	You feel resistance at about 30 degrees of abduction and, if there is a dislocation, a click as the dislocation is reduced.
Barlow's test To identify hip instability in infants	With the infant in the same position as for Ortolani's test (above), stabilize the pelvis between the symphysis and sacrum with one hand. With the thumb of the other hand, attempt to dislocate the hip with gentle but firm posterior pressure.	The hip dislocates.
True leg length test To detect a difference in leg length, secondary to bony inequality of the pelvis, femur, or tibia	With the patient supine, carefully check that his pelvis is level, his body is relatively straight, and his legs are approximately 6" to 8" (15 to 20 cm) apart and parallel to each other. If contracture is present in one hip, assess the opposite hip in a similar position to ensure accuracy of measurement. Also, be sure to be consistent in choosing the specific point of the landmarks to measure for discrepancy; otherwise, comparison will yield inaccurate information. Take the initial measurement from the ASIS to the medial malleolus. If excessive hypertrophy or atrophy of one thigh is present, you may choose to use the lateral malleolus, rather than the medial malleo-	Differences between limbs of more than ⅜" (1 cm) are abnormal, indicating leg-length inequality due to skeletal differences. The specific measurements listed above may allow you to identify the skeletal component responsible for the discrepancy. You also can visually assess for a difference in limb length at the femur or the tibia by flexing the subject's hips and knees, making sure that the feet are lined up evenly and symmetrically with each (continued)

ORHOPEDIC TESTS (continued)

Test and purpose	Procedure	Positive result
Hip True leg length test (continued)	lus, for measurement to minimize error due to circumferential soft-tissue differences. If you find a leg-length discrepancy, take and compare these specific measurements from various landmarks: • ASIS to greater trochanter to assess hip varus or valgus • greater trochanter to the lateral joint line of the femur to assess length of the femoral shaft • medial joint line of the knee to medial malleolus to assess tibial shaft length.	other; a longer femur will cause the ipsilateral knee to project more distally than the other knee when viewed from the side, while a longer tibia will cause the tibia to lie more proximal than the opposite one.
Thomas test To test for contracture of the hip flexor muscles	With the patient supine, ask him to flex one hip and hold it flexed against his chest.	The other thigh doesn't remain flat against the surface.
Ober's test To detect a shortened iliotibial band	With the patient lying on one side, ask him to flex the side-lying (non-test) leg. Then abduct and extend the other leg while you flex that knee to 90 degrees and allow it to drop.	The limb doesn't drop, indicating a shortened (tight) iliotibial band.
Hamstring length test To determine excessive hamstring length or tightness	With the patient supine, ask him to extend his knees while keeping his lower back and sacrum flat on the surface of the table. If the hip flexors are tight, place a roll or pillow under the nontest leg to allow the lower back to lie flat on the table; the pelvis must remain neutral in the sagittal plane. Next, holding the nontest leg down on the table, flex the test hip with the knee joint still extended and the ankle joint relaxed. Use a goniometer to measure the degree of hip joint flexion.	Less than 70 degrees of hip flexion in an adult indicates that the hamstring or gluteus maximus muscle is too tight. Greater than 80 degrees indicates excessive hamstring length. (Note that a posterior pelvic tilt increases actual hamstring muscle length, and an anterior pelvic tilt or a hyperextended low back makes the hamstring muscles appear too short.
Wrist and hand Finkelstein test To detect tenosynovitis of the abductor pollicis longus and extensor pollicis brevis tendons; (commonly) to detect de Quervain's disease	Ask the patient to make a fist with his thumb inside his fingers and then have him try to deviate ulnarly the first metacarpal and extend the primal joint of the thumb.	Pain occurs.

ORTHOPEDIC TESTS *(continued)*

Test and purpose	Procedure	Positive result
Wrist and hand *(continued)* Bunnel-Littler test To detect intrinsic muscle or joint contractures at the PIP joints	Flex the patient's PIP joint maximally while maintaining the MCP joint in slight extension.	The PIP joint can't be flexed, indicating a joint capsule contracture, or the MCP flexes slightly and the PIP flexes fully, indicating intrinsic muscle contracture.
Tinel's sign To detect carpal tunnel syndrome	Tap over the carpal tunnel of the patient's wrist.	Paresthesia occurs distal to the wrist.
Phalen's test To detect carpal tunnel syndrome	Flex the patient's wrists maximally and hold them together in this position for 1 minute.	Paresthesia occurs in the thumb, index finger, and the middle and lateral half of the ring finger.
Reverse Phalen's test To assess carpal tunnel syndrome in conjunction with Phalen's test	Ask the patient to squeeze your hand while you extend his wrist. Keeping the wrist extended, apply direct pressure over the carpal tunnel and maintain that pressure for 1 minute.	Symptoms noted with Phalen's test are present.
Allen test To determine patency of the vascular communication in the hand	Palpate and occlude the patient's radial and ulnar arteries. Then ask the patient to open and close his fingers rapidly three to five times to cause the palmar skin to blanch. Release the pressure from either the radial or ulnar artery and note the speed with which the hand regains color. Repeat the test, this time releasing the other artery.	The hand remains pale or white, indicating diminished or absent communication between the superficial ulnar arch and the deep radial arch.
Knee Lachman's test To identify injury to the anterior cruciate ligament	With the patient supine, stabilize the distal femur with one hand and grasp the proximal tibia with the other hand. Holding the knee slightly flexed, move the tibia forward on the femur.	You note a soft end-feel and excessive movement of the tibia.
Anterior drawer sign test To detect anterior instability of the knee	With the patient supine and his knee flexed 90 degrees, sit across the forefoot of his flexed leg. Keeping the patient's foot in neutral rotation, pull forward on the proximal part of the calf. Then test the other leg.	You note excessive anterior movement of the tibia compared to the femur.

(continued)

ORTHOPEDIC TESTS *(continued)*

Test and purpose	Procedure	Positive result
Knee *(continued)* Posterior drawer sign test To detect posterior cruciate ligament tear	With the patient supine, flex the test knee to 90 degrees and rest the foot on the table. Then, sitting on the foot to stabilize it, grasp the proximal tibia and push the tibia posteriorly on the femur.	You note excessive posterior translation of the tibia backward on the femur, indicating damage to any of the following structures: posterior cruciate or posterior oblique ligament, arcuate complex, or anterior cruciate ligament.
Varus stress test (Adduction test) To identify lateral instability of the knee	With the patient's ankle stabilized in full extension, apply a varus stress to the knee. Then repeat the test with the patient's knee in 20 to 30 degrees of flexion.	Gapping or pain with the knee extended suggests a major disruption of the knee ligaments; with the knee flexed, it suggests damage to the lateral collateral ligament.
Valgus stress test (Abduction test) To identify medial instability of the knee	With the patient's ankle fully extended and stabilized in slight lateral rotation, apply a valgus stress to the knee. Then repeat the test with the patient's knee at 20 degrees of flexion and stabilized in slight lateral rotation.	Excessive movement of the tibia away from the femur with the knee fully extended indicates major disruption of the knee ligaments. Excessive movement with the flexed knee indicates damage to the medial collateral ligament.
McMurray's test To identify meniscal lesions	With the patient supine, grasp his foot with one hand and palpate the joint line with the other. Fully flex the knee and rotate the tibia back and forth. Then hold the knee alternately in internal and external rotation as you extend the knee.	As the knee extends, you feel a click or crepitation over the joint line, indicating a posterior meniscal lesion.
Appley's (grinding) test To detect meniscal lesions	With the patient prone and his knees flexed 90 degrees, apply a compressive force through the foot and rotate the tibia back and forth with one hand as you palpate the joint line and feel for crepitation with the other hand.	Pain occurs, or you feel crepitation, indicating meniscal injury. Repeat the test by applying a distractive force to the leg. Pain occurs, indicating a ligament injury rather than a meniscal injury.

ORTHOPEDIC TESTS (continued)

Test and purpose	Procedure	Positive result
Foot and ankle Subtalar joint neutral test To determine structural or functional ability and prevent compensation of the foot	Hold the fourth and fifth metatarsal heads with one hand and palpate the talar heads with the other hand. While palpating the talar heads, gently dorsiflex the fourth and fifth metatarsal heads to the point of slight resistance. This bending ensures locking of the forefoot when the subtalar joint is in the neutral position. Maintaining dorsiflexion of the metatarsal heads, move the foot medially and laterally until congruence of the talar heads is apparent or neither head is prominent. This position is identified as the subtalar joint neutral position of the foot, the position in which the foot is neither pronated nor supinated and in which maximal function can occur. Another method of distinguishing subtalar joint neutral position is to observe the concavities superior and inferior to the lateral malleolus. When both concavities appear symmetrical and equal in size, the subtalar joint is in the neutral position. Objective assessment of the subtalar joint neutral position is performed with one arm of a goniometer aligned with the bisection of the distal third of the leg and the other arm aligned with the bisection of the calcaneus. A normal rearfoot position is one in which the angle created by these two goniometric alignments is 0 to 4 degrees of varus.	In the subtalar joint neutral position, the calcaneus is inverted more than 4 degrees compared to the tibia, indicating rearfoot varus, or it's everted relative to the tibia, indicating rearfoot valgus. (Objective assessment of maximal rearfoot pronation and supination should also be performed, because measurement will provide an indication of the patient's ability to compensate for rearfoot and forefoot problems. Measuring from the subtalar joint neutral position, the normal subtalar range of motion should demonstrate a 2:1 ratio of calcaneal inversion to eversion.)
Anterior drawer sign test To identify anterior ankle instability	With the patient supine, stabilize the distal tibia and fibula with one hand while you hold the foot in 20 degrees of plantar flexion with the other hand. Then draw the talus forward in the ankle mortise. Repeat the procedure on the nontest leg.	Straight anterior translation of the test leg exceeds that of the nontest leg.
Talar tilt test To identify lesions of the calcaneofibular ligament	Position the patient supine or lying on one side with his knee flexed to 90 degrees. With the foot in a neutral position, tilt the talus medially.	The amount of adduction on the involved side is excessive.

(continued)

ORTHOPEDIC TESTS (continued)

Test and purpose	Procedure	Positive result
Foot and ankle *(continued)*		
Thompson test To detect rupture of the Achilles tendon	With the patient prone or on his knees with his feet extended over the edge of the bed, squeeze the middle third of the calf muscle.	Normal plantar flexion doesn't occur, indicating Achilles tendon rupture.
Lateral pull test To help determine the role of excessive lateral pull of the quadriceps on patellofemoral pain	Position the patient supine with his leg extended and relaxed. Ask him to perform a quadriceps set as you observe for symmetrical patellar movement in a superior or superior and lateral direction.	Excessive lateral patellar movement occurs.

pain experience; and entries 17 to 20 are miscellaneous descriptors.

The questionnaire can be scored in various ways but in clinical practice the most common method is the Pain Rating Index. Within each column the words are numbered from top to bottom, with the first word valued at 1, the second at 2, and so forth. The values of the words chosen by the patient are added to obtain a score for each category. A total score is obtained by adding the scores in all categories. (See *McGill pain questionnaire.*)

A pain drawing, on which a patient can indicate where the pain is located as well as the type of pain, can help to show the spatial distribution of a patient's pain symptoms. (See *Using a pain drawing or scale,* page 38.)

Assessing sensation

If there is evidence of sensory involvement, evaluate and note the patient's ability to perceive the sensation being tested and the difference, if any, in the affected and unaffected sides.
• Ask the patient to close his eyes as you apply stimuli to both proximal and distal areas.

• Begin by running relaxed fingers or hands over the area and asking the patient to describe what he feels. If there is a problem area, map it and arrange for further testing.
• Check hot and cold sensations.
• Test superficial sensation to determine the response to sharp and dull by using a pin and a blunt object such as a pencil eraser. Because of referred pain, the sensation may come from any structure supplied by the affected nerve root. Assess which dermatomes are affected.
• Squeeze a tendon, muscle, or bony area to test deep pressure sensation.
• Ask the patient to identify letters or numbers written with a finger or blunt object on his hand or another body part.

Dermatomal testing

Your examination of the patient's sensory system includes testing his ability to feel pain and light touch. You can test most of the major dermatomes for pain by applying a sterile needle or pin, and you can test for light touch by using a wisp of cotton. (See *Dermatomal testing*, pages 39 and 40.)

MCGILL PAIN QUESTIONNAIRE

Tell your patient that there are many words to describe pain, and some of these are grouped in this list. Ask him to look at each group of words and circle a word that describes the pain he's experiencing right now. He should choose only one word from *each* word group, but he doesn't have to choose a word from *every* word group. If none of the words in a particular word group describe his pain, he can go to the next word group.

1 Flickering Quivering Pulsing Throbbing Beating Pounding	2 Jumping Flashing Shooting	3 Pricking Boring Drilling Stabbing Lancinating	4 Sharp Cutting Lacerating
5 Pinching Pressing Gnawing Cramping Crushing	6 Tugging Pulling Wrenching	7 Hot Burning Scalding Searing	8 Tingling Itchy Smarting Stinging
9 Dull Sore Hurting Aching Heavy	10 Tender Taut Rasping Splitting	11 Tiring Exhausting	12 Sickening Suffocating
13 Fearful Frightful Terrifying	14 Punishing Grueling Cruel Vicious Killing	15 Wretched Binding	16 Annoying Troublesome Miserable Intense Unbearable
17 Spreading Radiating Penetrating Piercing	18 Tight Numb Drawing Squeezing Tearing	19 Cool Cold Freezing	20 Nagging Nauseating Agonizing Dreadful Torturing

Adapted with permission from R. Melzak. "The McGill pain questionnaire: Major properties and scoring," *Pain* 1:277-99, 1975.

Assessing proprioception

The proprioceptive senses include both position sense and movement sense. Position sense is the awareness of the position of a joint at rest; movement sense is the awareness of movement.

To evaluate proprioception:

• Instruct the patient to close his eyes as you move a toe, arm, or hand in various directions.
• Ask the patient to describe the sensation, for example, if the toe is up or the arm is extended to the right side.

Finger-to-nose test
• Instruct the patient to close his eyes and then touch his nose with one of his fingers.

USING A PAIN DRAWING OR SCALE

On these drawings, indicate pain location by shading in the area involved. Refer to the key and place numbers that correspond to the pain's character over the appropriate shaded area. Also indicate areas of numbness. Don't indicate preexisting pain or numbness; show only pain related to the present injury or condition.

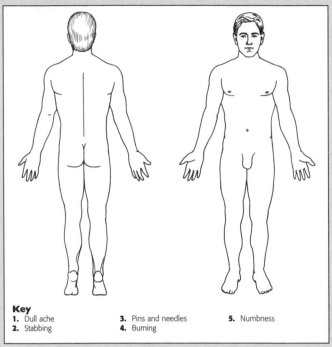

Key
1. Dull ache
2. Stabbing
3. Pins and needles
4. Burning
5. Numbness

A visual analog scale may be used to determine the intensity of a patient's pain. Ask the patient to assign a number to his pain from 0 (no pain) to 10 (maximum pain). Be sure to explain that the word "pain" covers a variety of descriptors, such as "aching," "burning," and "sharp." Then plot the patient's response on a 10-cm scale like the one shown below.

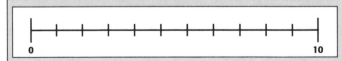

0   10

• Repeat with the other hand.

Proprioceptive space test
• Instruct the patient to close his eyes.
• Place one of the patient's hands or feet in a selected position in space and then ask him to imitate that position with the other hand or foot.
• True proprioceptive loss will prevent the patient from properly positioning or finding the normal limb.

DERMATOMAL TESTING

The body is divided into dermatomes, each of which represents an area of the skin supplied with afferent (sensory) nerve fibers that transmit pain, temperature, and touch from an individual spinal root — cervical (C), thoracic (T), lumbar (L), or sacral (S). Examination of the integrity of a dermatomal distribution should be performed in all apparent or suspected cases of peripheral nerve or nerve-root pathology and central nervous system involvement. The illustrations below show the dermatomes of the body.

Anterior view

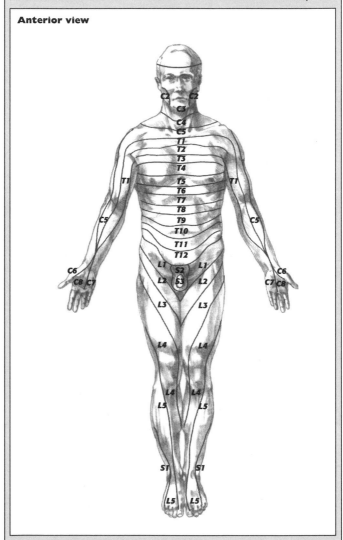

(continued)

DERMATOMAL TESTING *(continued)*

Posterior view

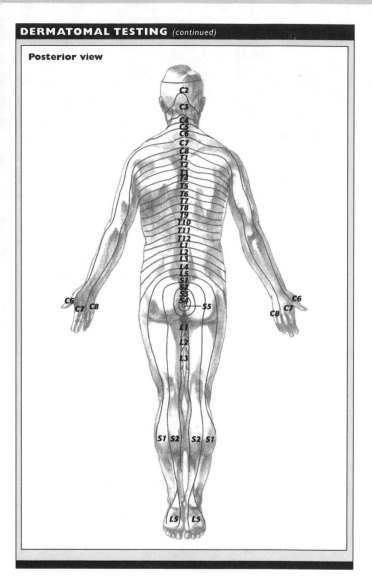

Assessing coordination

You should perform one of the following tests to evaluate coordination:

Heel-to-knee test
• Ask the patient to lie supine with his eyes open.

• Instruct him to take the heel of one foot and place it on the opposite knee and then slide the foot down the shin.
• Ask him to repeat the procedure with his eyes closed.
• Test both sides.

Finger-to-nose test
• Instruct the patient to stand or sit with his eyes open and touch his nose with one of his fingers.
• Ask him to repeat the same activity with his eyes closed and then again with the other side.

Finger-thumb test
• Ask the patient to quickly touch his thumb to each finger on his hand.
• Test both sides.

Hand-thigh test
• Instruct the patient to pat his thigh as quickly as possible with his hand. Then ask him to supinate and pronate his hand between pats.
• Watch timing and coordination.
• Test both sides.

Assessing reflexes

Assessment of deep tendon and superficial reflexes provides information about the intactness of the sensory receptor organ. It also evaluates how well the afferent nerve relays sensory messages to the spinal cord, the spinal cord or brain stem segment mediates the reflex, the lower motor neurons transmit messages to the muscles, and the muscles respond to the motor message.

To evaluate your patient's reflexes, you'll need to test deep tendon and superficial reflexes as well as observe for primitive reflexes.

Deep tendon reflexes
Before you test a deep tendon reflex, be sure the limb is relaxed and the joint is in midposition; for instance, the knee or elbow should be flexed at a 45-degree angle. Next, distract the patient by asking him to focus on an object across the room. If he focuses on his performance, the cerebral cortex may dampen his response. You can also distract the patient by using

Jendrassik's maneuver — simply instruct him to clench his teeth or to squeeze his thigh. Be sure to document which technique you used to distract the patient.

You should always move from head to toe in testing deep tendon reflexes and also compare contralateral reflexes. To elicit the reflex, tap the tendon lightly but firmly with the reflex hammer. Then grade the briskness of the response: 0 (no response), 1+ (hypoactive), 2+ (normal), 3+ (hyperactive), or 4+ (clonic).

Biceps reflex
Position the patient's arm so that his elbow is flexed at a 45-degree angle and his arm is relaxed. Next, place your thumb or index finger over the biceps tendon and your remaining fingers loosely over the triceps muscle, as shown below. Strike your thumb or index finger with the pointed tip of the reflex hammer, and watch and feel for contraction of the biceps muscle and flexion of the forearm.

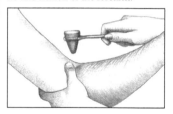

Triceps reflex
Ask the patient to abduct his arm and place his relaxed forearm across his chest. Strike the triceps tendon about 2″ (5.1 cm) above the olecranon on the extensor surface of the upper arm, as shown at top of next page. Watch for contraction of the triceps muscle and extension of the forearm.

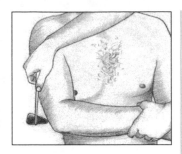

Brachioradialis reflex
Instruct the patient to rest the ulnar surface of his hand on his knee and partially flex his elbow. With the tip of the hammer, strike the radius about 2″ proximal to the radial styloid, as shown below. Watch for supination of the hand and flexion of the forearm at the elbow.

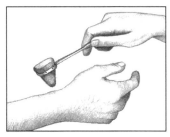

Patellar reflex
Ask the patient to sit on the side of the bed with his legs dangling freely. If he can't sit up, flex his knee at a 45-degree angle and place your nondominant hand behind it for support. Strike the patellar tendon just below the patella, as shown below. Look for contraction of the quadriceps muscle in the anterior thigh and for extension of the leg.

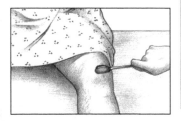

Achilles tendon reflex
Slightly flex the patient's foot and support the plantar surface. Using the pointed end of the reflex hammer, strike the Achilles tendon, as shown below. Watch for plantar flexion of the foot at the ankle.

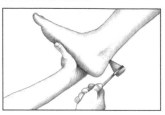

Superficial reflexes
These reflexes include the abdominal, cremasteric, and plantar reflexes. To elicit these reflexes, you should stimulate the patient's skin or mucous membranes. To document your findings, use a plus sign (+) to indicate that a reflex is present and a minus sign (−) to indicate that it's absent.

Abdominal reflex
Place the patient in the supine position, with his arms at his sides and his knees slightly flexed. Using the tip of the reflex hammer, a key, or an applicator stick, briskly stroke both sides of the abdomen above and below the umbilicus, moving from the periphery toward the midline, as shown below. After each stroke, watch for abdominal muscle contraction and movement of the umbilicus toward the stimulus. If you're evaluating an

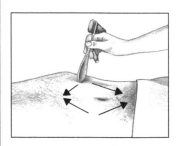

obese patient, retract the umbilicus to the side opposite the stimulus and note whether it pulls toward the stimulus. Aging and diseases of the upper and lower motor neurons cause an absent abdominal reflex.

Cremasteric reflex

With a male patient, use an applicator stick to lightly stimulate the inner thigh. Watch for contraction of the cremaster muscle in the scrotum and prompt elevation of the testicle on the side of the stimulus. This reflex may be absent in upper or lower motor neuron disease.

Plantar reflex

Using an applicator stick, a tongue blade, or a key, slowly stroke the lateral side of the patient's sole from the heel to the great toe, as shown below. The normal response is plantar flexion of the toes. In an elderly patient, this normal response may be diminished because of arthritic deformities of the toe or foot.

In patients with disorders of the pyramidal tract (such as cerebrovascular accident), Babinski's reflex, which is an abnormal response, is elicited. The patient responds to the stimulus by dorsiflexion of his great toe. You may also see a more pronounced response in which the other toes extend and abduct. In some cases, you may even see dorsiflexion of the ankle, knee, and hip.

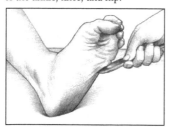

Primitive reflexes

Although normal in infants, primitive reflexes are pathologic in adults.

Grasp reflex

Apply gentle pressure to the patient's palm with your fingers, as shown below. If he grasps your fingers between his thumb and index finger, suspect cortical (premotor cortex) damage.

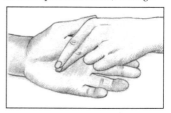

Snout reflex

Tap lightly on the patient's upper lip, as shown below. Lip pursing indicates frontal lobe damage.

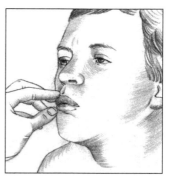

Sucking reflex

If the patient begins sucking while you're feeding him or suctioning his mouth, as shown below, you've elicited a reflex that indicates cortical damage characteristic of advanced dementia.

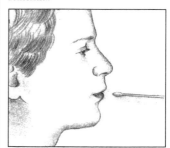

ASSESSING THE CRANIAL NERVES

Cranial nerve (CN) assessment provides valuable information about the condition of the central nervous system, particularly the brain stem. Because disorders can affect any of the CNs, knowing how to test each nerve is important. The techniques vary according to the nerve being tested.

Cranial nerve and assessment technique	Normal findings
Olfactory (CN 1) After checking the patency of the patient's nostrils, have him close both eyes. Then occlude one nostril and hold a familiar, pungent substance, such as coffee, tobacco, soap, or peppermint, under the patient's nose and ask its identity. Repeat this technique with the other nostril.	The patient should be able to detect and identify the smell correctly. If he reports detecting the smell but can't name it, offer a choice, such as, "Do you smell lemon, coffee, or peppermint?"
Optic (CN II) and oculomotor (CN III) To assess the optic nerve, check visual acuity, visual fields, and the retinal structures. To assess the oculo-motor nerve, check pupil size, pupil shape, and pupil-lary response to light.	The pupils should be equal, round, and reactive to light. When assessing pupil size, be especially alert for any trends. For example, watch for a grad-ual increase in the size of one pupil or the appearance of unequal pupils in a patient whose pupils were previously equal.
Oculomotor (CN III), trochlear (CN IV), and abducent (CN VI) To test the coordinated function of these three nerves, assess them simultaneously by evaluating the patient's extraocular eye movement.	The eyes should move smoothly and in a coordinated manner through all six direc-tions of eye movement. Observe each eye for rapid oscillation (nystagmus), move-ment not in unison with that of the other eye, or inability to move in certain directions (ophthalmoplegia). Also note any complaint of double vision (diplopia).
Trigeminal (CN V) To assess the sensory portion of the trigeminal nerve, gently touch the right side, then the left side of the patient's forehead with a cotton ball while his eyes are closed. Instruct him to announce the moment the cot-ton touches the area. Compare the patient's response on each side. Repeat the technique on the right and left cheek and on the right and left jaw. Next, repeat the entire procedure using a sharp object. The cap of a disposable ballpoint pen can be used to test light touch (dull end) and sharp stimuli (sharp end). If an abnor-mality appears, test for temperature sensation by touch-ing the patient's skin with test tubes filled with hot and cold water and asking him to differentiate between them.	The patient with a normal trigeminal nerve should report feeling both light touch and sharp stimuli in all three areas (forehead, cheek, and jaw) on both sides of his face.

ASSESSING THE CRANIAL NERVES *(continued)*

Cranial nerve and assessment technique	Normal findings

Trigeminal (CN V) *(continued)*

To assess the motor portion of the trigeminal nerve, ask the patient to clench his jaws. Palpate the temporal and masseter muscles bilaterally, checking for symmetry. Try to open the patient's clenched jaws. Next, watch for symmetry as the patient opens and closes his mouth.

The jaws should clench symmetrically and remain closed against resistance.

Then assess the corneal reflex.

The lids of both eyes should close when a wisp of cotton is lightly stroked across a cornea.

Facial (CN VII)

To test the motor portion of the facial nerve, ask the patient to wrinkle his forehead, raise and lower his eyebrows, smile and show his teeth, and puff out his cheeks. Also, with the patient's eyes tightly closed, attempt to open the eyelids. With each of these movements, observe closely for symmetry.

Normal facial movements are symmetrical.

To test the sensory portion of the facial nerve, which supplies taste sensation to the anterior two-thirds of the tongue, first prepare four marked, closed containers: one containing salt; another, sugar; a third, vinegar (or lemon); and a fourth, quinine (or bitters). Then, with the patient's eyes closed, place salt on the anterior two-thirds of his tongue using a cotton swab or dropper. Ask him to identify the taste as sweet, salty, sour, or bitter. Rinse the patient's mouth with water. Repeat this procedure, alternating flavors and sides of the tongue until all four flavors have been tested on both sides. Taste sensations to the posterior third of the tongue are supplied by the glossopharyngeal nerve (CN IX) and are usually tested at the same time.

Normal taste sensations are symmetrical.

Acoustic (CN VIII)

To assess the acoustic portion of this nerve, test the patient's hearing acuity.

The patient should be able to hear a whispered voice or a watch tick.

To assess the vestibular portion of this nerve, observe for nystagmus and disturbed balance and note reports of dizziness or vertigo.

The patient should display normal eye movement and balance and have no dizziness or vertigo.

Glossopharyngeal (CN IX) and vagus (CN X)

To assess these nerves, which have overlapping functions, first listen to the patient's voice for indications of a hoarse or nasal quality. Then watch the patient's soft palate when he says "ah." Next, test the gag reflex but warn the patient first. To evoke this reflex, touch the posterior wall of the pharynx with a cotton swab or tongue depressor.

The patient's voice should sound strong and clear. The soft palate and the uvula should rise when he says "ah," and the uvula should remain midline. The palatine arches should remain symmetrical during movement and at rest. The gag reflex should be intact. If the gag reflex appears decreased or the pharynx moves asymmetrically, evaluate each side of the posterior wall of the pharynx to confirm integrity of both cranial nerves.

(continued)

ASSESSING THE CRANIAL NERVES *(continued)*

Cranial nerve and assessment technique   **Normal findings**

Cranial nerve and assessment technique	Normal findings
Spinal accessory (CN XI) To assess this nerve, press down on the patient's shoulders while he attempts to shrug against the resistance. Note shoulder strength and symmetry while inspecting and palpating his trapezius muscle. Then apply resistance to the patient's turned head while he attempts to return it to a midline position. Note neck strength while inspecting and palpating the sternocleidomastoid muscle. Repeat for the opposite side.	Normally, both shoulders should be able to overcome the resistance equally well. The neck should overcome resistance in both directions.
Hypoglossal (CN XII) To assess this nerve, observe the patient's protruded tongue for deviation from midline, atrophy, or fasciculations, which are very fine muscle flickering indicative of lower motor neuron disease. Next, ask the patient to move the tongue rapidly from side to side with the mouth open. Then ask him to curl the tongue up toward the nose, then down toward the chin. Then use a tongue depressor or folded gauze pad to apply resistance to the patient's protruded tongue and ask him to try to push the depressor to one side. Repeat on the other side and note tongue strength. Listen to the patient's speech for *d, l, n,* and *t* sounds, which require use of the tongue. If general speech suggests a problem, have the patient repeat a phrase or series of words containing these sounds.	Normally, the tongue should be midline and the patient should be able to move it right to left, as well as up and down, equally. Pressure exerted by the tongue on the tongue depressor should be equal on either side. Speech should be clear.

Glabellar reflex
Repeatedly tap the bridge of the patient's nose. A persistent blinking response indicates diffuse cortical dysfunction.

Flexor withdrawal
Apply a noxious stimulus to the sole of the foot. Toe extension, foot dorsiflexion, and uncontrollable flexing of the entire leg indicate central nervous system damage.

Crossed extension
With the patient's leg fixed in extension, apply a noxious stimulus to the ball of the foot. Flexion followed by adduction and extension of the opposite lower leg indicates central nervous system damage.

Moro reflex
Drop the patient backward from a sitting position to create a sudden change in position of the head in relation to the trunk. Full extension and abduction of the arms and opening of the hands indicates central nervous system damage.

Startle reflex
Make a sudden loud or harsh noise. Sudden extension or abduction of the arms indicates central nervous system damage.

Assessing the cranial nerves

There are 12 pairs of cranial nerves that transmit motor and sensory messages between the brain and the head and neck. These nerves are designated by both a name, which indicates their function, and a Roman numeral. (See *Assessing the cranial nerves*, pages 44 to 46.)

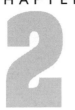
Signs and symptoms
Evaluating their significance

Common signs and symptoms

Arm pain

Arm pain usually results from musculoskeletal disorders; however, it can also result from neurovascular or cardiovascular disorders. Its location, onset, and character provide clues to its cause. The pain may affect the entire arm or only the upper arm or forearm. It may arise suddenly or gradually and be constant or intermittent. Arm pain can be described as sharp or dull, burning or numbing, and shooting or penetrating. Diffuse arm pain, though, may be difficult to describe, especially if it isn't associated with injury.

Medical causes

• *Angina.* This disorder may cause inner arm pain as well as chest and jaw pain. Typically, the pain follows exertion and persists for a few minutes. Accompanied by dyspnea, diaphoresis, and apprehension, the pain is relieved by rest or vasodilators such as nitroglycerin.

• *Biceps rupture.* Rupture of the biceps after excessive weight lifting or osteoarthritic degeneration of bicipital tendon insertion at the shoulder can cause pain in the upper arm. Forearm flexion and supination aggravate the pain. Other signs include muscle weakness, deformity, and edema.

• *Cellulitis.* Typically, this disorder affects the legs, but it can also affect the arms. It produces pain as well as redness, tenderness, edema and, at times, fever, chills, tachycardia, headache, and hypotension.

• *Cervical nerve root compression.* Compression of the cervical nerves supplying the upper arm produces chronic arm and neck pain, which may worsen with movement or prolonged sitting. The patient may also experience muscle weakness, paresthesia, and decreased reflex response.

• *Compartment syndrome.* Severe pain with passive muscle stretching is the cardinal sign of this syndrome. It may also impair distal circulation and cause muscle weakness, decreased reflex response, paresthesia, and edema. Ominous signs include paralysis and absent pulse.

• *Fractures.* In fractures of the cervical vertebrae, humerus, scapula, clavicle, radius, or ulna, pain can occur at the injury site and radiate throughout the entire arm. Pain at a fresh fracture site is intense and worsens with movement. Associated signs and symptoms include crepitus, which is felt and heard from bone ends rubbing together (don't attempt to elicit this sign); deformity, if bones are unaligned; local ecchymosis and edema; impaired distal circulation; paresthesia; and decreased sensation distal to the injury site.

• *Muscle contusion.* This disorder may cause generalized pain in the area of injury. It may also cause local swelling and ecchymosis.

• *Muscle strain.* Acute or chronic muscle strain causes mild to severe pain with movement. The resulting reduction in arm movement may cause muscle weakness and atrophy.

• *Myocardial infarction.* In this life-threatening disorder, the patient may complain of left arm pain as well as the characteristic deep and crushing chest pain. He may display weakness, pallor, nausea, vomiting, diaphoresis, altered blood pressure, tachycardia, dyspnea, and feelings of apprehension or impending doom.

• *Neoplasms of the arm.* This disorder produces continuous, deep, and penetrating arm pain that worsens at night. Occasionally, redness and swelling accompany the arm pain.

Later, skin breakdown, impaired circulation, and paresthesia may occur.
• *Osteomyelitis.* This disorder typically begins with the sudden onset of localized arm pain and fever. It's accompanied by local tenderness, painful and restricted movement and, later, swelling. Associated findings include malaise and tachycardia.

ALERT In children, arm pain commonly results from fractures, muscle sprain, muscular dystrophy, and rheumatoid arthritis. In young children especially, the exact location of the pain may be difficult to establish. Watch for nonverbal clues, such as wincing and guarding.

Ataxia

Classified as cerebellar or sensory, ataxia refers to incoordination and irregularity of voluntary, purposeful movements. Cerebellar ataxia is a result of disease of the cerebellum and its pathways to and from the cerebral cortex, brain stem, and spinal cord. It causes disorders of gait, trunk, limbs and, possibly, speech. Sensory ataxia is a result of impaired position sense (proprioception) caused by interruption of afferent nerve fibers in the peripheral nerves, posterior roots, posterior columns of the spinal cord, or medial lemnisci. It can also be caused by a lesion in the parietal lobes, which causes gait disorders.

Ataxia occurs in acute and chronic forms. Acute ataxia may result from hemorrhage or a large tumor in the posterior fossa. In this life-threatening condition, the cerebellum may herniate downward through the foramen magnum behind the cervical spinal cord or upward through the tentorium upon the cerebral hemispheres. Herniation may also compress the brain stem. Acute ataxia may also result from drug toxicity or

SUDDEN ATAXIA: WHAT TO DO
If ataxic movements suddenly develop, increased intracranial pressure and impending herniation may be the cause. Quick evaluation of level of consciousness, pupillary changes, motor weakness or paralysis, neck stiffness or pain, and vomiting is indicated. Vital signs must be assessed, especially respirations; abnormal respiratory patterns may quickly lead to respiratory arrest. The head of the bed should be elevated. Emergency resuscitation equipment must be readily available. The patient may require a computed tomography scan or surgery.

poisoning. Chronic ataxia can be progressive and can result from acute disease. It can also occur in metabolic and chronic degenerative neurologic disease.

Emergency interventions

See *Sudden ataxia: What to do.*

Medical causes

• *Cerebellar abscess.* This disorder commonly causes limb ataxia on the same side as the lesion as well as gait and truncal ataxia. The initial symptom is typically headache localized behind the ear or in the occipital region, which is followed by ocular motor palsy, fever, vomiting, altered level of consciousness (LOC), and coma.
• *Cerebellar hemorrhage.* In this life-threatening disorder, ataxia usually occurs acutely but is transient. Unilateral or bilateral ataxia affects the trunk, gait, or limbs.

The patient initially experiences repeated vomiting, an occipital headache, vertigo, ocular motor palsy, dysphagia, and dysarthria. Later signs, such as decreased LOC and coma, signal impending herniation.

• *Cerebrovascular accident (CVA).* In this disorder, occlusions in the vertebrobasilar arteries halt blood flow and cause infarction in the medulla, pons, or cerebellum that may lead to ataxia. The ataxia may occur at the onset of CVA and remain as a residual deficit. Worsening ataxia during the acute phase may indicate extension of the CVA or severe swelling. The ataxia may be accompanied by unilateral or bilateral motor weakness, altered LOC, sensory loss, vertigo, nausea, vomiting, ocular motor palsy, and dysphagia.

• *Diabetic neuropathy.* Peripheral nerve damage caused by diabetes mellitus may cause sensory ataxia as well as extremity pain, slight leg weakness, skin changes, and bowel and bladder dysfunction.

• *Guillain-Barré syndrome.* Peripheral nerve involvement usually follows this mild viral infection, but rarely leads to sensory ataxia. This syndrome can also cause ascending paralysis and possible respiratory distress.

• *Hyperthermia.* In this disorder, cerebellar ataxia occurs if the patient survives the coma and seizures characteristic of the acute phase. Subsequent findings include slowly resolving confusion, dementia, and spastic paralysis.

• *Metastatic carcinoma.* Carcinoma that metastasizes to the cerebellum may cause gait ataxia accompanied by headache, dizziness, nystagmus, decreased LOC, nausea, and vomiting.

• *Multiple sclerosis.* Nystagmus and cerebellar ataxia often occur in this disorder, but limb weakness and spasticity don't always accompany them. Speech ataxia (especially scanning) may occur as well as sensory ataxia from spinal cord involvement. During remissions, ataxia may subside or even disappear. During exacerbations, it may reappear, worsen, or even become permanent.

Multiple sclerosis also causes optic neuritis, optic atrophy, numbness and weakness, diplopia, dizziness, and bladder dysfunction.

• *Olivopontocerebellar atrophy.* This disease produces gait ataxia and later, limb and speech ataxia. Rarely, it produces intention tremor. It's accompanied by choreiform movements, dysphagia, and loss of sphincter tone.

• *Polyarteritis nodosa (PAN).* Acute or subacute PAN may cause sensory ataxia, abdominal and limb pain, hematuria, fever, and elevated blood pressure.

• *Polyneuropathy.* Carcinomatous and myelomatous polyneuropathy may occur before detection of the primary tumor in carcinoma, multiple myeloma, or Hodgkin's disease. Signs and symptoms include ataxia, severe motor weakness, muscle atrophy, and sensory loss in the limbs. Pain and skin changes may also occur.

• *Posterior fossa tumor.* Gait, truncal, or limb ataxia is an early sign of a posterior fossa tumor and may worsen as the tumor enlarges. This sign is accompanied by vomiting, headache, papilledema, vertigo, ocular motor palsy, decreased LOC, and motor and sensory impairments on the same side as the lesion.

• *Wernicke's disease.* The result of thiamine deficiency, this disease produces gait ataxia and, rarely, intention tremor and speech ataxia. In severe ataxia, the patient may be unable to stand or walk. Ataxia decreases with thiamine therapy. Associated signs include nystagmus, diplopia, ocular palsies, confusion, tachycardia, exertional dyspnea, and postural hypotension.

Other causes

• *Drugs.* Toxic levels of anticonvulsants, especially phenytoin, may result in gait ataxia. Toxic levels of anticholinergics and tricyclic antidepressants may also result in ataxia. Aminoglutethimide causes ataxia in about 10% of patients; however, this effect usually disappears 4 to 6 weeks after the cessation of drug therapy.

 ALERT In children, ataxia occurs in acute and chronic forms, resulting from congenital or acquired disease. Acute ataxia may stem from febrile infection, brain tumors, mumps, and other disorders. Chronic ataxia may stem from Gaucher's disease, Refsum's disease, and other inborn errors of metabolism.

When assessing a child for ataxia, consider his level of motor skills and emotional state. Your examination may be limited to observing the child in spontaneous activity and carefully questioning his parents about changes in his motor activity, such as increased unsteadiness and falling. If you suspect ataxia, the child may need to be referred for a neurologic evaluation to rule out brain tumor.

Babinski's reflex

Babinski's reflex (extensor plantar reflex) refers to dorsiflexion of the great toe with extension and fanning of the other toes. It's an abnormal reflex elicited by firmly stroking the lateral aspect of the sole of the foot with a blunt object. In some patients, this reflex can be triggered by noxious stimuli, such as pain, noise, and even bumping of the bed. An indicator of corticospinal damage, Babinski's reflex may occur unilaterally or bilaterally. It may also be temporary or permanent. A temporary Babinski's reflex commonly occurs during the postictal phase of a seizure, whereas a permanent Babinski's reflex occurs with corticospinal damage. A positive Babinski's reflex is normal in neonates and in infants less than 12 months old. (See *How to elicit Babinski's reflex,* page 52.)

Medical causes

• *Amyotrophic lateral sclerosis (ALS).* In this progressive motor neuron disorder, bilateral Babinski's reflex may occur with hyperactive DTRs and spasticity. Typically, ALS produces fasciculations accompanied by muscle atrophy and weakness. Incoordination makes carrying out activities of daily living difficult for the patient. Associated signs and symptoms include impaired speech; difficulty chewing, swallowing, and breathing; urinary frequency and urgency; and occasionally, choking and excessive drooling. Although his mental status should remain intact, the patient's poor prognosis may cause periods of depression. Progressive bulbar palsy involves the brain stem and may cause episodes of crying or inappropriate laughter.

• *Brain tumor.* When it involves the corticospinal tract, a brain tumor may produce Babinski's reflex. The reflex may be accompanied by hyperactive DTRs (unilateral or bilateral), spasticity, seizures, cranial nerve dysfunction, hemiparesis or hemiplegia, decreased pain sensation, unsteady gait, incoordination, headache, emotional lability, and decreased level of consciousness (LOC).

• *Cerebrovascular accident (CVA).* Babinski's reflex varies with the site of the CVA. If the CVA involves the cerebrum, it produces unilateral Babinski's reflex accompanied by hemiplegia or hemiparesis, unilateral hyperactive DTRs, hemianopia, and aphasia. If it involves the brain stem, it produces bilateral Babinski's reflex

HOW TO ELICIT BABINSKI'S REFLEX

To elicit Babinski's reflex, stroke the lateral aspect of the sole of the patient's foot with your thumbnail or another moderately sharp object. Normally, this elicits flexion of all toes (a negative Babinski's reflex). In a positive Babinski's reflex, the great toe extends and the other toes fan out.

Negative Babinski's reflex

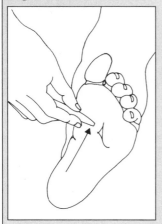

Positive Babinski's reflex

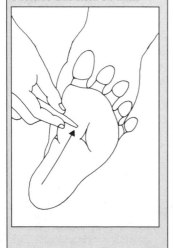

accompanied by bilateral weakness or paralysis, bilateral hyperactive DTRs, cranial nerve dysfunction, incoordination, and unsteady gait. Generalized signs and symptoms of CVA may include headache, vomiting, fever, disorientation, nuchal rigidity, seizures, and coma.

• *Head trauma.* Unilateral or bilateral Babinski's reflex may occur as a result of primary corticospinal damage or secondary injury associated with increased intracranial pressure. Hyperactive deep tendon reflexes and spasticity commonly occur with Babinski's reflex. The patient may also have weakness and incoordination. Other signs and symptoms vary with the type of head trauma. There may be headache, vomiting, behavior changes, altered vital signs, and decreased LOC with abnormal pupillary size and response to light.

• *Multiple sclerosis (MS).* In most patients with this demyelinating disorder, Babinski's reflex eventually occurs bilaterally. It follows the initial signs and symptoms of MS, which are most commonly paresthesia, nystagmus, blurred vision, and double vision. Associated signs and symptoms include scanning speech, dysphagia, intention tremor, weakness, incoordination, spasticity, gait ataxia, seizures, paraparesis or paraplegia, bladder incontinence and, occasionally, loss of pain and temperature sensation and proprioception. Emotional lability is also characteristic.

• *Spinal cord injury.* In an acute injury, spinal shock temporarily erases all reflexes. As shock resolves, Babinski's reflex occurs unilaterally when injury affects only one side of the spinal cord (Brown-Séquard's syndrome), and bilaterally when the injury affects both sides. Rather than signaling the return of neurologic function, this reflex confirms corticospinal damage. It's accompanied by hyperactive DTRs, spasticity, and variable or total loss of pain and temperature sensation, proprioception, and motor function. Horner's syndrome, marked by unilateral ptosis, pupillary constriction, and facial anhidrosis, may occur with lower cervical cord injury.

• *Spinal cord tumor.* In this disorder, bilateral Babinski's reflex occurs with variable loss of pain and temperature sensation, proprioception, and motor function. Spasticity, hyperactive DTRs, absent abdominal reflexes, and incontinence are also characteristic of this disorder. Diffuse pain may occur at the level of the tumor.

• *Syringomyelia.* In this disorder, bilateral Babinski's reflex occurs with muscle atrophy and weakness that may progress to paralysis. It's accompanied by spasticity, ataxia and, occasionally, deep pain. DTRs may be hypoactive or hyperactive. Cranial nerve dysfunction, such as dysphagia and dysarthria, commonly appears late in the disorder.

 ALERT Babinski's reflex occurs normally in children under age 2 and reflects immaturity of the corticospinal tract. After age 2, Babinski's reflex is pathologic and may result from hydrocephalus or any of the causes more commonly seen in adults.

Back pain

Back pain affects an estimated 80% of the population; in fact, it's second only to the common cold as a cause of lost time from work. Although this symptom may herald a spondylogenic disorder, it may also result from genitourinary, GI, cardiovascular, and neoplastic disorders. Postural imbalance associated with pregnancy may also cause back pain.

The onset, location, and distribution of pain and its response to activity and rest provide important clues about the causative disorder. Pain may be acute or chronic and constant or intermittent. It may remain localized in the back or radiate along the spine or down one or both legs. Pain may be exacerbated by activities, such as bending, stooping, and lifting and alleviated by rest, or it may be unaffected by both.

Intrinsic back pain results from muscle spasm nerve root irritation, fracture, or a combination of these mechanisms. It most commonly occurs in the lower back, or lumbosacral area. Back pain may also be referred from the abdomen or flank, possibly signaling life-threatening perforated ulcer, acute pancreatitis, or dissecting abdominal aortic aneurysm.

Emergency interventions

See *Severe back pain: What to do*, page 54.

Medical causes

• *Abdominal aortic aneurysm (dissecting).* Life-threatening dissection of this aneurysm may initially cause lower back pain or dull abdominal pain. More often, it produces constant upper abdominal pain. A pulsating abdominal mass may be palpated in the epigastrium. Although after a rupture, it no longer pulses. Aneurysmal dissection can also cause mottled skin below the waist, absent femoral and pedal pulses, lower blood pressure in the legs than in the arms, mild to moderate tenderness with guarding, and abdominal rigidity. Signs of shock, such as cool, clammy skin, will appear if blood loss is significant.

• *Ankylosing spondylitis.* This chronic, progressive disorder causes sacroiliac pain that radiates up the spine and is aggravated by lateral pressure on the pelvis. The pain is

If the patient reports acute, severe back pain, vital signs should be assessed and a rapid evaluation performed to rule out life-threatening causes. You should ask him when the pain began. Ask if he can relate it to any causes. For example, did the pain occur after eating? After falling on ice? Then ask the patient to describe the pain. Is it burning, stabbing, throbbing, or aching? Is it constant or intermittent? Does it radiate to the buttocks or legs? Is there any leg weakness? Does the pain seem to originate in the abdomen and radiate to the back? What makes it feel better and worse? Is it affected by activity and rest? Is it worse in the morning or evening? Typically, visceral referred back pain is unaffected by activity and rest. In contrast, pain of spondylogenic origin worsens with activity and improves with rest. Pain of neoplastic origin is frequently relieved by walking and worsens at night.

If the patient describes deep lumbar pain unaffected by activity, refer him to a doctor for evaluation. If this sign is present along with a pulsating abdominal mass, you should suspect a dissecting abdominal aortic aneurysm.

If the patient describes severe epigastric pain that radiates through the abdomen to the back, assessment for absent bowel sounds and for abdominal rigidity and tenderness by a doctor is indicated. If these assessments are found, a perforated ulcer or acute pancreatitis should be suspected.

fatigue, fever, anorexia, weight loss, and occasional iritis.

• *Endometriosis.* This disorder causes deep sacral pain and severe, cramping pain in the lower abdomen. The pain worsens just before or during menstruation and may be aggravated by defecation. It's accompanied by constipation, abdominal tenderness, dysmenorrhea, and dyspareunia.

• *Intervertebral disk rupture.* This disorder produces gradual or sudden lower back pain with or without leg pain (sciatica). It also rarely produces leg pain alone. More often, pain begins in the back and radiates to the buttocks and leg. The pain is exacerbated by activity, coughing, and sneezing and is eased by rest. It's accompanied by paresthesia (most commonly, numbness or tingling in the lower leg and foot); paravertebral muscle spasm; and decreased reflexes on the affected side. This disorder also affects posture and gait. The patient's spine is slightly flexed and he leans toward the painful side. He walks slowly and rises from a sitting to standing position with extreme difficulty.

• *Lumbosacral sprain.* This disorder causes aching and localized pain and tenderness associated with muscle spasm on lateral motion. The recumbent patient will typically flex his knees and hips to help ease the pain. Flexion of the spine intensifies the pain, whereas rest helps to relieve it.

• *Metastatic tumors.* These tumors commonly spread to the spine, causing lower back pain in at least 25% of patients. Typically, the pain begins abruptly, is accompanied by cramping muscular pain, and isn't relieved by rest.

• *Myeloma.* Back pain caused by this primary malignant tumor frequently begins abruptly and worsens with exercise. It may be accompanied by arthritic symptoms, such as achi-

usually most severe in the morning or after a period of inactivity and isn't relieved by rest. Abnormal rigidity of the lumbar spine with forward flexion is also characteristic. This disorder can also cause local tenderness,

ness, joint swelling, and tenderness. Other clinical effects include fever, malaise, peripheral paresthesia, and weight loss.

• *Prostatic carcinoma.* Chronic, aching back pain may be the only symptom of prostatic carcinoma. This disorder may also produce hematuria.

• *Pyelonephritis (acute).* This disorder produces progressive flank and lower abdominal pain accompanied by back pain or tenderness (especially over the costovertebral angle). Other signs and symptoms include high fever, chills, nausea, vomiting, flank and abdominal tenderness, and urinary frequency and urgency.

• *Renal calculi.* The colicky pain of this disorder usually results from irritation of the ureteral lining, and increases the frequency and force of peristaltic contractions. The pain travels from the costovertebral angle to the flank, suprapubic region, and external genitalia. Its intensity varies but may become excruciating if calculi travel down a ureter. If calculi are in the renal pelvis and calyces, dull and constant flank pain may occur. Renal calculi also cause nausea, vomiting, urinary urgency (if a calculus lodges near the bladder), hematuria, and agitation due to pain.

• *Sacroiliac strain.* This disorder causes sacroiliac pain that may radiate to the buttock, hip, and lateral aspect of the thigh. The pain is aggravated by weight bearing on the affected extremity and by abduction with resistance of the leg. Associated signs and symptoms include tenderness of the symphysis pubis and a limp or Trendelenburg lurch.

• *Spinal neoplasm (benign).* Typically, this disorder causes severe, localized back pain and scoliosis.

• *Spinal stenosis.* Resembling a ruptured intervertebral disk, this disorder produces back pain with or without sciatica. Frequently, sciatica affects both legs and is accompanied by claudication. The pain may progress to numbness or weakness unless the patient rests for relief.

• *Spondylolisthesis.* A major structural disorder characterized by forward slippage of one vertebra onto another, spondylolisthesis may be asymptomatic or cause lower back pain with or without nerve root involvement. Associated symptoms of nerve root involvement include paresthesia, buttock pain, and pain radiating down the leg. Palpation of the lumbar spine may reveal a "step-off" of the spinous process. Flexion of the spine may be limited.

• *Transverse process fracture.* This fracture causes severe localized back pain with muscle spasm and hematoma.

• *Vertebral compression fracture.* Initially, this fracture may be painless. Several weeks later, it causes back pain aggravated by weight bearing and local tenderness. Fracture of a thoracic vertebra may cause referred pain in the lumbar area.

• *Vertebral osteomyelitis.* Initially, this disorder causes insidious back pain. As it progresses, the pain may become constant, more pronounced at night, and aggravated by spinal movement. Accompanying symptoms include vertebral and hamstring spasms, tenderness of the spinous processes, fever, and malaise.

• *Vertebral osteoporosis.* This disorder causes chronic, aching back pain that is aggravated by activity and somewhat relieved by rest. Tenderness may also occur.

Carpopedal spasm

Carpopedal spasm is the violent, painful contraction of the muscles in the hands and feet. (See *Identifying carpopedal spasm,* page 56.) It's an important sign of tetany, a potentially

IDENTIFYING CARPOPEDAL SPASM

In the hand, carpopedal spasm involves adduction of the thumb over the palm, followed by flexion of the metacarpophalangeal joints, extension of the interphalangeal joints (fingers together), adduction of the hyperextended fingers, and flexion of the wrist and elbow joints. Similar effects occur in the joints of the feet.

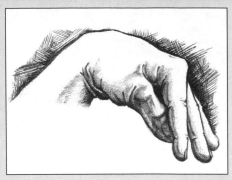

life-threatening condition characterized by increased neuromuscular excitation and sustained muscle contraction that is commonly associated with hypocalcemia.

Carpopedal spasm requires prompt evaluation and intervention; if left untreated, it can cause laryngospasm, seizures, cardiac arrhythmias, and cardiac and respiratory arrest.

Emergency interventions

See *Carpopedal spasm: What to do*.

Medical causes

• *Hypocalcemia*. Carpopedal spasm is an early sign of hypocalcemia. It's usually accompanied by paresthesia of the fingers, toes, and perioral area; muscle weakness, twitching, and cramping; hyperreflexia; chorea; fatigue; and palpitations. Positive Chvostek's and Trousseau's signs can be elicited. Laryngospasm, stridor, and seizures may appear in severe hypocalcemia.

Chronic hypocalcemia may be accompanied by mental status changes; cramps; dry, scaly skin; brittle nails; and thin, patchy hair and eyebrows.

Other causes

• *Treatments*. Multiple blood transfusions and parathyroidectomy may cause hypocalcemia, resulting in carpopedal spasm. Surgical procedures that impair calcium absorption, such as ileostomy formation and gastric resection with gastrojejunostomy, may also cause hypocalcemia.

Chest pain

This symptom most often results from disorders that affect thoracic or abdominal organs, including the heart, pleurae, lungs, esophagus, rib cage, gallbladder, pancreas, or stomach. It's an important indicator of several acute and life-threatening cardiopulmonary and GI disorders. However, it can also result from musculoskeletal and hematologic disorders, anxiety, and drug therapy.

The cause of chest pain may initially be difficult to distinguish. Chest pain can arise suddenly or gradually. It can radiate to the arms, neck, jaw, and back. It can be steady or intermittent and mild or acute. It can also range in character from a sharp shooting sensation to a feeling of heaviness, fullness, and even indigestion. It can be provoked or aggravated by stress, anxiety, exertion, deep breathing, and eating certain foods.

Emergency interventions

See *Chest pain: What to do,* page 58.

Medical causes

• *Angina.* In angina pectoris, the patient may experience a feeling of tightness or pressure in the chest that he describes as pain or a sensation of indigestion or expansion. Usually, the pain occurs in the retrosternal region over a palm-sized or larger area. It may radiate to the neck, jaw, and arms — typically, the inner aspect of the left arm. Anginal pain tends to begin gradually, build to its maximum, and then slowly subside. Provoked by exertion, emotional stress, or a heavy meal, the pain typically lasts 2 to 10 minutes. Associated findings may include dyspnea, nausea, vomiting, tachycardia, dizziness, diaphoresis, belching, palpitations, and an atrial gallop (S_4) or murmur during an anginal episode.

In Prinzmetal's angina, chest pain occurs when the patient is at rest or it may awaken him. It may occur with shortness of breath, nausea, vomiting, dizziness, and palpitations. During an attack, an atrial gallop may be present.

• *Anxiety.* Acute anxiety can produce intermittent, sharp, stabbing pain, often located in the left breast. This pain isn't related to exertion and lasts only a few seconds, but the patient may experience a precordial ache or a sensation of heaviness that lasts for hours or days. Associated signs and symptoms may include precordial tenderness, palpitations, fatigue, headache, insomnia, breathlessness, nausea, vomiting, diarrhea, and tremors.

CARPOPEDAL SPASM: WHAT TO DO

If you detect carpopedal spasm, quickly examine the patient for signs of respiratory distress, such as laryngospasm, stridor, loud crowing noises, and cyanosis, or cardiac arrhythmias, which indicate hypocalcemia. Notify the primary care provider or call for emergency services. An I.V. calcium preparation should be administered and emergency respiratory and cardiac support provided if necessary. If calcium infusion doesn't control the seizures, the administration of a sedative such as chloral hydrate may be necessary.

• *Aortic aneurysm (dissecting).* The chest pain associated with this disorder usually begins suddenly and is most severe at its onset. The patient describes an excruciating tearing, ripping, and stabbing pain in his chest and neck that radiates to his upper back, abdomen, and lower back. He may also have abdominal tenderness, a palpable abdominal mass, tachycardia, murmurs, syncope, blindness, loss of consciousness, weakness or transient paralysis of the arms or legs, a systolic bruit, systemic hypotension, asymmetrical brachial pulses, lower blood pressure in the legs than in the arms, and weak or absent femoral or pedal pulses. His skin may be pale, cool, diaphoretic, and mottled below the waist. Capillary refill time is prolonged in the toes, and palpation reveals decreased pulsation of one or both carotid arteries.

• *Cardiomyopathy.* In hypertrophic cardiomyopathy, angina-like chest pain may occur with dyspnea, a cough, dizziness, syncope, gallops, murmurs, and arrhythmias.

CHEST PAIN: WHAT TO DO

You should ask the patient when his chest pain began. Did it arise suddenly or gradually? Is it more severe or frequent now than when it first started? Sudden, severe chest pain requires prompt evaluation and treatment by a doctor because it may herald a life-threatening disorder.

• *Costochondritis.* Pain and tenderness occur at the costochondral junctions, especially at the second costicartilage.

• *Interstitial lung disease.* As this disease advances, the patient may have pleuritic chest pain along with progressive dyspnea, cellophane-type crackles, nonproductive cough, fatigue, weight loss, clubbing, and cyanosis.

• *Lung abscess.* Pleuritic chest pain develops insidiously in this disorder along with a pleural friction rub and a cough that raises copious amounts of purulent, foul-smelling, blood-tinged sputum. The affected side is dull to percussion, and decreased breath sounds and crackles may be heard. The patient will also display diaphoresis, anorexia, weight loss, fever, chills, fatigue, weakness, dyspnea, and clubbing.

• *Lung cancer.* The chest pain associated with lung cancer is often described as an intermittent aching felt deep within the chest. If the tumor metastasizes to the ribs or vertebrae, the pain becomes localized, continuous, and gnawing. Associated findings may include a cough that is sometimes bloody, wheezing, dyspnea, fatigue, anorexia, weight loss, and fever.

• *Mitral prolapse.* Typically, the patient with a prolapsed mitral valve will experience sharp, stabbing precordial chest pain or precordial ache. The pain can last for seconds or for hours and occasionally mimics the pain of ischemic heart disease. The characteristic sign of mitral prolapse is a midsystolic click followed by a systolic murmur at the apex. The patient may experience cardiac awareness, migraine headache, dizziness, weakness, episodic severe fatigue, dyspnea, tachycardia, mood swings, and palpitations.

• *Muscle strain.* Strained chest, arm, or shoulder muscles may cause a superficial and continuous ache or "pulling" sensation in the chest. Lifting, pulling, or pushing heavy objects may aggravate this discomfort. In acute muscle strain, the patient may experience fatigue, weakness, and rapid swelling of the affected area.

• *Myocardial infarction (MI).* The chest pain in MI can last from 15 minutes to hours. It's typically a crushing substernal pain, unrelieved by rest or nitroglycerin. It may radiate to the patient's left arm, jaw, neck, or shoulder blades. The patient may have pallor, clammy skin, dyspnea, diaphoresis, nausea, vomiting, anxiety, restlessness, and a feeling of impending doom. He may develop hypotension or hypertension, an atrial gallop, murmurs, and crackles. A low-grade fever may also arise within 4 days.

• *Peptic ulcer.* In this disorder, sharp and burning pain usually arises in the epigastric region. This pain characteristically arises hours after food intake, often occurring during the night. It lasts longer than angina-like pain and can be relieved by food or antacids. Other findings may include nausea, vomiting, melena, and epigastric tenderness.

• *Pericarditis.* This disorder produces precordial or retrosternal pain aggravated by deep breathing, coughing, position changes and, occasionally, swallowing. Frequently, the pain is sharp or cutting and radiates to the shoulder and neck. Associated signs and symptoms may include pericardial friction rub, fever, tachycardia, and dyspnea.

• *Pleurisy.* The chest pain of pleurisy arises abruptly and reaches maximum intensity within a few hours. It's sharp, even knifelike, usually unilateral, and located in the lower and lateral aspects of the chest. Deep breathing, coughing, or thoracic movement characteristically aggravates it. Auscultation over the painful area may reveal decreased breath sounds, inspiratory crackles, and a pleural friction rub. Other effects may include dyspnea, cyanosis, fever, fatigue, and rapid, shallow breathing.

• *Pneumonia.* This disorder produces pleuritic chest pain that increases with deep inspiration and is accompanied by shaking chills and fever. The patient will have a dry cough that later becomes productive. Other signs and symptoms may include crackles, rhonchi, tachycardia, tachypnea, myalgias, fatigue, headache, dyspnea, abdominal pain, anorexia, cyanosis, decreased breath sounds, and diaphoresis.

• *Pneumothorax.* Spontaneous pneumothorax, a life-threatening disorder, causes sudden sharp chest pain that is severe, often unilateral, and rarely localized, which increases with chest movement. When it's located centrally and radiates to the neck, pneumothorax may mimic an MI. After the onset of pain, dyspnea and cyanosis progressively worsen. Breath sounds are decreased or absent on the affected side with hyperresonance or tympany, subcutaneous crepitation, and decreased vocal fremitus. Asymmetrical chest expansion, accessory muscle use, a nonproductive cough, tachypnea, tachycardia, anxiety, and restlessness also occur.

• *Pulmonary embolism.* This acute, life-threatening disorder produces chest pain or a choking sensation. Typically, the patient first experiences sudden dyspnea with intense angina-like or pleuritic pain aggravated by deep breathing and thoracic movement. Other findings may include tachycardia; tachypnea; cough, which may be nonproductive or productive of blood-tinged sputum; a low-grade fever; restlessness; diaphoresis; crackles; a pleural friction rub; diffuse wheezing; dullness to percussion; signs of circulatory collapse, including weak, rapid pulse and hypotension; signs of cerebral ischemia, including transient unconsciousness, coma, and seizures; signs of hypoxia, including restlessness; and particularly in the elderly, hemiplegia and other focal neurologic deficits. Less common signs include massive hemoptysis, chest splinting, and leg edema. A patient with a large embolus may have cyanosis and distended neck veins.

• *Rib fracture.* The chest pain due to fractured ribs is usually sharp, severe, and aggravated by inspiration, coughing, or pressure on the affected area. Besides dyspnea, cough, and shallow, splinted respirations, the patient experiences tenderness and slight edema at the fracture site.

• *Thoracic outlet syndrome.* Often causing paresthesia along the ulnar distribution of the arm, this syndrome can be confused with angina. The patient usually experiences angina-like pain after lifting his arms above his head, working with his hands above his shoulders, or lifting a weight. The pain disappears immediately when he lowers his arms. Other signs and symptoms may include a difference in blood pressure between each arm and cool, pale skin.

Other causes

• *Drugs.* Abrupt withdrawal of beta-adrenergic blockers can cause rebound angina in patients with coronary heart disease, especially those who have received high doses for a prolonged period.

Cogwheel rigidity

This cardinal sign of Parkinson's disease is marked by muscle rigidity that reacts with superimposed ratchetlike movements when the muscle is passively stretched. This sign can be elicited by stabilizing the patient's forearm and then moving his hand through the range of motion. (Cogwheel rigidity most often appears in the arms but can sometimes be elicited in the ankle.) Both the patient and examiner can see and feel these characteristic movements, thought to be a combination of rigidity and tremor.

Medical causes

• *Parkinson's disease.* In this disorder, cogwheel rigidity occurs together with an insidious tremor, which usually begins in the fingers (unilateral pill-roll tremor), increases during stress or anxiety, and decreases with purposeful movement and sleep.

Bradykinesia, or slowness of voluntary movements and speech, also occurs. The patient walks with short, shuffling steps; his gait lacks normal parallel motion and may be retropulsive or propulsive. He may have a monotone way of speaking and a masklike facial expression and may experience drooling; loss of posture control, causing him to walk with his body bent forward; dysphagia; and dysarthria. An oculogyric crisis (eyes fixed upward and involuntary tonic movements) or blepharospasm (complete eyelid closure) may also occur.

Other causes

• *Drugs.* Phenothiazines and other antipsychotic drugs, such as haloperidol, thiothixene, and loxapine can also cause cogwheel rigidity. Metoclopramide infrequently causes it.

Confusion

An umbrella term for puzzling or inappropriate behavior or responses, confusion reflects the inability to think quickly and coherently. Depending on its cause, confusion may arise suddenly or gradually and may be temporary or irreversible. Aggravated by stress and sensory deprivation, confusion often occurs in hospitalized patients, especially the elderly, in whom it may be mistaken for senility.

When severe confusion arises suddenly and the patient also has hallucinations and psychomotor hyperactivity, his condition is classified as delirium. Long-term, progressive confusion with deterioration of all cognitive functions is classified as dementia.

Confusion can result from fluid and electrolyte imbalance or hypoxemia due to pulmonary disorders. However, it can also have a metabolic, neurologic, cardiovascular, cerebrovascular, or nutritional origin. It can also result from a severe systemic infection or the effects of toxins, drugs, or alcohol. Confusion may signal worsening of an underlying and perhaps irreversible disease.

Medical causes

• *Brain tumor.* In the early stages of a brain tumor, confusion is usually mild and difficult to detect. As the tumor impinges on cerebral structures, however, the patient's confusion worsens, and he may display personality changes, bizarre behavior, or sensory and motor deficits. He may also have visual field deficits and aphasia.

• *Cerebrovascular disorders.* These disorders produce confusion due to tissue hypoxia and ischemia. Confusion may be insidious and fleeting, as in a transient ischemic attack, or acute and permanent, as in cerebrovascular accident.

• *Dementia.* This group of progressive brain diseases, such as Alzheimer's disease, eventually produces severe and irreversible confusion along with memory loss and intellectual deterioration. Disorientation, tremors, and gait disturbances may also occur.

• *Fluid and electrolyte imbalance.* The extent of imbalance determines the severity of the patient's confusion. Typically, a patient will show signs of dehydration, such as lassitude, poor skin turgor, dry skin and mucous membranes, and oliguria. He may also have hypotension and a low-grade fever.

• *Head trauma.* Concussion, contusion, and brain hemorrhage may produce confusion at the time of injury, shortly afterward, or even months or years afterward. The patient may be delirious, with periodic loss of consciousness. Vomiting, severe headache, pupillary changes, and sensory and motor deficits are also common.

• *Hypoxemia.* Acute pulmonary disorders that result in hypoxemia produce confusion that can range from mild disorientation to delirium. Chronic pulmonary disorders produce persistent confusion.

• *Infection.* Severe generalized infection, such as sepsis, often produces delirium. Central nervous system (CNS) infections, such as meningitis, cause varying degrees of confusion along with headache and nuchal rigidity.

• *Low perfusion states.* Mild confusion is an early sign of decreased cerebral perfusion. Associated findings usually include hypotension, tachycardia or bradycardia, irregular pulse, ventricular gallop, edema, and cyanosis.

• *Metabolic encephalopathy.* Both hyperglycemia and hypoglycemia can produce a sudden onset of confusion. A patient with hypoglycemia may also experience transient delirium and seizures. Uremic and hepatic encephalopathies produce a gradual confusion that may progress to seizures and coma. Usually, the patient experiences tremors and restlessness, as well.

• *Nutritional deficiencies.* Inadequate dietary intake of thiamine, niacin, or vitamin B_{12} produces insidious, progressive confusion and possible mental deterioration.

• *Seizure disorders.* Mild to moderate confusion may immediately follow any type of seizure. The confusion usually disappears within several hours.

Other causes

• *Drugs.* Large doses of CNS depressants produce confusion that can persist for several days after the drug is discontinued. Narcotic and barbiturate withdrawal also causes acute confusion, possibly with delirium. Other drugs that commonly cause confusion include lidocaine, digoxin, indomethacin, cycloserine, chloroquine, atropine, and cimetidine.

Crepitation, bony

Bony crepitation is a palpable vibration or an audible crunching sound that results when one bone grates against another. It often results from a fracture. It can also happen when bones that have been stripped of their protective articular cartilage grind against each other as they articulate, for example, in advanced arthritic or degenerative joint disorders.

Eliciting bony crepitation can help confirm diagnosis of a fracture. However, it can also cause further soft-tissue, nerve, or vessel injury. In addition, rubbing fractured bone ends together can convert a closed fracture into an open one if a bone end penetrates the skin; therefore, after initial detection of crepitation in a patient with a fracture, you should avoid subsequent elicitation of this sign.

Medical causes

• *Fracture.* In addition to bony crepitation, a fracture causes acute local pain, hematoma, edema, and decreased ROM. Other findings may include deformity, point tenderness, discoloration of the limb, and loss of limb function. Neurovascular damage may cause prolonged capillary refill time, diminished or absent pulses, mottled cyanosis, paresthesia, and decreased sensation (all distal to the fracture site). An open fracture produces an obvious skin wound.
• *Osteoarthritis.* In advanced cases of this disorder, joint crepitation may be elicited during ROM testing. The cardinal symptom of osteoarthritis is joint pain, especially during motion and weight bearing. Other findings include joint stiffness that typically occurs after resting and subsides within a few minutes after the patient begins moving.
• *Rheumatoid arthritis.* In advanced cases of this disorder, bony crepitation is heard when the affected joint is rotated. However, rheumatoid arthritis usually develops insidiously, producing nonspecific signs and symptoms, such as fatigue, malaise, anorexia, a persistent low-grade fever, weight loss, lymphadenopathy, and vague arthralgias and myalgias. Lat-

er, more specific and localized articular signs develop, frequently at the proximal finger joints. These signs usually occur bilaterally and symmetrically and may extend to the wrists, knees, elbows, and ankles. The affected joints may stiffen after inactivity. The patient also has increased warmth, swelling, and tenderness of affected joints, and limited ROM.

Deep tendon reflexes, hyperactive

A hyperactive deep tendon reflex (DTR) is an abnormally brisk muscle contraction in response to a sudden stretch that may be induced by sharply tapping the muscle's tendon of insertion. This elicited sign may be graded as brisk or pathologically hyperactive. Hyperactive reflexes are often accompanied by clonus.

The corticospinal and other descending tracts govern the reflex arc, which is the relay cycle that produces any reflex response. A corticospinal lesion above the level of the reflex arc being tested may result in a hyperactive DTR. Abnormal neuromuscular transmission at the end of the reflex arc may also cause a hyperactive DTR. For example, deficiency of calcium or magnesium may cause a hyperactive DTR because these electrolytes regulate neuromuscular excitability.

Although hyperactive DTRs frequently accompany other neurologic findings, they usually lack specific diagnostic value. For example, hyperactive DTRs are an early, cardinal sign of hypocalcemia.

Medical causes

• *Amyotrophic lateral sclerosis.* This disorder produces generalized hyperactive DTRs. Weakness of the hands and forearms and spasticity of the legs accompany these DTRs. Eventually, the patient develops atrophy of the neck and tongue muscles, fasciculations, occasional weakness of the legs, and possible bulbar signs, including dysphagia, dysphonia, facial weakness, and dyspnea.

• *Brain tumor.* A cerebral tumor causes hyperactive DTRs on the side opposite the lesion. Associated signs and symptoms develop slowly and may include unilateral paresis or paralysis, anesthesia, visual field deficits, spasticity, and a positive Babinski's reflex.

• *Cerebrovascular accident (CVA).* Any CVA that affects the origin of the corticospinal tracts causes sudden onset of hyperactive DTRs on the side opposite the lesion. There may also be unilateral paresis or paralysis, anesthesia, visual field deficits, spasticity, and a positive Babinski's reflex.

• *Hypocalcemia.* This disorder may produce sudden or gradual onset of generalized hyperactive DTRs with paresthesia, muscle twitching and cramping, positive Chvostek's and Trousseau's signs, carpopedal spasm, and tetany.

• *Hypomagnesemia.* This disorder results in gradual onset of generalized hyperactive DTRs accompanied by muscle cramps, hypotension, tachycardia, paresthesia, ataxia, tetany, and possible seizures.

• *Hypothermia.* Mild hypothermia (90° to 94° F [32.2° to 34.4° C]) produces generalized hyperactive DTRs. Other signs and symptoms include shivering, fatigue, weakness, lethargy, slurred speech, ataxia, muscle stiffness, tachycardia, diuresis, bradypnea, hypotension, and cold, pale skin.

• *Multiple sclerosis.* Typically, hyperactive DTRs are preceded by weakness and paresthesia in one or both arms or legs. Associated signs include clonus and a positive Babinski's re-

flex. Passive flexion of the patient's neck may cause a tingling sensation down his back. Later, ataxia, diplopia, vertigo, vomiting, and urine retention or urinary incontinence may occur.

• *Preeclampsia.* Occurring in pregnancies of at least 20 weeks' duration, preeclampsia may cause the gradual onset of generalized hyperactive DTRs. Accompanying signs and symptoms include increased blood pressure; abnormal weight gain; edema of the face, fingers, and abdomen after bed rest; oliguria; severe headache; blurred or double vision; epigastric pain; nausea and vomiting; irritability; cyanosis; shortness of breath; and crackles. If preeclampsia progresses to eclampsia, the patient will have seizures.

• *Spinal cord lesion.* Incomplete spinal cord lesions cause hyperactive DTRs below the level of the lesion. In a traumatic lesion, hyperactive DTRs follow the resolution of spinal shock. In a neoplastic lesion, hyperactive DTRs gradually replace normal DTRs. Other signs and symptoms are paralysis and sensory loss below the level of the lesion, urine retention with overflow incontinence, and alternating constipation and diarrhea. In a lesion above T6, there may also be autonomic hyperreflexia with diaphoresis and flushing above the level of the lesion, headache, nasal congestion, nausea, increased blood pressure, and bradycardia.

ALERT Hyperreflexia may be a normal sign in neonates. After age 6, reflex responses are similar to those of adults. When testing DTRs in small children, use distraction techniques to promote reliable results.

Cerebral palsy frequently causes hyperactive DTRs in children. Reye's syndrome causes generalized hyperactive DTRs in Stage II; in Stage V, DTRs are absent. Adult causes of hyperactive DTRs may also appear in children.

Deep tendon reflexes, hypoactive

A hypoactive deep tendon reflex (DTR) is an abnormally diminished muscle contraction in response to a sudden stretch that may be induced by sharply tapping the muscle's tendon of insertion. It may be graded as minimal (+) or absent (0). (See *Documenting deep tendon reflexes.*)

Normally, a DTR operates via the reflex arc, which is governed by the corticospinal and other descending tracts. A hypoactive DTR may result from damage to the reflex arc involving the specific muscle, the peripheral nerve, the nerve roots, or the spinal cord at that level. Hypoactive DTRs are an important sign of many disorders, especially when they appear with other neurologic signs and symptoms.

Medical causes

• *Cerebellar dysfunction.* This disorder may produce hypoactive DTRs by increasing the level of inhibition through long tracts upon spinal motor neurons. Associated clinical findings vary depending on the cause and location of the dysfunction.
• *Eaton-Lambert syndrome.* This disorder produces generalized hypoactive DTRs. Early signs include difficulty in rising from a chair, climbing stairs, and walking. The patient may also complain of achiness, paresthesia, and muscle weakness that is most severe in the morning. Weakness improves with mild exercise and worsens with strenuous exercise.
• *Guillain-Barré syndrome.* This disorder causes bilateral hypoactive

DTRs that progress rapidly from hypotonia to areflexia in several days. Typically, this disorder causes muscle weakness that begins in the legs and then extends to the arms and possibly to the trunk and neck muscles. Occasionally, weakness may progress to total paralysis. Other clinical features include cranial nerve palsies, pain, paresthesia, and signs of brief autonomic dysfunction, such as sinus tachycardia or bradycardia, flushing, fluctuating blood pressure, and anhidrosis or episodic diaphoresis.

Typically, muscle weakness and hypoactive DTRs peak in severity within 10 to 14 days; then symptoms begin to clear. However, there may be residual hypoactive DTRs and motor weakness in severe cases.
• *Peripheral neuropathy.* Characteristic in end-stage diabetes mellitus, renal failure, and alcoholism, peripheral neuropathy results in progressive hypoactive DTRs. Other effects include motor weakness, sensory loss, paresthesia, tremors, and possible autonomic dysfunction, such as orthostatic hypotension and incontinence.
• *Polymyositis.* In this disorder, hypoactive DTRs accompany muscle weakness, pain, stiffness, spasms and, possibly, increased size or atrophy. These effects are usually temporary, and their location varies with the affected muscles.
• *Spinal cord lesions.* Spinal cord injury or complete transection produces spinal shock, resulting in hypoactive DTRs or areflexia below the level of the lesion. Associated signs and symptoms may include quadriplegia or paraplegia, flaccidity, loss of sensation below the level of the lesion, and dry, pale skin. Also characteristic are urine retention with overflow incontinence, hypoactive bowel sounds, constipation, and genital reflex loss. Hypoactive DTRs and flaccidity are usually transient; reflex ac-

tivity may return within several weeks.

• *Syringomyelia.* Permanent bilateral hypoactive DTRs occur early in this slowly progressive disorder. Other clinical features are muscle weakness and atrophy; loss of sensation, usually extending in a capelike fashion over the arms, shoulders, neck, back, and occasionally the legs; deep, boring pain (despite an anesthestic) in the limbs; and signs of brain stem involvement, including nystagmus, facial numbness, unilateral vocal cord paralysis or weakness, and unilateral tongue atrophy.

Other causes

• *Drugs.* Barbiturates and paralyzing drugs, such as pancuronium and curare, may cause hypoactive DTRs.

ALERT Hypoactive DTRs frequently occur in muscular dystrophy, Friedreich's ataxia, syringomyelia, and spinal cord injury. They also accompany progressive muscular atrophy, which affects preschoolers and adolescents.

You should use distraction techniques to test DTRs. Assess motor function by watching the infant or child at play.

Dizziness

A common symptom, dizziness is a sensation of imbalance or faintness, sometimes associated with giddiness, weakness, confusion, and blurred or double vision. Episodes of dizziness are usually brief. They may be mild or severe with abrupt or gradual onset. Dizziness may be aggravated by standing up quickly and alleviated by lying down and by resting.

Typically, dizziness results from inadequate blood flow and oxygen supply to the cerebrum and spinal cord. It may occur in anxiety, respiratory

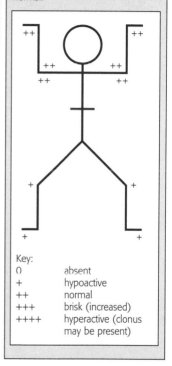

DOCUMENTING DEEP TENDON REFLEXES

Record your patient's deep tendon reflex scores by drawing a stick figure and entering the grades from the scale below at the proper location. The figure shown here indicates hypoactive deep tendon reflexes in the legs; other reflexes are normal.

Key:
0	absent
+	hypoactive
++	normal
+++	brisk (increased)
++++	hyperactive (clonus may be present)

and cardiovascular disorders, and postconcussion syndrome. It's a key symptom in certain serious disorders, such as hypertension and vertebrobasilar artery insufficiency.

Dizziness is often confused with vertigo, a sensation of the body revolving in space or the surroundings revolving about oneself. However, unlike dizziness, vertigo is often accompanied by nausea, vomiting, nystagmus, staggering gait, and tinnitus or hearing loss. Dizziness and vertigo

---

DIZZINESS: WHAT TO DO

If your patient complains of dizziness, you should first determine the severity and onset. Ask the patient to describe the dizziness and ask if it's associated with headache or blurred vision. Take his vital signs and ask about a history of high blood pressure. Notify the doctor or, if necessary, call for emergency services. You may be asked to recheck vital signs every 15 minutes. An I.V. line may need to be started and medications administered as ordered.

---

may occur together, as in postconcussion syndrome.

Emergency interventions

See *Dizziness: What to do.*

Medical causes

• *Anemia.* Typically, this disorder causes dizziness that is aggravated by postural changes or exertion. Other clinical features include pallor, dyspnea, fatigue, tachycardia, and bounding pulse. Capillary refill time will be prolonged.

• *Cardiac arrhythmias.* Dizziness lasts for several minutes or longer with this disorder and may precede fainting. The patient may experience palpitations; irregular, rapid, or thready pulse; and possible hypotension. He may also experience weakness, blurred vision, paresthesia, and confusion.

• *Generalized anxiety disorder.* This disorder produces continuous dizziness that may intensify as the disorder worsens. Associated signs and symptoms are persistent anxiety (for at least 1 month), insomnia, difficulty concentrating, and irritability. The patient may also show signs of

motor tension, for example, twitching or fidgeting, muscle aches, furrowed brow, and a tendency to be startled. He may also display signs of autonomic hyperactivity, for example, diaphoresis, palpitations, cold and clammy hands, dry mouth, paresthesia, indigestion, hot or cold flashes, frequent urination, diarrhea, a lump in the throat, pallor, and increased pulse and respirations.

• *Hypertension.* In this disorder, dizziness may precede fainting. However, it may also be relieved by rest. Other common signs and symptoms include headache and blurred vision. Retinal changes include hemorrhage, sclerosis of retinal blood vessels, exudate, and papilledema.

• *Hyperventilation syndrome.* Episodes of hyperventilation cause dizziness that usually lasts a few minutes; however, if these episodes occur frequently, dizziness may persist between them. Other effects include apprehension, diaphoresis, pallor, dyspnea, chest tightness, palpitations, trembling, fatigue, and peripheral and circumoral paresthesia.

• *Orthostatic hypotension.* This condition produces dizziness that may terminate in fainting or disappear with rest. Related findings include dim vision, spots before the eyes, pallor, diaphoresis, hypotension, tachycardia, and possibly signs of dehydration.

• *Postconcussion syndrome.* Occurring 1 to 3 weeks after a head injury, this syndrome is marked by dizziness; headache that may be throbbing, aching, bandlike, or stabbing; emotional lability; alcohol intolerance; fatigue; anxiety; and vertigo. Dizziness and other symptoms are intensified by mental or physical stress. The syndrome may persist for years, but symptoms eventually abate.

• *TIA.* Lasting from a few seconds to 24 hours, a TIA frequently signals impending stroke and may be triggered by turning the head to the side. Dizziness of varying severity occurs during an attack. It's accompanied by unilateral or bilateral diplopia, blindness or visual field deficits, ptosis, tinnitus, hearing loss, paresis, and numbness. Other findings include dysarthria, dysphagia, vomiting, hiccups, confusion, decreased LOC, and pallor.

Other causes

• *Drugs.* Antianxiety drugs, central nervous system depressants, narcotics, decongestants, antihistamines, antihypertensives, and vasodilators frequently cause dizziness.

Dystonia

Dystonia is marked by slow involuntary movements of large muscle groups of the limbs, trunk, and neck. This extrapyramidal sign may involve flexion of the foot, hyperextension of the legs, extension and pronation of the arms, arching of the back, and extension and rotation of the neck (spasmodic torticollis). (See *Recognizing dystonia.*)

Dystonia is typically aggravated by walking and emotional stress and relieved by sleep. It may be intermittent, lasting just a few minutes, or continuous and painful. Occasionally, it causes permanent contractures, resulting in a grotesque posture. Although dystonia may be hereditary or idiopathic, it results more often from extrapyramidal disorders or drugs.

Medical causes

• *Alzheimer's disease.* Dystonia is a late sign of this disorder, which is marked by slowly progressive dementia. The patient typically displays a decreased attention span, amnesia, agitation, inability to carry out activi-

RECOGNIZING DYSTONIA

Dystonia, chorea, and athetosis may occur simultaneously. To differentiate between them, keep the following points in mind:

• *Dystonic* movements are slow and twisting and involve large-muscle groups in the head, neck (as shown below), trunk, and limbs. They may be intermittent or continuous.
• *Choreiform* movements are rapid, highly complex, and jerky.
• *Athetoid* movements are slow, sinuous, and writhing but *always* continuous. They typically affect the hands and extremities.

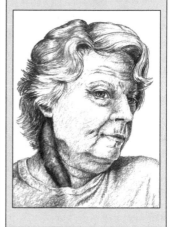

ties of daily living, dysarthria, and emotional lability.

• *Dystonia musculorum deformans.* Prolonged, generalized dystonia is the hallmark of this disorder, which usually develops in childhood and worsens with age. Initially, it causes foot inversion followed by growth retardation and scoliosis. Late signs include twisted, bizarre postures, limb contractures, and dysarthria.
• *Huntington's disease.* Dystonic movements mark the preterminal stage of Huntington's disease. Characterized by progressive intellectual

decline, this disorder leads to dementia and emotional lability. The patient displays choreoathetosis accompanied by dysarthria, dysphagia, facial grimacing, and wide-based prancing gait.

• *Parkinson's disease.* Dystonic spasms are common in this disorder. Other classic features include uniform or jerky rigidity, "pill-rolling" tremor, bradykinesia, dysarthria, dysphagia, drooling, a masklike facies, monotone voice, stooped posture, and propulsive gait.

Other causes

• *Drugs.* All three types of phenothiazines may cause dystonia. Piperazine phenothiazines, such as fluphenazine and trifluoperazine, produce this sign most frequently; aliphatics such as chlorpromazine cause it less often; and piperidines rarely cause it.

Haloperidol, loxapine, and other antipsychotics usually produce acute facial dystonia. Antiemetic doses of metoclopramide, excessive doses of levodopa, and metyrosine do as well.

ALERT Children don't exhibit dystonia until after they can walk. Even then, it rarely occurs until after age 10. Common causes include Fahr's disease, dystonia musculorum deformans, athetoid cerebral palsy, and the residual effects of anoxia at birth.

Edema of the arm

The result of excess interstitial fluid in the arm, this edema may be unilateral or bilateral and may develop gradually or abruptly. It may be aggravated by immobility and alleviated by arm elevation and exercise.

Arm edema signals localized fluid imbalance between vascular and interstitial spaces. It commonly results from trauma, venous disorders, toxins, and treatments.

Medical causes

• *Angioneurotic edema.* This common reaction is characterized by the sudden onset of painless, nonpruritic edema affecting the hands, feet, eyelids, lips, face, neck, genitalia, or viscera. Although these swellings usually don't itch, they may burn and tingle. If edema spreads to the larynx, signs of respiratory distress may occur.

• *Arm trauma.* Shortly after a crush injury, severe edema may affect the entire arm. Ecchymoses, superficial bleeding, pain or numbness and, possibly, paralysis may occur.

• *Burns.* Two days or less after injury, arm burns may cause mild to severe edema, pain, and tissue damage.

• *Superior vena cava syndrome.* Bilateral arm edema usually progresses slowly and is accompanied by facial and neck edema. Dilated veins mark the edematous areas. The patient may also complain of headache, vertigo, and visual disturbances.

• *Thrombophlebitis.* This disorder may cause arm edema, pain, and warmth. Deep vein thrombophlebitis can also produce cyanosis, fever, chills, and malaise; superficial thrombophlebitis can also cause redness, tenderness, and induration along the vein.

Other causes

• *Treatments.* Localized arm edema may result from infiltration of I.V. fluid into the interstitial tissue. A radical or modified radical mastectomy that disrupts lymphatic drainage may cause edema of the entire arm. Also, radiation therapy for breast cancer may produce arm edema immediately after treatment or months later.

Edema of the leg

This edema results when excess interstitial fluid accumulates in one or both legs. It may affect just the foot and ankle or extend to the thigh. This common sign may be slight or dramatic and pitting or nonpitting.

Leg edema may result from venous disorders, trauma, and certain bone and cardiac disorders that disturb normal fluid balance. However, several nonpathologic mechanisms may also cause it. For example, prolonged sitting, standing, or immobility may cause bilateral orthostatic edema. Usually, this pitting edema affects the foot and disappears with rest and leg elevation. Increased venous pressure late in pregnancy may also cause ankle edema.

Medical causes

• *Burns.* Two days or less after injury, leg burns may cause mild to severe edema, pain, and tissue damage.
• *Heart failure.* Bilateral leg edema is an early sign in right-sided heart failure. Other effects may include weight gain (despite anorexia), nausea, chest tightness, hypotension, pallor, tachypnea, palpitations, ventricular gallop, and inspiratory crackles. Pitting ankle edema signals more advanced heart failure, as do hepatomegaly, hemoptysis, and cyanosis.
• *Leg trauma.* Mild to severe localized edema may form around the trauma site.
• *Osteomyelitis.* When this bone infection affects the lower leg, it usually produces localized, mild to moderate edema, which may spread to the adjacent joint.
• *Thrombophlebitis.* Both deep and superficial vein thromboses may cause onset of unilateral mild to moderate edema. Deep vein thrombophlebitis may be asymptomatic or cause mild to severe pain, warmth,

and cyanosis in the affected leg as well as fever, chills, and malaise. Superficial thrombophlebitis typically causes pain, warmth, redness, tenderness, and induration along the affected vein.
• *Venous insufficiency (chronic).* Unilateral or bilateral leg edema occurs and is moderate to severe in this disorder. Initially, the edema is soft and pitting; later, it becomes hard as tissues thicken. Other signs include darkened skin and painless, easily infected stasis ulcers that develop around the ankle.

Other causes

• *Diagnostic tests.* Venography is a rare cause of leg edema.
• *Coronary artery bypass surgery.* Unilateral venous insufficiency may follow saphenous vein retrieval.

Fasciculations

Fasciculations are local muscle contractions representing the spontaneous discharge of a muscle fiber bundle that is innervated by a single motor nerve filament. These contractions cause visible dimpling or wave-like twitching of the skin but aren't strong enough to produce joint movement. They occur irregularly at frequencies ranging from once every several seconds to two or three times per second. Infrequently, myokymia — continuous, rapid fasciculations that cause a rippling effect — may occur. Because fasciculations are brief and painless, they often go undetected or are ignored.

Benign, nonpathologic fasciculations are common and normal. They often occur in tense, anxious, or overtired persons and typically affect the eyelid, thumb, or calf. However, fasciculations may also indicate a severe neurologic disorder, most no-

tably a diffuse motor neuron disorder
that causes loss of control over muscle fiber discharge. They're also an
early sign of pesticide poisoning.

Emergency interventions

See *Fasciculations: What to do.*

Medical causes

• *Amyotrophic lateral sclerosis.*
Coarse fasciculations usually begin in
the small muscles of the hands and
feet, then spread to the forearms and
legs. Widespread, symmetrical muscle
atrophy and weakness may result in
dysarthria; difficulty chewing, swallowing, and breathing; and occasionally choking and drooling.
• *Bulbar palsy.* Fasciculations of the
face and tongue commonly appear
early. Progressive signs include
dysarthria, dysphagia, hoarseness,
and drooling. Eventually, weakness
spreads to the respiratory muscles.
• *Guillain-Barré syndrome.* Fasciculations may occur, but the dominant neurologic sign is muscle weakness, which typically begins in the
legs and spreads quickly to the arms
and face. Other findings include
paresthesia, incontinence, footdrop,

tachycardia, dysphagia, and respiratory insufficiency.
• *Herniated disk.* Fasciculations of
the muscles innervated by compressed nerve roots may be widespread and profound in this disorder,
but the overriding symptom is severe
lower back pain that may radiate
unilaterally to the leg. Coughing,
sneezing, bending, and straining exacerbate the pain. Related effects include muscle weakness, atrophy, and
spasms; paresthesia; footdrop; steppage gait; and hypoactive deep tendon reflexes in the leg.
• *Spinal cord tumors.* Fasciculations may develop, along with muscle
atrophy and cramps, asymmetrically
at first and then bilaterally as cord
compression progresses. Motor and
sensory changes distal to the tumor
include weakness or paralysis, areflexia, paresthesia, and a tightening
band of pain. Bowel and bladder control may also be lost.
• *Syringomyelia.* Fasciculations
may occur along with Charcot's
joints, deep aching pain, areflexia,
and muscle atrophy. Additional findings may include thoracic scoliosis
and the loss of pain and temperature
sensation over the neck, shoulders,
and arms.

Footdrop

Footdrop, which is plantar flexion of
the foot with the toes bent toward the
instep, results from weakness or paralysis of the dorsiflexor muscles of
the foot and ankle. A characteristic
and important sign of certain peripheral nerve or motor neuron disorders,
it may also stem from prolonged immobility when inadequate support,
improper positioning, or infrequent
passive exercises produce shortening
of the Achilles tendon. Unilateral
footdrop can result from compression

of the common peroneal nerve against the head of the fibula.

Footdrop can range in severity from slight to complete, depending on the extent of muscle weakness or paralysis. It develops slowly in progressive muscle degeneration and suddenly in spinal cord injury.

Medical causes

• *Cerebrovascular accident (CVA).* Unilateral footdrop often appears with arm and leg weakness or paralysis in CVA. Other effects depend on the site and severity of vascular damage. Sensorimotor disturbances may include paresthesia, dysphagia, visual field deficits, diplopia, and bowel and bladder dysfunction. Personality changes, amnesia, aphasia, dysarthria, and decreased level of consciousness may also occur.

• *Guillain-Barré syndrome.* Unilateral or bilateral footdrop and steppage gait may result from profound muscle weakness. This weakness usually begins in the legs and extends to the arms and face within 72 hours. It can progress to total motor paralysis with respiratory failure. The patient may also have transient paresthesia, hypoactive DTRs, hypernasality, dysphagia, diaphoresis, tachycardia, orthostatic hypotension, and incontinence.

• *Herniated lumbar disk.* Footdrop and steppage gait may result from leg muscle weakness and atrophy. However, the most pronounced symptom is severe lower back pain, which may radiate to the buttocks, legs, and feet, usually unilaterally. Sciatic pain follows, often with muscle spasms and sensorimotor loss. Paresthesia, hypoactive DTRs, and fasciculations may also occur.

• *Multiple sclerosis.* Footdrop may develop suddenly or slowly, producing steppage gait. It typically fluctuates in severity with this disorder's cycle of periodic exacerbation and remission. Muscle weakness most commonly affects the legs and ranges from minor fatigability to paraparesis with urinary urgency and constipation. Related findings include facial pain, visual disturbances, paresthesia, incoordination, and loss of vibration and position sensation in the ankle and toes.

• *Myasthenia gravis.* Footdrop and related limb weakness are common manifestations of this disorder, which is often heralded by weak eye closure, ptosis, and diplopia. Skeletal muscle weakness and fatigability may progress to paralysis. Typically, muscle function worsens throughout the day and with exercise and improves with rest. Involvement of respiratory muscles can cause breathing difficulty.

• *Peroneal muscle atrophy.* Bilateral footdrop, ankle instability, and steppage gait occur early in this chronic disorder. Other early signs and symptoms include paresthesia, aching, and cramping in the feet and legs, along with coldness, swelling, and cyanosis. As the disease progresses, all leg muscles become weak and atrophic, with hypoactive or absent DTRs. Later, atrophy and sensory losses spread to the hands and forearms.

• *Peroneal nerve trauma.* Footdrop may occur suddenly but it's temporary and resolves with the release of peroneal nerve compression. It's associated with ipsilateral steppage gait, muscle weakness, and sensory loss over the lateral surface of the calf and foot.

• *Polio.* Unilateral or bilateral footdrop may develop, producing steppage gait. Initially, fever precedes asymmetrical muscle weakness, coarse fasciculations, paresthesia, hypoactive or absent DTRs, and permanent muscle paralysis and atrophy. Dysphagia, urine retention, and respiratory difficulty may occur.

• *Polyneuropathy.* Footdrop and steppage gait may accompany muscle weakness, which usually affects distal areas of the extremities and can progress to flaccid paralysis. Muscle atrophy and hypoactive or absent DTRs may occur, along with paresthesia, hyperesthesia, or anesthesia and loss of vibration sensation in the hands and feet. Cutaneous manifestations include glossy, red skin and anhidrosis.

• *Spinal cord trauma.* Unilateral or bilateral footdrop can occur suddenly and may be permanent. In the ambulatory patient, it also produces steppage gait. Other findings vary and may include neck and back pain; paresthesia, sensory loss, and muscle weakness; atrophy or paralysis distal to the injury; asymmetrical or absent DTRs; and fecal and urinary incontinence.

ALERT Common causes of footdrop in children include spinal birth defects such as spina bifida and degenerative disorders such as muscular dystrophy. To aid ambulation, the child should be fitted with supportive shoes and possibly in-shoe splints or braces.

Intermittent claudication

Most common in the legs, intermittent claudication is cramping limb pain brought on by exercise and relieved by 1 or 2 minutes of rest. It may be acute or chronic. When it's acute, it may signal acute arterial occlusion. Intermittent claudication occurs most often in men ages 50 to 60 with a history of diabetes mellitus, hyperlipidemia, hypertension, or tobacco use. Without treatment, it may progress to pain at rest. In chronic arterial occlusion, limb loss is uncommon because collateral circulation usually develops.

In occlusive artery disease, intermittent claudication results from an inadequate blood supply. Pain in the calf (the most common area) or foot indicates disease of the femoral or popliteal arteries, and pain in the buttocks and upper thigh indicates disease of the aortoiliac arteries. During exercise, the pain typically results from the release of lactic acid due to anaerobic metabolism in the ischemic segment, secondary to obstruction. When exercise stops, the lactic acid clears and the pain subsides.

Intermittent claudication may also have a neurologic cause, narrowing of the vertebral column at the level of the cauda equina. This creates pressure on the nerve roots of the lower extremities. Walking stimulates circulation to the cauda equina, causing increased pressure on those nerves and pain.

Emergency interventions

See *Sudden intermittent claudication: What to do.*

Medical causes

• *Acute arterial occlusion.* This disorder produces intense intermittent claudication, which is sudden severe or aching leg pain aggravated by exercise. A saddle embolus may affect both legs. Associated findings include paresthesia, paresis, and sensations of cold in the affected limb. The limb is cool, pale, and cyanotic (mottled) with absent pulses below the occlusion. Capillary refill time is prolonged.

• *Aortic arteriosclerotic occlusive disease.* In this disorder, intermittent claudication occurs in the buttock, hip, thigh, and calf, along with absent or diminished femoral pulses.

Bruits can be auscultated over the femoral and iliac arteries. Examination reveals pallor of the affected limb on elevation and profound limb weakness. The leg may be cool to the touch.

• *Arteriosclerosis obliterans.* This disorder usually affects the femoral and popliteal arteries, causing intermittent claudication (the most common symptom) in the calf. Typical associated findings include diminished or absent popliteal and pedal pulses, coolness in the affected limb, pallor on elevation, and profound limb weakness with continuing exercise. Other possible findings include numbness, paresthesia and, in severe disease, pain in the toes or foot while at rest, ulceration, and gangrene.

• *Buerger's disease.* Typically, this disorder produces intermittent claudication of the instep. Early signs include migratory superficial nodules and erythema along extremity blood vessels (nodular phlebitis) and a migratory venous phlebitis. With exposure to cold, the feet initially become cold, cyanotic, and numb. Later, they redden, become hot, and tingle. Occasionally, Buerger's disease also affects the hands and can cause painful fingertip ulcerations. Other characteristic findings include impaired peripheral pulses, paresthesia of the hands and feet, and migratory superficial thrombophlebitis.

• *Leriche's syndrome.* Arterial occlusion causes intermittent claudication of the hip, thigh, and buttock. It also causes impotence in men. Examination reveals bruits, global atrophy, and absent or diminished pulses. The leg becomes cool and pale when elevated.

• *Neurogenic claudication.* Neurospinal disease causes pain from intermittent claudication that requires a longer rest time than the 2 to 3 minutes needed in vascular claudication. Associated findings include

---

SUDDEN INTERMITTENT CLAUDICATION: WHAT TO DO

If your patient has sudden intermittent claudication with severe or aching leg pain at rest, check the leg's temperature and palpate pulses. Then check its color. Ask about numbness and tingling. Suspect acute arterial occlusion if pulses are absent and the leg feels cold and looks pale, cyanotic, or mottled or if paresthesia and pain are present. Don't elevate the leg. Protect it and let nothing press on it. Refer the patient for medical intervention.

---

paresthesia, weakness and clumsiness when walking, and hypoactive DTRs after walking. However, in this disorder, pulses aren't affected.

• *Thoracic outlet syndrome.* Activity that requires raising the hands above the shoulders, lifting a weight, or abducting the arm can cause intermittent pain along the ulnar distribution of the arm and forearm along with paresthesia and weakness. This isn't true claudication pain because it's position-related, not exercise-related. Signs and symptoms disappear when the arm is lowered. Other features may include asymmetrical blood pressure and cool, pale skin.

Leg pain

Although leg pain often signifies a musculoskeletal disorder, this symptom can also result from more serious vascular or neurologic disorders. The pain may arise suddenly or gradually and may be localized or affect the entire leg. Constant or intermittent, it may feel dull, burning, sharp, shooting, or tingling. Leg pain often affects locomotion, limiting weight bearing. Severe leg pain that follows cast application for a fracture may

COMMON CAUSES OF LOCAL LEG PAIN

Various disorders — such as those listed below — cause hip, knee, ankle, or foot pain, which may radiate to surrounding tissues and be reported as leg pain. Local pain is commonly accompanied by tenderness, swelling, and deformity in the affected area.

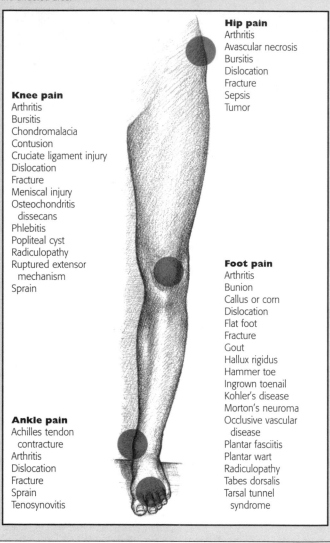

Hip pain
Arthritis
Avascular necrosis
Bursitis
Dislocation
Fracture
Sepsis
Tumor

Knee pain
Arthritis
Bursitis
Chondromalacia
Contusion
Cruciate ligament injury
Dislocation
Fracture
Meniscal injury
Osteochondritis
  dissecans
Phlebitis
Popliteal cyst
Radiculopathy
Ruptured extensor
  mechanism
Sprain

Foot pain
Arthritis
Bunion
Callus or corn
Dislocation
Flat foot
Fracture
Gout
Hallux rigidus
Hammer toe
Ingrown toenail
Kohler's disease
Morton's neuroma
Occlusive vascular
  disease
Plantar fasciitis
Plantar wart
Radiculopathy
Tabes dorsalis
Tarsal tunnel
  syndrome

Ankle pain
Achilles tendon
  contracture
Arthritis
Dislocation
Fracture
Sprain
Tenosynovitis

signal limb-threatening compartment syndrome. Sudden onset of severe leg pain in a patient with underlying vascular insufficiency may signal acute deterioration, possibly requiring an arterial graft or amputation. (See *Common causes of local leg pain.*)

Emergency interventions

See *Acute leg pain: What to do*.

Medical causes

• *Bone neoplasm.* Continuous deep or boring pain, often worse at night, may be the first symptom. Later, skin breakdown and impaired circulation may occur, along with cachexia, fever, and impaired mobility.

• *Compartment syndrome.* Progressive, intense, lower leg pain that increases with passive muscle stretching is a cardinal sign of this limb-threatening disorder. Restrictive dressings or traction may aggravate the pain, which typically worsens despite analgesia. Other findings may include muscle weakness and paresthesia, but apparently normal distal circulation. With irreversible muscle ischemia, you'll also find paralysis and absent pulse.

• *Fracture.* Severe, acute pain accompanies swelling and ecchymosis in the affected leg. Movement produces extreme pain, and the leg may be unable to bear weight. Neurovascular status distal to the fracture may be impaired, causing paresthesia, absent pulse, mottled cyanosis, and cool skin. Deformity, muscle spasms, and bony crepitation may also occur.

• *Infection.* Local leg pain, erythema, swelling, and warmth characterize both soft tissue and bone infections. Fever and tachycardia may be present with other systemic signs.

• *Occlusive vascular disease.* Continuous cramping pain in the legs and feet may worsen with walking, inducing claudication. The patient may report increased pain at night and complain of cold feet and cold intolerance. Examination may reveal ankle and lower leg edema, decreased or absent pulses, and decreased capillary refill time.

> ### ACUTE LEG PAIN: WHAT TO DO
>
> If your patient has acute leg pain and a history of trauma, you should quickly take his vital signs and determine the leg's neurovascular status. You should observe the leg position and check for swelling, gross deformities, or abnormal rotation. Also, be sure to check distal pulses and note skin color and temperature. Impaired circulation may be indicated if the affected leg is pale, cool, and pulseless. Emergency surgery may be required.

• *Sciatica.* Pain radiates down the back of the leg along the sciatic nerve. Pain may be described as shooting, aching, or tingling. Typically, activity exacerbates the pain and rest relieves it. The patient may limp to avoid aggravating the leg pain and may have difficulty moving from a sitting to a standing position.

• *Strain or sprain.* Acute strain causes sharp, transient pain and rapid swelling, followed by leg tenderness and ecchymosis. Chronic strain produces stiffness, soreness, and generalized leg tenderness several hours after the injury. Active and passive motion may be painful or impossible. A sprain causes local pain, especially during joint movement. Ecchymosis and possibly local swelling and loss of mobility may also develop.

• *Thrombophlebitis.* Discomfort may range from calf tenderness to severe pain accompanied by swelling, warmth, and a feeling of heaviness in the affected leg. The patient may also have fever, chills, malaise, muscle cramps, and a positive Homans' sign. Assessment may reveal visibly engorged, palpable superficial veins.

• *Varicose veins.* Mild to severe leg symptoms may develop, including nocturnal cramping, a feeling of heaviness, aching during menses, and diffuse, dull aching after prolonged standing or walking. Assessment may reveal palpable nodules, orthostatic edema, and stasis pigmentation of the calves and ankles.

• *Venous stasis ulcers.* Localized pain and bleeding arise from infected ulcerations on the calves. Mottled, bluish pigmentation is characteristic, and local edema may also occur.

Lymphadenopathy

Lymphadenopathy, or enlargement of one or more lymph nodes, may result from increased production of lymphocytes or reticuloendothelial cells, or from the infiltration of cells not normally present. This sign may be generalized (involving three or more node groups) or localized. Generalized lymphadenopathy may be caused by an inflammatory process, such as bacterial or viral infection, connective tissue disease, endocrine disorder, and neoplasm. Localized lymphadenopathy most commonly results from infection or trauma affecting the area drained by the specific lymph nodes. (See *Common causes of local lymphadenopathy,* pages 78 and 79.)

Normally, lymph nodes range from 0.5 to 2.5 cm and are discrete, mobile, nontender and, except in children, nonpalpable. Nodes that exceed 3 cm are cause for concern. They may be tender and erythematous, suggesting a draining lesion. Alternatively, they may be hard and fixed and tender or nontender, suggesting malignancy.

Medical causes

• *Acquired immunodeficiency syndrome.* Besides lymphadenopathy, findings include a history of fatigue, night sweats, afternoon fevers, diarrhea, weight loss, and cough with several concurrent infections appearing soon afterward.

• *Brucellosis.* Generalized lymphadenopathy most often affects cervical and axillary lymph nodes, making them tender. The disease usually begins insidiously with easy fatigability, headache, backache, anorexia, and arthralgias. It may also begin abruptly with chills, fever, and diaphoresis.

• *Chronic fatigue syndrome.* Lymphadenopathy may occur with incapacitating fatigue, sore throat, myalgia, and cognitive dysfunction. The cause of this syndrome is unknown.

• *Cytomegalovirus infection.* Generalized lymphadenopathy occurs in the immunocompromised patient. It's accompanied by fever, malaise, rash, and hepatosplenomegaly.

• *Hodgkin's disease.* The extent of lymphadenopathy determines the stage of malignancy — from stage-I involvement of a single lymph node region to stage-IV generalized lymphadenopathy. Usually, nodes in the neck enlarge first and become hard, swollen, movable, nontender, and discrete. Other common early signs and symptoms include pruritus and, in older patients, fatigue, weakness, night sweats, malaise, weight loss, and unexplained fever (usually up to 101° F [38.3° C]). Also, if mediastinal lymph nodes enlarge, tracheal and esophageal pressure produces dyspnea and dysphagia.

• *Infectious mononucleosis.* Characteristic, painful lymphadenopathy involves cervical, axillary, and inguinal nodes. Prodromal symptoms (headache, malaise, and fatigue) typically occur 3 to 5 days before the appearance of the classic triad of lymphadenopathy, sore throat, and temperature fluctuations with an evening peak of about 102° F (38.9° C).

Hepatosplenomegaly may develop, along with findings of stomatitis, exudative tonsillitis, or pharyngitis.

• *Leukemia (acute lymphocytic).* Generalized lymphadenopathy is accompanied by fatigue, malaise, pallor, and low-grade fever. The patient also experiences prolonged bleeding time, swollen gums, weight loss, bone or joint pain, and hepatosplenomegaly.

• *Leukemia (chronic lymphocytic).* Generalized lymphadenopathy appears early, along with fatigue, malaise, and fever. As the disease progresses, hepatosplenomegaly, severe fatigue, and weight loss occur. Other late findings include bone tenderness, edema, pallor, dyspnea, tachycardia, palpitations, bleeding, and often macular or nodular lesions.

• *Lyme disease.* Spread by the bite of certain ticks, Lyme disease begins with a skin lesion called erythema chronicum migrans. As the disease progresses, the patient may suffer from lymphadenopathy, constant malaise and fatigue, and intermittent headache, fever, chills, and aches. The patient may go on to develop neurologic and cardiac abnormalities and, eventually, arthritis.

• *Malignant lymphoma.* Painless enlargement of one or more peripheral lymph nodes is the most common sign of this cancer, with generalized lymphadenopathy characterizing stage IV. Dyspnea, cough, and hepatosplenomegaly also occur, along with systemic complaints of fever up to 101° F (38.3° C), night sweats, fatigue, malaise, and weight loss.

• *Mycosis fungoides.* Lymphadenopathy occurs in stage III of this rare, chronic malignant lymphoma. It's accompanied by ulcerated, brownish red tumors that are painful and itchy.

• *Rheumatoid arthritis.* Lymphadenopathy is an early, nonspecific finding associated with fatigue, malaise, continuous low fever, weight loss, and vague arthralgias and myalgias. Later, the patient develops joint tenderness, swelling, and warmth; joint stiffness after inactivity; and subcutaneous nodules on the elbows. Eventually, joint deformity, muscle weakness, and atrophy may occur.

• *Sarcoidosis.* Generalized, bilateral hilar and right paratracheal lymphadenopathy with splenomegaly are common. Initial findings are arthralgia, fatigue, malaise, and weight loss. Other findings vary with the site and extent of fibrosis. Typical cardiopulmonary findings include breathlessness, cough, substernal chest pain, and arrhythmias. Musculoskeletal and cutaneous features may include muscle weakness and pain, phalangeal and nasal mucosal lesions, and subcutaneous skin nodules. Common ophthalmic findings include eye pain, photophobia, and nonreactive pupils. Central nervous system involvement may produce cranial or peripheral nerve palsies and seizures.

• *Systemic lupus erythematosus.* Generalized lymphadenopathy often accompanies the hallmark butterfly rash, photosensitivity, Raynaud's phenomenon, and joint pain and stillness. Pleuritic chest pain and cough may appear with systemic findings, such as fever, anorexia, and weight loss.

Other causes

• *Drugs.* Phenytoin may cause generalized lymphadenopathy.
• *Immunizations.* Typhoid vaccination may also cause generalized lymphadenopathy.

COMMON CAUSES OF LOCAL LYMPHADENOPATHY

When you detect an enlarged lymph node, palpate the entire lymph node system to determine the extent of lymphadenopathy. Include the lymph nodes indicated below in your examination.

Localized lymphadenopathy may be caused by a variety of disorders, but it usually results from infection or trauma affecting the drained area. The list at right matches some common causes with the areas they affect.

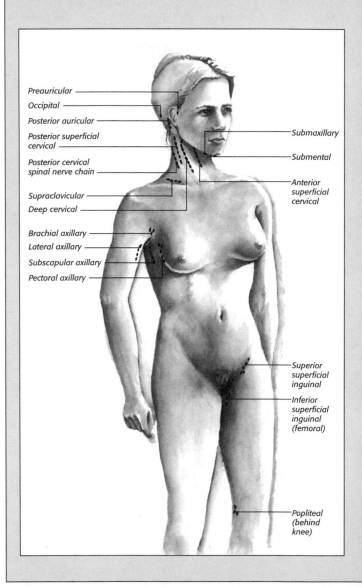

Preauricular

Occipital

Posterior auricular

Posterior superficial cervical

Posterior cervical spinal nerve chain

Supraclavicular

Deep cervical

Brachial axillary

Lateral axillary

Subscapular axillary

Pectoral axillary

Submaxillary

Submental

Anterior superficial cervical

Superior superficial inguinal

Inferior superficial inguinal (femoral)

Popliteal (behind knee)

Occipital
Roseola
Scalp infection
Seborrheic dermatitis
Tick bite
Tinea capitis

Auricular
Erysipelas
Herpes zoster ophthalmicus
Infection
Mastoiditis
Otitis media
Rubella
Squamous cell carcinoma
Styes or chalazion
Tularemia

Cervical
Cat scratch fever
Facial or oral cancer
Infection
Mucocutaneous lymph node
   syndrome
Rubella
Rubeola
Thyrotoxicosis
Tonsilitis
Tuberculosis
Varicella

**Submaxillary and
   submental**
Cystic fibrosis
Dental infection
Gingivitis
Glossitis

Supraclavicular
Neoplastic disease

Axillary
Breast cancer
Lymphoma

Inguinal and femoral
Carcinoma
Chancroid
Lymphogranuloma venereum
Syphilis

Popliteal
Infection

McMurray sign

Frequently an indicator of medial meniscal injury, McMurray sign is a palpable, audible click or pop elicited by manipulating the leg. It results when gentle manipulation of the leg traps torn cartilage and then lets it snap free.

Because eliciting this sign forces the surface of the tibial plateau against the femoral condyles, it's contraindicated in patients with suspected fractures of the tibial plateau or femoral condyles.

A positive McMurray sign augments other findings commonly associated with meniscal injury, such as severe knee pain and decreased range of motion (ROM). (See *Eliciting McMurray sign*, page 80.)

Medical cause

• *Meniscal tear.* In this injury, a McMurray sign can frequently be elicited. Associated signs and symptoms may also include acute knee pain at the medial or lateral joint line (depending on injury site) and decreased ROM or locking of the knee joint. Quadriceps weakening and atrophy frequently occur.

Muscle flaccidity

Flaccid muscles are profoundly weak and soft. They have with decreased resistance to movement, increased mobility, and greater than normal range of motion. The result of disrupted muscle innervation, muscle flaccidity (or hypotonicity) can be localized to a limb or muscle group or generalized over the entire body. Its onset may be acute, as in trauma, or chronic, as in neurologic disease.

ELICITING MCMURRAY SIGN

Eliciting this sign requires special training and gentle manipulation of the patient's leg to avoid extending a meniscal tear or locking the knee. If you've been trained to elicit a McMurray sign, follow these steps:

Place the patient in a supine position and flex his affected knee until his heel nearly touches his buttock. Place your thumb and index finger on

either side of the knee joint space and grasp his heel with your other hand. Then rotate the foot and lower leg laterally to test the posterior meniscus. Keeping his foot in a lateral position, extend the knee to a 90-degree angle to test the anterior meniscus. A palpable or audible click — a positive McMurray sign — indicates a meniscal tear.

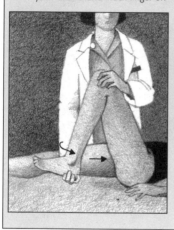
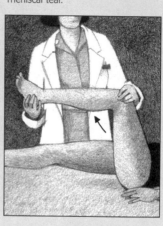

Emergency interventions

See *Flaccidity: What to do*.

Medical causes

• *Amyotrophic lateral sclerosis.* Progressive muscle weakness and paralysis are accompanied by generalized flaccidity. Typically these effects begin in one hand, spread to the arm, and then develop in the other hand and arm. Eventually, they spread to the trunk, neck, tongue, larynx, pharynx, and legs. Progressive respiratory muscle weakness leads to respiratory insufficiency. Other findings may include muscle cramps and coarse fasciculations, hyperactive DTRs, slight leg muscle spasticity, dysphagia, dysarthria, excessive drooling, and depression.

• *Brain lesions.* Frontal and parietal lobe lesions may cause contralateral flaccidity, weakness or paralysis, and even eventually spasticity. Other findings may include hyperactive DTRs, positive Babinski's sign, loss of proprioception, analgesia, anesthesia, and thermanesthesia.

• *Cerebellar disease.* Here, generalized muscle flaccidity or hypotonia is accompanied by ataxia, dysmetria, intention tremor, slight muscle weakness, fatigue, and dysarthria.

• *Guillain-Barré syndrome.* This disorder causes muscle flaccidity. Progression is typically symmetrical and ascending, moving from the feet to the arms and facial nerves within 24 to 72 hours of onset. Associated findings include sensory loss or paresthesia, absent DTRs, tachycardia (or, less often, bradycardia), fluctuating hypertension and postural hypotension, diaphoresis, incontinence, dysphagia, dysarthria, hypernasality, and facial diplegia. Weakness may progress to total motor paralysis and respiratory failure.

• *Huntington's disease.* Besides flaccidity, progressive mental status changes and choreiform movements are major symptoms. Others include poor balance, hesitant or explosive speech, dysphagia, impaired respirations, and incontinence.

• *Peripheral nerve trauma.* Flaccidity, paralysis, and loss of sensation and reflexes in the innervated area can occur.

• *Peripheral neuropathy.* Flaccidity most commonly occurs in the legs due to chronic progressive muscle weakness and paralysis. It may also cause mild to sharp burning pain, glossy red skin, anhidrosis, and loss of vibration sensation. Paresthesia, hyperesthesia, or anesthesia may affect the hands and feet. DTRs may be hypoactive or absent.

• *Polio.* Damage to the anterior horn cells in the spinal cord and brain stem causes flaccid weakness and loss of reflexes.

• *Seizure disorder.* Brief periods of syncope and generalized flaccidity commonly follow a generalized tonic-clonic seizure.

• *Spinal cord injury.* Spinal shock can result in acute muscle flaccidity or spasticity below the level of injury. Associated signs and symptoms also occur below the level of injury and may include paralysis; absent DTRs; analgesia; thermanesthesia; loss of proprioception and vibration, touch, and pressure sensation; and anhidrosis (usually unilateral). Hypotension, bowel and bladder dysfunction, and impotence or priapism may also occur. Injury in the C1 to C5 region can produce respiratory paralysis and bradycardia.

FLACCIDITY: WHAT TO DO

If your patient's flaccidity results from trauma, ensure that his cervical spine has been stabilized. Quickly determine his respiratory status and then call for emergency services. If you note signs of respiratory insufficiency, such as dyspnea, shallow respirations, nasal flaring, and cyanosis, you should administer oxygen by nasal cannula or mask. Intubation and mechanical ventilation may also be necessary.

Muscle spasms

Muscle spasms (or muscle cramps) are strong, painful contractions. They can occur in virtually any muscle but are most common in the calf and foot. Muscle spasms typically result from simple muscle fatigue, from exercise, and during pregnancy. However, they may also occur in electrolyte imbalances and neuromuscular disorders or as the result of certain drugs. They're often precipitated by movement and can usually be relieved by slow stretching.

Emergency interventions

See *Muscle spasms: What to do,* page 82.

Medical causes

• *Amyotrophic lateral sclerosis.* In this disorder, muscle spasms may accompany progressive muscle weariness and atrophy that typically begin in one hand, spread to the arm, and then spread to the other hand and arm. Eventually, muscle weakness and atrophy affect the trunk, neck, tongue, larynx, pharynx, and legs. Progressive respiratory muscle weakness leads to respiratory insufficiency. Other findings may include muscle flaccidity progressing to spasticity, coarse fasciculations, hyperactive deep tendon reflexes (DTRs), dysphagia, impaired speech, excessive drooling, and depression.

• *Arterial occlusive disease.* Arterial occlusion typically produces spasms and intermittent claudication in the leg, with residual pain. Associated findings are usually localized to the legs and feet and include loss of peripheral pulses, pallor or cyanosis, decreased sensation, hair loss, dry or scaling skin, edema, and ulcerations.

• *Dehydration.* Sodium loss may produce limb and abdominal cramps. Other findings may include a slight fever, decreased skin turgor, dry mucous membranes, tachycardia, postural hypotension, muscle twitching, seizures, nausea, vomiting, and oliguria.

• *Fracture.* Localized spasms and pain are mild if the fracture is nondisplaced and intense if it's severely displaced. Other findings may include swelling, limited mobility, and bony crepitation.

• *Hypocalcemia.* The classic feature of this disorder is tetany, a syndrome of muscle cramps and twitching, carpopedal and facial muscle spasms, and seizures, possibly with stridor.

Both Chvostek's and Trousseau's signs may be elicited. Related findings include choreiform movements, hyperactive DTRs, fatigue, palpitations, cardiac arrhythmias, and paresthesia of the lips, fingers, and toes.

• *Hypothyroidism.* Muscle involvement may produce spasms and stiffness, along with leg muscle hypertrophy or proximal limb weakness and atrophy. Other findings include forgetfulness and mental instability; fatigue; cold intolerance; dry, pale, cool, doughy skin; puffy face, hands, and feet; periorbital edema; dry, sparse, brittle hair; bradycardia; and weight gain (despite anorexia).

• *Muscle trauma.* Excessive muscle strain may cause mild to severe spasms. The injured area may be painful, swollen, reddened, and warm.

• *Spinal injury or disease.* Muscle spasms can result from spinal injury, such as cervical extension injury and spinous process fracture, or from spinal disease, such as infection.

Other causes

• *Drugs.* Common spasm-producing drugs include diuretics, corticosteroids, and estrogens.

Muscle spasticity

Spasticity is a state of excessive muscle tone manifested by increased resistance to stretching and heightened reflexes. It's commonly detected by evaluating a muscle's response to passive movement. A spastic muscle offers more resistance when the passive movement is performed quickly.

Caused by an upper motor neuron lesion, muscle spasticity (or hypertonicity) most commonly occurs in arm and leg muscles. Long-term spasticity results in muscle fibrosis and contractures.

Medical causes

• *Amyotrophic lateral sclerosis.* This disorder commonly produces spasticity, spasms, coarse fasciculations, hyperactive deep tendon reflexes (DTRs), and a positive Babinski's sign. Earlier effects include progressive muscle weakness and flaccidity that typically begin in the hands and arms and eventually spread to the trunk, neck, larynx, pharynx, and legs. Progressive respiratory muscle weakness leads to respiratory insufficiency. Other findings may include dysphagia, dysarthria, excessive drooling, and depression.

• *Cerebrovascular accident (CVA).* Spastic paralysis may develop on the affected side following the acute stage of CVA. Associated findings vary with the site and extent of vascular damage and may include dysarthria, aphasia, ataxia, apraxia, agnosia, ipsilateral paresthesia or sensory losses, visual disturbances, altered level of consciousness, amnesia and poor judgment, personality changes, emotional lability, bowel and bladder dysfunction, headache, vomiting, and seizures.

• *Epidural hemorrhage.* In this disorder, bilateral limb spasticity is a late and ominous sign. Other findings may include a momentary loss of consciousness after head trauma, followed by a lucid interval, and then a rapid deterioration in consciousness. The patient may also have unilateral hemiparesis or hemiplegia; seizures; fixed, dilated pupils; high fever; decreased, bounding pulse; widened pulse pressure; elevated blood pressure; irregular respiratory pattern; and decerebrate posture. A positive Babinski's sign can be elicited.

• *Multiple sclerosis.* Muscle spasticity, hyperreflexia, and contractures may eventually develop. Earlier muscle changes include progressive weakness and atrophy. Associated signs and symptoms often fluctuate and may include diplopia, blurring or loss of vision, nystagmus, sensory loss or paresthesia, dysarthria, dysphagia, incoordination, ataxic gait, intention tremors, emotional lability, impotence, and urinary dysfunction.

• *Spinal cord injury.* Spasticity commonly results from cervical and high thoracic spinal cord injury, especially from incomplete lesions. Spastic paralysis in the affected limbs follows initial flaccid paralysis. Typically, spasticity and muscle atrophy increase for 1½ to 2 years after the injury, then gradually regress to flaccidity. Associated signs and symptoms vary with the level of the injury but may include respiratory insufficiency or paralysis, sensory losses, bowel and bladder dysfunction, hyperactive DTRs, positive Babinski's sign, sexual dysfunction, priapism, hypotension, anhidrosis, and bradycardia.

• *Tetanus.* This rare, life-threatening disease produces varying degrees of spasticity. In generalized tetanus, the most common form, early signs and symptoms include jaw and neck stiffness, trismus, headache, irritability, restlessness, low-grade fever with chills, tachycardia, diaphoresis, and hyperactive DTRs. As the disease progresses, painful involuntary spasms may spread and cause boardlike abdominal rigidity, opisthotonos, and a characteristic grotesque grin known as risus sardonicus. Reflex spasms may occur in any muscle group with the slightest stimulus. Glottal, pharyngeal or respiratory muscle involvement can cause death by asphyxia or cardiac failure.

Muscle weakness

Muscle weakness is detected by observing and measuring the strength of an individual muscle or muscle group. It can result from a malfunction in the cerebral hemispheres, brain stem, spinal cord, nerve roots, peripheral nerves, or myoneural junctions and within the muscle itself. Muscle weakness occurs in certain neurologic, musculoskeletal, metabolic, endocrine, and cardiovascular disorders; as a response to certain drugs; and after prolonged immobilization.

Medical causes

• *Amyotrophic lateral sclerosis.* This disorder typically begins with muscle weakness and atrophy in one hand that rapidly spreads to the arm and then to the other hand and arm. Eventually, these effects spread to the trunk, neck, tongue, larynx, pharynx, and legs. Progressive respiratory muscle weakness leads to respiratory insufficiency.

• *Anemia.* Varying degrees of muscle weakness and fatigue are exacerbated by exertion and temporarily relieved by rest. Other signs and symptoms may include pallor, tachycardia, paresthesia, and bleeding tendencies.

• *Brain tumor.* Signs and symptoms of muscle weakness vary with the location of the tumor. Other associated findings include headache, vomiting, diplopia, decreased visual acuity, decreased level of consciousness (LOC), pupillary changes, decreased motor strength, hemiparesis, hemiplegia, diminished sensations, ataxia, seizures, and behavioral changes.

• *Cerebrovascular accident (CVA).* Depending on the site and extent of damage, a CVA may produce contralateral or bilateral weakness of the arms, legs, face, and tongue, possibly progressing to hemiplegia and atrophy. Associated effects may include dysarthria, aphasia, ataxia, apraxia, agnosia, ipsilateral paresthesia or sensory losses, visual disturbances, altered LOC, amnesia, poor judg-

ment, personality changes, bowel and bladder dysfunction, headache, vomiting, and seizures.

• *Guillain-Barré syndrome.* Rapidly progressive, symmetrical weakness ascends from the feet to the arms and facial nerves and may progress to total motor paralysis and respiratory failure. Associated findings include sensory loss or paresthesia, muscle flaccidity, loss of DTRs, tachycardia or bradycardia, fluctuating hypertension and postural hypotension, diaphoresis, bowel and bladder incontinence, facial diplegia, dysphagia, dysarthria, and hypernasality.

• *Head trauma.* Severe head injury can cause varying degrees of muscle weakness. Other findings may include decreased LOC, otorrhea or rhinorrhea, raccoon's eyes and Battle's sign, sensory disturbances, and signs of increased intracranial pressure.

• *Herniated disk.* Pressure on nerve roots leads to muscle weakness, disuse, and ultimately atrophy. The primary symptom is severe lower back pain, possibly radiating to the buttocks, legs, and feet and usually occurring on one side. Diminished reflexes and sensory changes may also occur.

• *Hodgkin's disease.* Muscle weakness may accompany the classic sign of lymphadenopathy. Other findings include paresthesia, fatigue, and weight loss.

• *Hypercortisolism.* This disorder may cause limb weakness and eventually atrophy. Related cushingoid features include buffalo hump, moonface, truncal obesity, purple striae, thin skin, acne, elevated blood pressure, fatigue, hyperpigmentation, easy bruising, poor wound healing, and diaphoresis. The male patient may be impotent; the female patient may have hirsutism and menstrual irregularities.

• *Hypothyroidism.* Reversible weakness and atrophy of proximal limb muscles may occur in hypothyroidism. Other signs and symptoms commonly include muscle cramps; cold intolerance; weight gain (despite anorexia); mental dullness; dry, pale, doughy skin; puffy face, hands, and feet; impaired hearing and balance; and bradycardia.

• *Multiple sclerosis.* Muscle weakness in one or more limbs may progress to atrophy, spasticity, and contractures. Other findings typically fluctuate and may include diplopia and blurred vision, vision loss, nystagmus, hyperactive DTRs, sensory loss or paresthesia, dysarthria, dysphagia, incoordination, ataxic gait, intention tremors, emotional lability, impotence, and urinary dysfunction.

• *Myasthenia gravis.* Gradually progressive skeletal muscle weakness and fatigue are the cardinal symptoms of this disorder. Typically, weakness is mild upon awakening but worsens during the day. Early signs may include weak eye closure, ptosis, and diplopia; a blank, masklike facies; difficulty chewing and swallowing; nasal regurgitation of fluid with hypernasality; and a hanging jaw and bobbing head. Respiratory muscle involvement may eventually lead to respiratory failure.

• *Osteoarthritis.* This chronic disorder causes progressive muscle disuse and weakness that leads to atrophy.

• *Paget's disease.* As this disease progresses, muscle weakness or paralysis may develop, along with paresthesia and pain.

• *Parkinson's disease.* Muscle weakness accompanies rigidity in this degenerative disorder. Related findings include a unilateral pill-rolling tremor, propulsive gait, dysarthria, bradykinesia, drooling, dysphagia, masklike facies, and a high-pitched, monotone voice.

• *Peripheral nerve trauma.* Prolonged pressure on or injury to a peripheral nerve causes muscle weakness and atrophy. Other findings may include paresthesia or sensory loss, pain, and loss of reflexes supplied by the damaged nerve.

• *Peripheral neuropathy.* In this disorder, muscle weakness progresses slowly to flaccid paralysis, generally affecting distal extremities first. It may be accompanied by the loss of vibration sense; paresthesia, hyperesthesia, or anesthesia in the hands and feet; hypoactive or absent DTRs; mild to sharp, burning pain; anhidrosis; and glossy, red skin.

• *Polio.* Rapidly developing asymmetrical muscle weakness that progresses to flaccid paralysis occurs in paralytic polio. Associated signs and symptoms include moderate fever, headache, vomiting, lethargy, irritability, and widespread pain. As the disorder progresses, it may produce a loss of superficial reflexes and DTRs, paresthesia, hyperalgesia, urine retention, constipation, abdominal distention, nuchal rigidity, and Hoyne's, Kernig's, and Brudzinski's signs. Bulbar paralytic polio produces symptoms of encephalitis along with facial weakness, dysphasia, dysphagia, and respiratory abnormalities.

• *Polymyositis.* This disorder produces insidious or acute onset of symmetrical limb and trunk muscle weakness and tenderness. Weakness may progress to facial, neck, pharyngeal, and laryngeal muscles. Associated findings may also include hypoactive DTRs, dysphagia, and dysphonia.

• *Potassium imbalance.* In hypokalemia, temporary generalized muscle weakness may be accompanied by nausea, vomiting, diarrhea, decreased mentation, leg cramps, diminished reflexes, malaise, polyuria, dizziness, hypotension, and arrhythmias. In hyperkalemia, weakness may progress to flaccid paralysis accompanied by irritability and confusion, hyperreflexia, paresthesia or anesthesia, oliguria, anorexia, nausea, diarrhea, abdominal cramps, tachycardia or bradycardia, and arrhythmias.

• *Rheumatoid arthritis*. In this disorder, muscle weakness may accompany increased warmth, swelling, and tenderness in involved joints; pain; and stiffness that restricts motion.

• *Seizure disorder*. Temporary generalized muscle weakness may occur after a generalized tonic-clonic seizure; other postictal findings include headache, muscle soreness, and profound fatigue.

• *Spinal trauma and disease*. Trauma can cause severe muscle weakness, leading to flaccidity or spasticity and, eventually, paralysis. Infection, tumor, and cervical spondylosis or stenosis can also cause muscle weakness.

Other causes

• *Drugs*. Generalized muscle weakness can result from prolonged corticosteroid use, digitalis toxicity, and excessive doses of dantrolene. Aminoglycoside antibiotics may worsen weakness in patients with myasthenia gravis.

• *Immobility*. Immobilization in a cast, splint, or traction can lead to muscle weakness in the involved extremity; prolonged bed rest or inactivity results in generalized muscle weakness.

Neck pain

Neck pain may originate from any neck structure, ranging from the meninges and cervical vertebrae to blood vessels, muscles, and lymphatic tissue. This symptom can also be referred from other areas of the body. The location, onset, and pattern of neck pain help to determine its origin and underlying causes. Neck pain most commonly results from trauma and degenerative, congenital, inflammatory, metabolic, and neoplastic disorders.

Medical causes

• *Ankylosing spondylitis*. Intermittent, moderate to severe neck pain and stiffness with severely restricted ROM is characteristic of this disorder. Related findings also occur intermittently and may include lower back pain and stiffness, arm pain, low-grade fever, limited chest expansion, malaise, anorexia, fatigue, and occasionally iritis.

• *Cervical extension injury*. Anterior or posterior neck pain may develop within hours or days following a whiplash injury (cervical extension). Anterior pain usually diminishes within several days, but posterior pain persists and may even intensify. Associated findings may include tenderness, swelling and nuchal rigidity, arm and back pain, occipital headache, muscle spasms, visual blurring, and unilateral miosis on the affected side.

• *Cervical fibrositis*. This disorder may produce anterior neck pain that radiates to one or both shoulders. Pain is intermittent and variable, often changing with weather patterns. Other findings are nonspecific but frequently include motor point tenderness over involved muscles.

• *Cervical spine fracture*. A fracture at C1 to C4 often causes sudden death; survivors may have severe neck pain that restricts all movement, an intense occipital headache, quadriplegia, deformity, and respiratory paralysis.

• *Cervical spine infection*. Acute infection can cause neck pain that restricts motion. Other findings may include fever, possible deformity, muscle spasms, local tenderness, dysphagia, paresthesia, and muscle weakness.

• *Cervical spine tumor.* Metastatic tumors typically produce persistent neck pain that increases with movement and isn't relieved by rest; primary tumors cause mild to severe pain along a specific nerve root. Other findings depend on the lesions and may include paresthesia, arm and leg weakness that progresses to atrophy and paralysis, and bladder and bowel incontinence.

• *Cervical spondylosis.* This degenerative process produces posterior neck pain that restricts movement and is aggravated by it. Pain may radiate down either arm and may accompany paresthesia and weakness.

• *Cervical stenosis.* This progressive disorder is frequently asymptomatic and may cause nonspecific neck and arm pain, paresthesia, muscle weakness or paralysis, and decreased ROM.

• *Herniated cervical disk.* This disorder characteristically causes variable neck pain that restricts movement and is aggravated by it. It also causes referred pain, paresthesia and other sensory disturbances, and arm weakness.

• *Hodgkin's disease.* This disorder may eventually result in generalized pain that may affect the neck. Lymphadenopathy, the classic sign, may accompany paresthesia, muscle weakness, fever, fatigue, weight loss, malaise, and hepatomegaly.

• *Laryngeal cancer.* Neck pain that radiates to the ear develops late in this disorder. The patient may also have dysphagia, dyspnea, hemoptysis, stridor, hoarseness, and cervical lymphadenopathy.

• *Lymphadenitis.* In this disorder, enlarged and inflamed cervical lymph nodes cause acute pain and tenderness. Fever, chills, and malaise may also occur.

• *Neck sprain.* Minor sprains typically produce pain, slight swelling, stiffness, and restricted ROM. Ligament rupture causes pain, marked swelling, ecchymosis, muscle spasms, and nuchal rigidity with head tilt.

• *Osteoporosis.* Neck pain occurs rarely in this disorder, which usually affects the thoracic and lumbar vertebrae. Cervical vertebral involvement produces tenderness and deformity.

• *Paget's disease.* This slowly developing disease is often asymptomatic in its early stages. As it progresses, cervical vertebral deformity may produce severe, persistent neck pain, along with paresthesia and arm weakness or paralysis.

• *Rheumatoid arthritis.* This disorder most often affects peripheral joints, but it can also involve the cervical vertebrae. Acute inflammation may cause moderate to severe pain that radiates along a specific nerve root; increased warmth, swelling, and tenderness in involved joints; stiffness restricting ROM; paresthesia and muscle weakness; low-grade fever; anorexia; malaise; fatigue; and neck deformity. Some pain and stiffness remain after the acute phase.

• *Spinous process fracture.* Fracture near the cervicothoracic junction produces acute pain radiating to the shoulders. Associated findings include swelling, exquisite tenderness, restricted ROM, muscle spasms, and deformity.

• *Torticollis.* In this neck deformity, severe neck pain accompanies recurrent unilateral stiffness and muscle spasms that produce a characteristic head tilt.

Paralysis

Paralysis, the total loss of voluntary motor function, results from severe cortical or pyramidal tract damage. It occurs in cerebrovascular disorders, degenerative neuromuscular disease, trauma, tumors, or central nervous system infection. Acute paralysis may be an early indicator of a life-threatening disorder, such as Guillain-Barré syndrome. Paralysis can be local or widespread, symmetrical or asymmetrical, transient or permanent, and spastic or flaccid. It's often classified according to location and severity as paraplegia (sometimes transient paralysis of the legs), quadriplegia (permanent paralysis of the arms, legs, and body below the level of the spinal lesion), or hemiplegia (unilateral paralysis of varying severity and permanence). Incomplete paralysis with profound weakness (paresis) may precede total paralysis in some patients.

Emergency interventions

See *Sudden paralysis: What to do*.

Medical causes

• *Amyotrophic lateral sclerosis.* This invariably fatal disorder produces spastic or flaccid paralysis in the major muscle groups, eventually progressing to total paralysis. Earlier findings include progressive muscle weakness, fasciculations, and muscle atrophy, often beginning in the arms and hands. Cramping and hyperreflexia are also common. Respiratory muscle and brain stem involvement produce dyspnea and possibly respiratory distress. Developing cranial nerve paralysis causes dysarthria, dysphagia, drooling, choking, and difficulty chewing.

• *Bell's palsy.* A disease of cranial nerve VII, Bell's palsy causes transient, unilateral facial muscle paralysis. The affected muscles sag and eyelid closure is impossible. Other signs include increased tearing, drooling, and a diminished or absent corneal reflex.

• *Brain abscess.* Advanced abscess in the frontal or temporal lobe can cause hemiplegia accompanied by other late findings, such as ocular disturbances, unequal pupils, decreased LOC, ataxia, tremors, and signs of infection.

• *Brain tumor.* A tumor affecting the motor cortex of the frontal lobe may cause contralateral hemiparesis that progresses to hemiplegia. Onset is gradual, but paralysis is permanent without treatment. In early stages, frontal headache and behavioral changes may be the only indicators. Eventually, seizures, aphasia, and signs of increased intracranial pressure (ICP), including decreased LOC and vomiting, develop.

• *Cerebrovascular accident (CVA).* A CVA involving the motor cortex can produce contralateral paresis or paralysis. Onset may be sudden or gradual, and paralysis may be transient or permanent. Associated signs and symptoms vary widely and may include headache, vomiting, seizures, decreased LOC and mental acuity, dysarthria, dysphagia, ataxia, contralateral paresthesia or sensory loss, apraxia, agnosia, aphasia, visual disturbances, emotional lability, and bowel and bladder dysfunction.

• *Conversion disorder.* Hysterical paralysis, a classic symptom of conversion disorder, is characterized by the loss of voluntary movement with no obvious physical cause. It can affect any muscle group, appears and disappears unpredictably, and may occur with histrionic behavior (manipulative, dramatic, vain, and irrational) or a strange indifference.

• *Encephalitis.* Variable paralysis develops in the late stages of this disorder. Earlier signs and symptoms include rapidly decreasing LOC (possibly coma), fever, headache, photophobia, vomiting, signs of meningeal irritation (including nuchal rigidity, positive Kernig's and Brudzinski's signs), aphasia, ataxia, nystagmus, ocular palsy, myoclonus, and seizures.

• *Guillain-Barré syndrome.* This syndrome is characterized by a rapidly developing, but reversible, ascending paralysis. It commonly begins as leg muscle weakness and progresses symmetrically, sometimes affecting even the cranial nerves, producing dysphagia, nasal speech, and dysarthria. Respiratory muscle paralysis may be life-threatening. Other effects may include transient paresthesia, orthostatic hypotension, tachycardia, diaphoresis, and bowel and bladder incontinence.

• *Head trauma.* Cerebral injury can cause paralysis due to cerebral edema and increased ICP. Onset is usually sudden. Location and extent vary, depending on the injury. Associated findings also vary but may include decreased LOC; sensory disturbances, such as paresthesia and loss of sensation; headache; blurred or double vision; nausea and vomiting; and focal neurologic disturbances.

• *Migraine headache.* Hemiparesis, scotomas, paresthesia, confusion, dizziness, photophobia, and other transient symptoms may precede the onset of a throbbing unilateral headache and may persist after it subsides.

• *Multiple sclerosis.* In this disorder, paralysis commonly fluctuates until the later stages, when it may become permanent. Its extent can range from monoplegia to quadriplegia. In most patients, visual and sensory disturbances, such as paresthesia, are the earliest symptoms. Later findings vary widely and may include muscle weakness and spasticity, nystagmus, hyperreflexia, intention tremor, gait ataxia, dysphagia, dysarthria, impotence, and constipation. Urinary frequency, urgency, and incontinence may also occur.

• *Myasthenia gravis.* In this neuromuscular disease, profound muscle weakness and abnormal fatigability may produce paralysis of certain muscle groups. Paralysis is usually transient in early stages but becomes more persistent as the disease progresses. Associated findings depend on the areas of neuromuscular involvement and may include weak eye closure, ptosis, diplopia, lack of facial mobility, dysphagia, nasal speech, and frequent nasal regurgitation of fluids. Neck muscle weakness may cause the patient's jaw to drop and his head to bob. Respiratory muscle involvement can lead to respiratory distress, including dyspnea, shallow respirations, and cyanosis.

• *Parkinson's disease.* Tremor, bradykinesia, and lead-pipe or cogwheel rigidity are the classic signs of Parkinson's disease. Extreme rigidity can progress to paralysis, particularly in the extremities. In most cases, paralysis resolves with prompt treatment of the disease.

• *Peripheral nerve trauma.* Severe injury to a peripheral nerve or group of nerves results in the loss of motor and sensory function in the innervated area. Muscles become flaccid and atrophied, and reflexes are lost. If transection isn't complete, paralysis may be temporary.

• *Peripheral neuropathy.* Typically, this syndrome produces muscle weakness that may lead to flaccid paralysis and atrophy. Related effects may include paresthesia, loss of vibration sensation, hypoactive or absent DTRs, neuralgia, and skin changes such as anhidrosis.

• *Polio.* This disorder can produce insidious, permanent flaccid paralysis and hyporeflexia. Sensory function remains intact, but the patient loses voluntary muscle control.

• *Rabies.* This acute disorder produces progressive flaccid paralysis, vascular collapse, coma, and death within 2 weeks of contact with an infected animal. Prodromal signs and symptoms develop almost immediately, including fever, headache, hyperesthesia, paresthesia, coldness and itching at the bite site, photophobia, tachycardia, shallow respirations, and excessive salivation, lacrimation, and perspiration. Within 10 days, a phase of excitement begins with agitation, cranial nerve dysfunction (pupil changes, hoarseness, facial weakness, ocular palsies), tachycardia or bradycardia, cyclic respirations, high fever, urine retention, drooling, and hydrophobia.

• *Seizure disorders.* Seizures, particularly focal seizures, can cause transient local paralysis (Todd's paralysis). Any part of the body may be affected, although paralysis tends to occur contralateral to the side of the irritable focus.

• *Spinal cord injury.* Complete spinal cord transection results in permanent spastic paralysis below the level of injury. Reflexes may return after resolution of spinal shock. Partial transection causes variable paralysis and paresthesia, depending on the location and extent of injury. (See

Understanding spinal cord syndromes.)

• *Spinal cord tumors.* Paresis, pain, paresthesia, and variable sensory loss may occur along the nerve distribution pathway served by the affected cord segment. Eventually, this may progress to spastic paralysis with hyperactive DTRs (unless the tumor is in the cauda equina, which produces hyporeflexia) and, perhaps, bladder and bowel incontinence. Paralysis is permanent without treatment.

• *Syringomyelia.* This degenerative spinal cord disease produces segmental paresis, leading to flaccid paralysis of the hands and arms. Reflexes are absent, and the loss of pain and temperature sensation are distributed over the neck, shoulders, and arms in a capelike pattern.

• *Transient ischemic attack (TIA).* Episodic TIAs may cause transient unilateral paresis or paralysis accompanied by paresthesia, blurred or double vision, dizziness, aphasia, dysarthria, decreased LOC, and other site-dependent effects.

Other causes

• *Drugs.* Therapeutic use of neuromuscular blocking agents, such as pancuronium and curare, produces paralysis.

• *Electroconvulsive therapy.* This therapy can produce acute, but transient, paralysis.

Paresthesia

Paresthesia is an abnormal sensation, often described as numbness, prickling, or tingling, that is felt along peripheral nerve pathways. These sensations generally aren't painful. Unpleasant or painful sensations are termed dysesthesia. Paresthesia may develop suddenly or grad-

UNDERSTANDING SPINAL CORD SYNDROMES

When the patient's spinal cord is incompletely severed, he will have partial motor and sensory loss. Most incomplete cord lesions fit into one of the syndromes described below. Dark-shaded areas in the illustrations indicate areas of lesions.

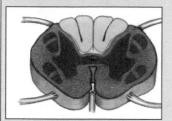

Anterior cord syndrome, most commonly resulting from a flexion injury, causes motor paralysis and loss of pain and temperature sensation below the level of injury. Touch, proprioception, and vibration sensation are usually preserved.

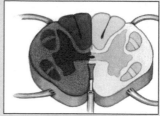

Brown-Sequard's syndrome can result from flexion, rotation, or penetration injuries. It's characterized by unilateral motor paralysis ipsilateral to the injury and loss of pain and temperature sensation contralateral to the injury.

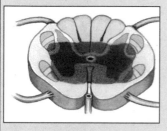

Central cord syndrome is caused by hyperextension or flexion injuries. Motor loss is variable and greater in the arms than in the legs; sensory loss is usually slight.

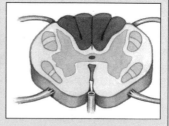

Posterior cord syndrome, produced by a cervical hyperextension injury, causes only a loss of proprioception and loss of light touch sensation. Motor function remains intact.

---

ually and may be transient or permanent.

A common symptom of many neurologic disorders, paresthesia may also result from certain systemic disorders or drug effects. It may reflect damage or irritation of the parietal lobe, thalamus, spinothalamic tract, or spinal or peripheral nerves.

Medical causes

• *Arterial occlusion (acute)*. In this disorder, sudden paresthesia and coldness may develop in one or both legs with a saddle embolus. Paresis, intermittent claudication, and aching pain at rest are also common. The extremity becomes mottled with a line of temperature and color demarcation at the level of occlusion. Pulses are absent below the occlusion, and capillary refill is diminished.

• *Arteriosclerosis obliterans.* This disorder produces paresthesia, intermittent claudication (the most common symptom), diminished or absent popliteal and pedal pulses, pallor, paresis, and coldness in the affected leg.

• *Arthritis.* Rheumatoid or osteoarthritic changes in the cervical spine may cause paresthesia in the neck, shoulders, and arms. Less frequently the lumbar spine is affected, causing paresthesia in one or both legs and feet.

• *Brain tumor.* Tumors affecting the sensory cortex in the parietal lobe may cause progressive contralateral paresthesia accompanied by agnosia, apraxia, agraphia, homonymous hemianopia, and loss of proprioception.

• *Buerger's disease.* In this smoking-related inflammatory occlusive disorder, exposure to cold makes the feet cold, cyanotic, and numb, Later, they become red and hot, and tingle. Intermittent claudication, which is aggravated by exercise and relieved by rest, is also common. Other findings include weak peripheral pulses, migratory superficial thrombophlebitis and, later, ulceration, muscle atrophy, and gangrene.

• *Cerebrovascular accident (CVA).* Although contralateral paresthesia may occur in CVA, sensory loss is more common. Associated features vary with the artery affected. There may be contralateral hemiplegia, decreased LOC, and homonymous hemianopia, among others.

• *Diabetes mellitus.* Glove and stocking paresthesia of diabetic neuropathy often give a burning sensation. Other findings may include insidious, permanent anosmia, fatigue, polyuria, polydipsia, weight loss, and polyphagia.

• *Guillain-Barré syndrome.* In this syndrome, transient paresthesia may precede muscle weakness, which usu-ally begins in the legs and ascends to the arms and facial nerves. Weakness may progress to total paralysis. Other clinical features may be dysarthria, dysphagia, nasal speech, orthostatic hypotension, bladder and bowel incontinence, diaphoresis, tachycardia, and possibly signs of life-threatening respiratory muscle paralysis.

• *Head trauma.* Unilateral or bilateral paresthesia may occur when head trauma causes concussion or contusion; however, sensory loss is more common. Other findings may include variable paresis or paralysis, decreased LOC, headache, blurred or double vision, nausea, vomiting, dizziness, and seizures.

• *Herniated disk.* Herniation of a lumbar or cervical disk may cause acute or gradual onset of paresthesia along the distribution pathways of affected spinal nerves. Other neuromuscular effects include severe pain, muscle spasms, and weakness that may progress to atrophy unless herniation is relieved.

• *Herpes zoster.* An early symptom of this disorder, paresthesia occurs in the dermatome supplied by the affected spinal nerve. Within several days, this dermatome is marked by a pruritic, erythematous, vesicular rash associated with sharp, shooting, or burning pain.

• *Hyperventilation syndrome.* Usually triggered by acute anxiety, this syndrome may produce transient paresthesia in the hands, feet, and circumoral area, accompanied by agitation, vertigo, syncope, pallor, muscle twitching and weakness, carpopedal spasm, and cardiac arrhythmias.

• *Hypocalcemia.* Early in this disorder, asymmetrical paresthesia usually occurs in the fingers, toes, and circumoral area. Other manifestations include muscle weakness, twitching, or cramps; palpitations; hyperactive DTRs; carpopedal spasm; and positive Chvostek's and Trousseau's signs.

• *Migraine headache.* Paresthesia in the hands, face, and perioral area may herald an impending migraine headache. Other prodromal symptoms may include scotomas, hemiparesis, confusion, dizziness, and photophobia. These effects may persist during the characteristic throbbing headache and continue after it subsides.

• *Multiple sclerosis (MS).* In this disorder, demyelination of the sensory cortex or spinothalamic tract may produce paresthesia, which is often one of the earliest symptoms of MS. Like other effects of MS, paresthesia commonly fluctuates until the later stages, when it may become permanent. Associated findings may include muscle weakness, spasticity, and hyperreflexia.

• *Peripheral nerve trauma.* Injury to any of the major peripheral nerves may cause paresthesia — often dysesthesias — in the area supplied by that nerve. Paresthesia begins shortly after trauma and may be permanent. Other effects may include flaccid paralysis or paresis, hyporeflexia, and variable sensory loss.

• *Peripheral neuropathy.* This syndrome may cause progressive paresthesia in all extremities. The patient also commonly displays muscle weakness, which may lead to flaccid paralysis and atrophy; loss of vibration sensation; diminished or absent DTRs; neuralgia; and cutaneous changes, such as glossy, red skin and anhidrosis.

• *Raynaud's disease.* Exposure to cold or stress makes the fingers turn pale, cold, and cyanotic; with rewarming, they become red and paresthetic. Ulceration may occur in chronic cases.

• *Seizure disorders.* Seizures originating in the parietal lobe usually cause paresthesia of the lips, fingers, and toes. This paresthesia may act as an aura that leads to generalized tonic-clonic seizures.

• *Spinal cord injury.* Paresthesia may occur in partial spinal cord transection after spinal shock resolves. It may be unilateral or bilateral, occurring at or below the level of the lesion. Associated sensory and motor loss varies. Spinal cord disorders may be associated with paresthesia on head flexion (Lhermitte's sign).

• *Spinal cord tumors.* Paresthesia, paresis, pain, and sensory loss along nerve pathways served by the affected cord segment result from such tumors. Eventually, paresis may cause spastic paralysis with hyperactive DTRs (unless the tumor is in the cauda equina, which produces hyporeflexia) and, possibly, bladder and bowel incontinence.

• *Systemic lupus erythematosus.* This disorder may cause paresthesia. Primary clinical features include nondeforming arthritis (usually of hands, feet, and large joints), photosensitivity, and a "butterfly" rash that appears across the nose and cheeks.

• *Thoracic outlet syndrome.* Paresthesia occurs suddenly in this syndrome when the affected arm is raised and abducted. The arm also becomes pale and cool with diminished pulses. Unequal blood pressure between arms may be noted.

• *Transient ischemic attack (TIA).* Typically, paresthesia occurs abruptly in a TIA and is limited to one arm or another isolated part of the body. TIAs usually last about 10 minutes and are accompanied by paralysis or paresis. Associated findings may include decreased LOC, dizziness, unilateral vision loss, nystagmus, aphasia, dysarthria, tinnitus, facial weakness, dysphagia, and ataxic gait.

• *Vitamin B deficiency.* Chronic thiamine or vitamin B_{12} deficiency may cause paresthesia and weakness in the arms and legs. Burning leg pain, hypoactive DTRs, and variable sensory loss are common in thiamine deficiency. Vitamin B_{12} deficiency also produces mental status changes and impaired vision.

Other causes

• *Drugs.* Phenytoin, chemotherapeutic agents (such as vincristine, vinblastine, and procarbazine), penicillamine, isoniazid, nitrofurantoin, chloroquine, and parenteral gold therapy may produce transient paresthesia that disappears when the drug is discontinued.

• *Radiation therapy.* Long-term radiation therapy may eventually cause peripheral nerve damage, producing paresthesia.

Romberg's sign

A positive Romberg's sign refers to a patient's inability to maintain balance when standing erect with his feet together and his eyes closed. It indicates a vestibular or proprioceptive disorder, which is a disorder of the spinal tracts (the posterior columns) that carry proprioceptive information — the perception of one's position in space and joint movements and of pressure sensations — to the brain. Insufficient vestibular or proprioceptive information causes an inability to execute precise movements and maintain balance without visual cues.

Medical causes

• *Multiple sclerosis.* Early features may include vision changes, diplopia, and paresthesia. Besides a positive Romberg's sign, other findings may include nystagmus, constipation, muscle weakness and spasticity, hyperreflexia, dysphagia, dysarthria, incontinence, urinary frequency and urgency, impotence, and emotional instability.

• *Peripheral nerve disease.* Besides a positive Romberg's sign, advanced disease may produce impotence, fatigue, and paresthesia, hyperesthesia, or anesthesia in the hands and feet. Related findings include incoordination, ataxia, burning pain in the affected area, progressive muscle weakness and atrophy, hypoactive DTRs, and loss of vibration sense.

• *Pernicious anemia.* A positive Romberg's sign and loss of proprioception in the lower limbs reflect peripheral nerve and spinal cord damage. Gait changes (usually ataxia), muscle weakness, impaired coordination, paresthesia, and sensory loss may also be present. DTRs may be hypoactive or hyperactive. Other findings include a sore tongue, a positive Babinski's reflex, fatigue, blurred vision, diplopia, and light-headedness.

• *Spinal cerebellar degeneration.* In this disorder, a positive Romberg's sign accompanies decreased visual acuity, fatigue, paresthesia, loss of vibration sense, incoordination, ataxic gait, and muscle weakness and atrophy. DTRs may be hypoactive.

• *Spinal cord disease.* A positive Romberg's sign may accompany fasciculations, muscle weakness and atrophy, and loss of proprioception, vibration, and other senses. DTRs may be hypoactive at the level of the lesion and hyperactive above it. Other features include pain and loss of sphincter tone.

• *Vestibular disorders.* In addition to a positive Romberg's sign, these disorders commonly cause vertigo. They also cause nystagmus, nausea, and vomiting.

Seizure, absence

Absence seizures (or generalized absence seizures) are benign, generalized tonic-clonic seizures thought to originate subcortically. These brief episodes of unconsciousness last 3 to 20 seconds and can occur 100 or more times a day, commonly causing periods of inattention. Absence seizures most often affect children between the ages of 4 and 12 and rarely persist beyond adolescence. Their first sign may be deteriorating schoolwork and behavior. Their cause isn't known.

Absence seizures occur without warning. The patient suddenly stops all purposeful activity and stares blankly ahead, as though daydreaming. Absence seizures may produce automatisms, such as repetitive lip smacking and mild clonic or myoclonic movements, including mild jerking of the eyelids. The patient may drop objects he's holding, and muscle relaxation may cause him to drop his head and arms or to slump. After the attack, the patient resumes activity, typically unaware of the episode.

Absence status, a rare form of absence seizure, occurs as a prolonged absence seizure or as repeated episodes of these seizures. Usually not life-threatening, it occurs most commonly in patients with preexisting absence seizures.

Medical cause

• *Idiopathic epilepsy.* Some forms of absence seizures are accompanied by automatisms and learning disability in this disorder.

Seizure, focal

Resulting from an irritable focus in the cerebral cortex, a focal seizure (or simple partial seizure) typically lasts about 30 seconds and doesn't alter the patient's level of consciousness (LOC). Its type and pattern reflect the location of the irritable focus. A focal seizure may be classified as motor or

somatosensory. A focal motor seizure includes a jacksonian seizure and epilepsia partialis continua. A somatosensory seizure involves visual, olfactory, and auditory areas.

A focal motor seizure is a series of unilateral clonic (muscle jerking) and tonic (muscle stiffening) movements of one part of the body. The patient's head and eyes characteristically turn away from the hemispheric focus, most commonly the frontal lobe near the motor strip. A tonic-clonic contraction of the trunk or extremities may follow.

A jacksonian motor seizure typically begins with a tonic contraction of a finger, the corner of the mouth, or a foot. Clonic movements follow, spreading to other muscles on the same side of the body, moving up the arm or leg, and eventually involving the whole side. Alternatively, clonic movements may spread to the opposite side, becoming generalized and leading to loss of consciousness. In the postictal phase, the patient may display paralysis (Todd's paralysis) in the affected limbs that usually resolves within 24 hours.

Epilepsia partialis continua causes clonic twitching of one muscle group, usually in the face, arm, or leg. Twitching occurs every few seconds and persists for hours, days, or months without spreading. Spasms affect the distal arm and leg muscles more frequently than the proximal ones. In the face, they affect the corner of the mouth, one or both eyelids and, occasionally, the neck or trunk muscles unilaterally.

A focal somatosensory seizure affects a localized body area on one side. Usually, this seizure initially causes numbness, tingling, or crawling or "electric" sensations; rarely, it may cause pain or burning sensations in the lips, fingers, or toes.

A visual seizure involves sensations of darkness or of stationary or moving lights or spots that are usually red at first and then change to blue, green, and yellow. It can affect both visual fields or just the visual field on the side opposite the lesion. The irritable focus is in the occipital lobe. In contrast, the irritable focus in an auditory or olfactory seizure is in the temporal lobe.

Medical causes

• *Brain abscess.* Seizures can occur in the acute stage of abscess formation or after resolution of the abscess. Decreased LOC varies from drowsiness to deep stupor. Early signs and symptoms reflect increased intracranial pressure and include constant, intractable headache, nausea, and vomiting. Later symptoms include ocular disturbances, such as nystagmus, decreased visual acuity, and unequal pupils. Other findings differ with the abscess site and may include aphasia, hemiparesis, and personality changes.

• *Brain tumor.* Focal seizures are commonly the earliest indicators of a brain tumor. The patient may report morning headache, dizziness, confusion, vision loss, and motor and sensory disturbances. He may also have aphasia, generalized tonic-clonic seizures, ataxia, decreased LOC, papilledema, vomiting, increased systolic blood pressure, and widening pulse pressure. Eventually, he may assume a decorticate posture.

• *Cerebrovascular accident (CVA).* A major cause of seizures in patients over age 50, a CVA may induce focal seizures within 6 months after its onset. Related effects depend on the type and extent of the CVA but may include decreased LOC, contralateral hemiplegia, dysarthria, dysphagia, ataxia, unilateral sensory loss, apraxia, agnosia, and aphasia. A CVA may also cause visual deficits, memory loss, poor judgment, personality

changes, emotional lability, headache, urine retention or urinary incontinence, and vomiting. It may cause generalized tonic-clonic seizures.

• *Head trauma.* Any head injury can cause seizures, but penetrating wounds are characteristically associated with focal seizures. These seizures most commonly arise 3 to 15 months after injury, decrease in frequency after several years, and eventually stop. The patient may have generalized tonic-clonic seizures and a decreased LOC that may progress to coma.

• *Multiple sclerosis.* Focal or generalized tonic-clonic seizures may occur, usually late in the course of this disorder. Other findings may include visual deficits, paresthesia, constipation, muscle weakness, spasticity, paralysis, hyperreflexia, intention tremor, gait ataxia, dysphagia, and dysarthria. There may also be emotional lability, impotence, and urinary frequency, urgency, and incontinence.

• *Neurofibromatosis.* Multiple brain lesions cause focal seizures and, at times, generalized tonic-clonic seizures. Inspection reveals café au lait spots, multiple skin tumors, scoliosis, and kyphoscoliosis. Related findings include dizziness, ataxia, progressive monocular blindness, nystagmus, and endocrine abnormalities.

• *Sarcoidosis.* Multiple lesions from this disorder affect the brain, producing focal and generalized tonic-clonic seizures. Associated findings include a nonproductive cough with dyspnea, substernal pain, malaise, fatigue, arthralgia, myalgia, weight loss, tachypnea, dysphagia, skin lesions, and impaired vision.

ALERT In children more often than in adults, focal seizures are likely to spread and become generalized. They typically cause the child's eyes, or his head and eyes, to turn to the side. In neonates, they cause mouth twitching, staring, or both.

Focal seizures in children can result from hemiplegic cerebral palsy, head trauma, child abuse, arteriovenous malformation, and Sturge-Weber syndrome. About 25% of febrile seizures may present as focal seizures.

Seizure, generalized tonic-clonic

Like other types of seizure, a generalized tonic-clonic seizure is caused by the paroxysmal, uncontrolled discharge of central nervous system (CNS) neurons, leading to neurologic dysfunction. *Unlike* most other types of seizure, this cerebral hyperactivity isn't confined to the original focus or a localized area but extends to the entire brain.

A generalized tonic-clonic seizure may begin with or without an aura. As seizure activity spreads to the subcortical structures, the patient loses consciousness, falls to the ground, and may utter a loud cry that is precipitated by air rushing from the lungs through the vocal cords. His body stiffens (tonic phase) and then undergoes rapid, synchronous muscle jerking and hyperventilation (clonic phase). Tongue biting, incontinence, diaphoresis, profuse salivation, and signs of respiratory distress may also occur. The seizure usually stops after 2 to 5 minutes. The patient then regains consciousness but displays confusion. He may complain of headache, fatigue, muscle soreness, and arm and leg weakness.

Generalized tonic-clonic seizures usually occur singly. The patient may be awake and active or sleeping. Possible complications include respiratory arrest due to airway obstruction from secretions, status epilepticus (occurring in 5% to 8% of patients), head or spinal injuries and bruises, Todd's paralysis and, rarely, cardiac arrest. Life-threatening status epilepticus is marked by prolonged seizure activity or by rapidly recurring seizures with no intervening periods of recovery. It's most commonly triggered by the abrupt discontinuation of anticonvulsant drugs.

Generalized tonic-clonic seizures may be caused by brain tumors, vascular disorders, head trauma, infections, metabolic and genetic defects, drug and alcohol withdrawal syndromes, and toxins. They may also result from a focal seizure. In recurring seizures, or epilepsy, the cause may be unknown.

Emergency interventions

See *Seizures: What to do,* page 98.

Medical causes

• *Alcohol withdrawal syndrome.* Sudden withdrawal from chronic alcohol dependence may cause seizures 7 to 48 hours later and status epilepticus. The patient may also be restless and have hallucinations, profuse diaphoresis, and tachycardia.

• *Arsenic poisoning.* Besides generalized tonic-clonic seizures, arsenic poisoning may cause a garlicky breath odor, increased salivation, and generalized pruritus. GI effects include diarrhea, nausea, vomiting, and severe abdominal pain. Related effects include diffuse hyperpigmentation; sharply defined edema of the eyelids, face, and ankles; numbness or tingling of the extremities; alopecia; irritated mucous membranes; weakness; muscle aches; and peripheral neuropathy.

• *Brain abscess.* Generalized tonic-clonic seizures may occur in the acute stage of abscess formation or after the abscess disappears. Depend-

SEIZURES: WHAT TO DO

If you witness the beginning of the seizure, stay with your patient and ensure a patent airway. Focus your care on observing the seizure and protecting the patient. Place a towel under his head to prevent injury, loosen his clothing, and move any sharp or hard objects out of his way. Never try to restrain him or force a hard object into his mouth; you may chip his teeth or fracture his jaw. Only at the start of the ictal phase can you safely insert a soft object into his mouth.

If possible during the seizure, turn the patient on one side to allow secretions to drain. Otherwise, do this at the end of the clonic phase when respirations return. If they fail to return, check for airway obstruction and suction the patient, if necessary. Intubation and mechanical ventilation may also be needed.

Protect the patient after the seizure by providing a safe area in which he can rest. As the patient awakens, you should reassure and reorient him. Check his vital signs and neurologic status. Be sure to carefully record these and observations you made during the seizure.

If the seizure lasts longer than 4 minutes or if a second seizure occurs before full recovery from the first, suspect status epilepticus. Turn the patient on his side, with his head in a semi-dependent position, to drain secretions and prevent aspiration.

ing on the size and location of the abscess, decreased level of consciousness (LOC) varies from drowsiness to deep stupor. Early signs and symptoms reflect increased intracranial pressure (ICP) and include constant headache, nausea, vomiting, and focal seizures. Later features typically include ocular disturbances, such as nystagmus, impaired vision, and unequal pupils. Other findings differ with the abscess site but may include aphasia, hemiparesis, abnormal behavior, and personality changes.

• *Brain tumor.* Generalized tonic-clonic seizures may occur, depending on the tumor's location and type. Other findings include a slowly decreasing LOC, morning headache, dizziness, confusion, focal seizures, vision loss, motor and sensory disturbances, aphasia, and ataxia. Later findings include papilledema, vomiting, increased systolic blood pressure, widening pulse pressure and, eventually, decorticate posture.

• *Cerebral aneurysm.* Occasionally, generalized tonic-clonic seizures may occur with an aneurysmal rupture. Premonitory signs and symptoms may last several days, but onset is typically abrupt with severe headache, nausea, vomiting, and decreased LOC. Depending on the site and amount of bleeding, related signs and symptoms vary but may include nuchal rigidity, irritability, hemiparesis, hemisensory defects, dysphagia, photophobia, diplopia, ptosis, and a unilateral dilated pupil.

• *Cerebrovascular accident (CVA).* Seizures (focal more often than generalized) occur within 6 months of an ischemic CVA. Associated signs and symptoms vary with the location and extent of brain damage. They include decreased LOC, contralateral hemiplegia, dysarthria, dysphagia, ataxia, unilateral sensory loss, apraxia, agnosia, and aphasia. There may also be visual deficits, memory loss, poor judgment, personality changes, emotional lability, urine retention or urinary incontinence, constipation, headache, and vomiting.

• *Eclampsia.* Generalized tonic-clonic seizures are a hallmark of this disorder. Related findings include severe frontal headache, nausea and vomiting, vision disturbances, increased blood pressure, peripheral edema, and sudden weight gain. The patient may also be irritable and have oliguria, hyperactive deep tendon reflexes (DTRs), and a decreased LOC.

• *Encephalitis.* Seizures are an early sign of this disorder and indicate a poor prognosis. They may also occur after recovery as a result of residual damage. Other findings include fever, headache, photophobia, nuchal rigidity, vomiting, aphasia, ataxia, hemiparesis, nystagmus, irritability, cranial nerve palsies (causing facial weakness, ptosis, dysphagia), and myoclonic jerks.

• *Head trauma.* In severe cases, generalized tonic-clonic seizures may occur at the time of injury. Months later, focal seizures may occur. Severe head trauma may also cause a decreased LOC that leads to coma; soft tissue injury of the face, head, or neck; clear or bloody drainage from the mouth, nose, or ears; facial edema; bony deformity of the face, head, or neck; Battle's sign; and lack of response to oculocephalic and oculovestibular stimulation. Motor and sensory deficits may occur along with altered respirations. Examination may reveal signs of increasing ICP, such as decreased response to painful stimuli, nonreactive pupils, bradycardia, increased systolic pressure, and widening pulse pressure. If the patient is conscious, he may have visual deficits, behavioral changes, and headache.

• *Hepatic encephalopathy.* Late in this disorder, generalized tonic-clonic seizures may occur. Associated late-stage findings in the comatose patient include fetor hepaticus, asterixis, hyperactive DTRs, and a positive Babinski's sign.

• *Hypertensive encephalopathy.* This life-threatening disorder may cause seizures, along with severely increased blood pressure, decreased LOC, intense headache, vomiting, transient blindness, paralysis and, eventually, Cheyne-Stokes respirations.

• *Hypoglycemia.* Generalized tonic-clonic seizures usually occur in severe hypoglycemia, accompanied by blurred or double vision, motor weakness, hemiplegia, trembling, excessive diaphoresis, tachycardia, myoclonic twitching, and decreased LOC.

• *Hyponatremia.* Seizures develop when serum sodium levels fall below 125 mEq/L, especially if the decrease is rapid. Hyponatremia also causes postural hypotension, headache, muscle twitching and weakness, fatigue, oliguria or anuria, cold and clammy skin, decreased skin turgor, irritability, lethargy, confusion, and stupor or coma. Excessive thirst, tachycardia, nausea, vomiting, and abdominal cramps may also occur. Severe hyponatremia may cause cyanosis and vasomotor collapse, with a thready pulse.

• *Hypoparathyroidism.* Worsening tetany causes generalized tonic-clonic seizures. Chronic hypoparathyroidism produces neuromuscular irritability and hyperactive DTRs.

• *Hypoxic-ischemic encephalopathy.* Besides generalized tonic-clonic seizures, this disorder may produce myoclonic jerks and coma. After the patient has recovered, dementia, visual agnosia, choreoathetosis, and ataxia may occur.

• *Idiopathic epilepsy.* In most cases, the cause of recurrent seizures is unknown.

• *Multiple sclerosis.* This disorder rarely produces generalized tonic-clonic seizures. Characteristic findings include vision deficits, paresthesia, constipation, muscle weakness, paralysis, spasticity, hyperreflexia, intention tremor, ataxic gait, dysphagia, dysarthria, impotence, and emotional lability. There may also be urinary frequency, urgency, and incontinence.

• *Neurofibromatosis.* Multiple brain lesions in this disorder cause focal and generalized tonic-clonic seizures. Inspection reveals café au lait spots, multiple skin tumors, scoliosis, and kyphoscoliosis. Related findings include dizziness, ataxia, monocular blindness, and nystagmus.

• *Sarcoidosis.* Lesions may affect the brain, causing generalized tonic-clonic and focal seizures. Associated findings include a nonproductive cough with dyspnea, substernal pain, malaise, fatigue, arthralgia, myalgia, weight loss, tachypnea, dysphagia, skin lesions, and impaired vision.

Other causes

• *Barbiturate withdrawal.* In chronically intoxicated patients, barbiturate withdrawal may produce generalized tonic-clonic seizures 2 to 4 days after the last dose. Status epilepticus is possible.

• *Drugs.* Toxic blood levels of some drugs, such as theophylline, lidocaine, meperidine, penicillins, and cimetidine, may cause generalized tonic-clonic seizures. Phenothiazines, tricyclic antidepressants, amphetamines, isoniazid, and vincristine may cause seizures in patients with preexisting epilepsy.

Vertigo

Vertigo is an illusion of movement in which the patient feels that he's revolving in space (subjective vertigo) or that his surroundings are revolving around him (objective vertigo). He may complain of feeling pulled sideways, as though drawn by a magnet.

A common symptom, vertigo usually begins abruptly and may be temporary or permanent and mild or severe. It may worsen when the patient moves and often subsides when he lies down. It's frequently confused with dizziness, which is a sensation of imbalance and light-headedness that is nonspecific. However, unlike dizziness, vertigo is often accompanied by nausea, vomiting, nystagmus, and tinnitus or hearing loss. Although the patient's limb coordination is unaffected, vertiginous gait may occur.

Vertigo may result from neurologic or otologic disorders that affect the equilibratory apparatus (the vestibule, semicircular canals, cranial nerve VIII, vestibular nuclei in the brain stem and their temporal lobe connections, and eyes). However, this symptom may also result from alcohol intoxication, hyperventilation, postural changes (benign postural vertigo), and the effects of certain drugs, tests, and procedures.

Medical causes

• *Acoustic neuroma.* This tumor of cranial nerve VIII causes mild, intermittent vertigo and unilateral sensorineural hearing loss. Other findings include tinnitus, postauricular or suboccipital pain and, with cranial nerve compression, facial paralysis.

• *Benign positional vertigo.* In this disorder, debris in a semicircular canal produces vertigo on head position change that lasts a few minutes. It's usually temporary and can be effectively treated with positional maneuvers.

• *Brain stem ischemia.* This condition produces sudden, severe vertigo that may become episodic and later persistent. Associated findings include ataxia, nausea, vomiting, increased blood pressure, tachycardia, nystagmus, and lateral deviation of the eyes toward the side of the lesion. Hemiparesis and paresthesia may also occur.

• *Head trauma.* Persistent vertigo, occurring soon after injury, accompanies spontaneous or positional nystagmus and, if the temporal bone is fractured, hearing loss. Associated findings include headache, nausea, vomiting, and decreased level of consciousness. Behavioral changes, diplopia or visual blurring, seizures, motor or sensory deficits, and signs of increased intracranial pressure may also occur.

• *Herpes zoster.* In this disorder, infection of cranial nerve VIII produces the sudden onset of vertigo accompanied by facial paralysis, hearing loss in the affected ear, and herpetic vesicular lesions in the auditory canal.

• *Labyrinthitis.* Severe vertigo begins abruptly with this inner ear infection. Vertigo may occur in a single episode or may recur over months or years. Associated findings may include nausea, vomiting, progressive sensorineural hearing loss, and nystagmus.

• *Ménière's disease.* In this disease, labyrinthine dysfunction causes the abrupt onset of vertigo, lasting minutes, hours, or days. Unpredictable episodes of severe vertigo and unsteady gait may cause the patient to fall. During an attack, any sudden motion of the head or eyes can precipitate nausea and vomiting.

• *Multiple sclerosis (MS).* Episodic vertigo may occur early and become persistent. Other early findings include diplopia, visual blurring, and paresthesia. MS may also produce nystagmus, constipation, muscle weakness, paralysis, spasticity, hyperreflexia, intention tremor, and ataxia.

• *Posterior fossa tumor.* In this disorder, positional vertigo lasts for a few seconds. The patient may also have papilledema, headache, memo-

ry loss, nausea, vomiting, nystagmus, apneustic or ataxic respirations, and increased blood pressure. He may also fall sideways.

• *Vestibular neuritis.* In this disorder, severe vertigo usually begins abruptly and lasts several days, without tinnitus or hearing loss. Other findings include nausea, vomiting, and nystagmus.

Other causes

• *Drugs and alcohol.* High or toxic doses of certain drugs and alcohol may produce vertigo. These drugs include salicylates, aminoglycosides, antibiotics, quinine, and oral contraceptives.

• *Surgery and other procedures.* Middle ear surgery may cause vertigo that lasts for several days. In addition, administration of overly warm or cold eardrops or irrigating solutions may cause vertigo.

 ALERT Ear infection is a common cause of vertigo in children. Vestibular neuritis may also cause this symptom.

Wristdrop

In wristdrop, the hand remains in a flexed position due to paresis of the extensor muscles of the hand, wrist, and fingers. This weakness may be slight or severe and temporary or permanent. Wristdrop may occur unilaterally and suddenly with a radial nerve injury, or bilaterally and gradually with neurologic disorders, such as myasthenia gravis, Guillain-Barré syndrome, and multiple sclerosis.

Medical causes

• *Guillain-Barré syndrome.* Wristdrop may occur in this syndrome, but the primary neurologic sign is diffuse muscle weakness that typically begins in the legs and ascends to the arms and facial nerves within 24 to 72 hours. Associated findings include paresthesia, diminished or absent corneal reflexes, dysarthria, hypernasality, dysphagia, respiratory insufficiency and, possibly, respiratory paralysis. Sympathetic nerve dysfunction, such as postural hypotension, loss of bladder and bowel control, sweating, and tachycardia, may also occur.

• *Lead intoxication.* A motor neuropathy, one that typically involves the radial nerve, may be seen in inorganic lead poisoning.

• *Multiple sclerosis.* This disorder may cause wristdrop, but the earliest symptoms are usually diplopia, blurred vision, and paresthesia. Other findings include nystagmus, constipation, muscle weakness, paralysis, spasticity, hyperreflexia, intention tremor, gait ataxia, dysphagia, dysarthria, urinary dysfunction, impotence, and emotional lability.

• *Myasthenia gravis.* In this disorder, weakness causes wristdrop. Associated findings vary with the muscle group affected and may include weak eye closure, ptosis, diplopia, masklike facies, difficulty chewing and swallowing, nasal regurgitation of fluids, and hypernasality. Weakened neck muscles may lead to head bobbing. Respiratory muscle weakness produces myasthenic crisis.

• *Radial nerve injury.* Compression, severance, or inflammation of the radial nerve causes a loss of motor and sensory function in the involved area. Wristdrop may occur; it may be temporary if injury is incomplete. Other findings in radial nerve injury include loss of finger and elbow extension, forearm supination, and thumb abduction as well as paresthesia and hand muscle atrophy.

 ALERT Radial nerve injury is the most common cause of wristdrop in children.

Outcome measurement

Documenting the path to recovery

Common documentation forms

Using outcome measurement tools

Rehabilitation focuses on restoring and improving the patient's ability to function. To achieve this overall goal, specific treatments are implemented based on the problem list generated by the clinician's assessment of the patient at the initial meeting. The patient is reassessed at intervals to evaluate the effectiveness of treatment and progress toward functional goals. Such an assessment involves the use of specific tools called *functional outcome measures*. When used in conjunction with physical examination findings and information from the patient interview, these tools can help to accomplish the following:

• setting goals
• directing treatment
• making prognoses for appropriate treatment, duration, and probable results
• serving as a mechanism for reimbursement of services provided
• justifying continuation of services to third-party payers.

Various tools for measuring functional outcomes are available, each with a specific purpose. The clinician must choose the most appropriate measurement tool for the specific patient.

To serve as an effective functional outcome measure, the tool must be:

• reliable — able to measure the patient's performance with consistent, replicable scoring over time that allows subsequent evaluations to truly reflect functional performance changes from baseline
• valid — able to measure exactly what is intended to be measured so

that inferences about treatment, prognosis, and outcomes can be made based on the assessment scores
• practical — designed to enhance the clinician's ability to use it to evaluate the patient's performance
• purposeful — developed specifically to measure the functional areas being assessed
• referenced — able to allow the clinician to judge the patient's performance compared to a normal peer group or standardized number in order to arrive at a determination of the patient's functional ability.

In the current managed-care environment, functional outcome measures play a key role. Appropriate selection of these tools provides objective information about the patient's overall well-being and ability, substantiating quality care through goal achievement.

This chapter briefly reviews a number of functional outcome measures commonly used to evaluate infants and children, the elderly, and patients requiring long-term care and rehabilitation, such as those recovering from serious injuries.

Barthel Index

The Barthel Index was developed to measure the level of functional independence in chronically disabled patients. This tool examines a variety of activities of daily living (ADLs) and household mobility activities to assess a patient's self-care ability.

The 10 ADLs evaluated in the Barthel Index are feeding, moving from wheelchair to bed and returning, performing personal toileting, getting on and off the toilet, bathing, walking on a level surface or propelling a wheelchair, going up and down stairs, dressing and undressing, maintaining bowel continence, and controlling the bladder. Each activity

USING THE BARTHEL INDEX

Date _February 7, 2000_   Patient's name _Fred Schumacher_
                                 Evaluator _Anne Farnesworth_

Action	With help	Independent
1. Feeding (if food needs to be cut up = help)	5	⑩
2. Moving from wheelchair to bed and return (includes sitting up in bed)	5 to 10	⑮
3. Personal toilet (wash face, comb hair, shave, clean teeth)	0	⑤
4. Getting on and off toilet (handling clothes, wipe, flush)	5	⑩ 5̸
5. Bathing self	0	
6. Walking on level surface (or, if unable to walk, propel wheelchair)	0*	5 or 15
7. Ascending and descending stairs	⑤	10
8. Dressing (includes tying shoes, fastening fasteners)	⑤	10
9. Controlling bowels	⑤	10
10. Controlling bladder	⑤	10

Total possible score = 100

Total score = 65

* Score only if unable to walk

Adapted with permission from Mahoney, F.I., and Barthel, D.W. "Functional Evaluation: The Barthel Index," *Maryland State Medical Journal* 14:62, 1965.

is scored on the patient's ability to complete the activity independently (scores of 5, 10, or 15) or with help (scores of 0, 5, or 10). A patient who can't perform a specific activity may be given a score of zero. During the evaluation, the patient may use assistive devices and adaptive equipment. (See *Using the Barthel Index*.)

Typically, the Barthel Index is used as a screening tool in rehabilitation, long-term care settings, and home care. Used repeatedly over time, this tool may reveal improvement or decline in a patient's functional levels.

The maximum score is 100, indicating that the patient is independent in the home with mobility and self-care activities. A score of 75 to 95 indicates a mild disability; a score of 50 to 70, moderate disability; a score of 20 to 45, severe disability; and a score of less than 20, very severe disability.

Because improvement in functional status isn't recorded until a level of independence is achieved, the Barthel

Index scoring system may not be as sensitive to someone who has minimal or moderate disability. Also, this tool doesn't address psychosocial aspects, safety, or cognition. However, research has shown that age-related Barthel index scores on urinary incontinence, functional ability, and sitting balance are prognostic indicators for persons recovering from cerebrovascular accident.

Berg Functional Balance Scale

The Berg Functional Balance Scale is a multidimensional tool for assessing a patient's risk of falling. It may be used as a one-time assessment but has also been used to monitor a patient's risk of falls over time. (See *Using the Berg Functional Balance Scale,* pages 106 to 109.)

(Text continues on page 110.)

USING THE BERG FUNCTIONAL BALANCE SCALE

Name _____Kevin Graves_____   Date ___2/2/2000___

Rater_____Sam Webber_____

General instructions

I.   Demonstrate each task and/or give instructions (as written). When scoring, record the lowest response category that applies for each item.

II. In most items, the subject is asked to maintain a given position for a specific amount of time. The subject should understand that he or she must maintain balance while attempting the tasks. The choices of which leg to stand on or how far to reach are left to the subject. Poor judgment will adversely influence the performance and scoring.

III. Progressively more points are deducted if:
1. the time or distance requirements are not met,
2. the subjects performance warrants supervision, or
3. the subject touches an external support or receives assistance from the examiner.

IV. Equipment required for testing includes:
1. a watch with a secondhand or a stopwatch;
2. a ruler or other indicator of 2, 5, and 10 inches;
3. 2 chairs of reasonable height, with and without armrests; and
4. a step stool of average height.

Score (0-4)	Item	Activity
4	1.	Sitting to standing
4	2.	Standing unsupported
4	3.	Sitting unsupported
4	4.	Standing to sitting
4	5.	Transfers
2	6.	Standing with eyes closed
2	7.	Standing with feet together
2	8.	Reaching forward with outstretched arm
3	9.	Retrieving object from floor
4	10.	Turning to look behind
2	11.	Turning 360 degrees
1	12.	Placing alternate foot on stool
0	13.	Standing with one foot in front
0	14.	Standing on one foot
36/56	**TOTAL**	

Berg balance and position tests

1. SITTING TO STANDING

INSTRUCTIONS: Please stand up. Try not to use your hands for support.

√	4	able to stand without using hands and stabilize independently
	3	able to stand independently using hands
	2	able to stand using hands after several tries
	1	needs minimal aid to stand or to stabilize
	0	needs moderate or maximal assist to stand

USING THE BERG FUNCTIONAL BALANCE SCALE
(continued)

Score (0-4)   Item   Activity

2. STANDING UNSUPPORTED

INSTRUCTIONS: Please stand for two minutes without holding on to the chair.

____√____	4	able to stand safely for 2 minutes
_____	3	able to stand 2 minutes with supervision
_____	2	able to stand 30 seconds unsupported
_____	1	needs several tries to stand 30 seconds unsupported
_____	0	unable to stand 30 seconds unassisted

If a subject is able to stand 2 minutes unsupported, score full points for sitting unsupported. Proceed to item #4.

3. SITTING WITH BACK UNSUPPORTED BUT FEET SUPPORTED ON FLOOR OR ON A STOOL.

INSTRUCTIONS: Please sit with arms folded for 2 minutes.

____√____	4	able to sit safely and securely for 2 minutes
_____	3	able to sit 2 minutes under supervision
_____	2	able to sit 30 seconds
_____	1	able to sit 10 seconds
_____	0	unable to sit 10 seconds without support

4. STANDING TO SITTING

INSTRUCTIONS: Please sit down.

____√____	4	sits safely with minimal use of hands
_____	3	controls descent by using hands
_____	2	uses back of legs against chair to control descent
_____	1	sits independently but has controlled descent
_____	0	needs assistance to sit

5. TRANSFERS

INSTRUCTIONS: Please transfer one way toward a seat with armrests and one way toward a seat without armrests. You may use two chairs (one with and one without armrests) or a bed and a chair.

____√____	4	able to transfer safely with minor use of hands
_____	3	able to transfer safely definite need of hands
_____	2	able to transfer with verbal cueing and/or supervision
_____	1	needs one person to assist
_____	0	needs two people to assist or supervise to be safe

6. STANDING UNSUPPORTED WITH EYES CLOSED

INSTRUCTIONS: Please close your eyes and stand still for 10 seconds.

_____	4	able to stand 10 seconds safely
_____	3	able to stand 10 seconds with supervision
____√____	2	able to stand 3 seconds
_____	1	unable to keep eyes closed 3 seconds but stays steady
_____	0	needs help to keep from falling

(continued)

Item	Activity

7. STANDING UNSUPPORTED WITH FEET TOGETHER

INSTRUCTIONS: Place your feet close together and stand without holding on to the chair.

_____	4	able to place feet together independently and stand safely for 1 minute
_____	3	able to place feet together independently and stand for 1 minute with supervision
___√___	2	able to place feet together independently but unable to hold for 30 seconds
_____	1	needs help to attain position but able to stand 15 seconds with feet together
_____	0	needs help to attain position and unable to hold for 15 seconds

8. REACHING FORWARD WITH OUTSTRETCHED ARM WHILE STANDING

INSTRUCTIONS: Lift arm to 90 degrees. Stretch out your fingers and reach forward as far as you can. (Examiner places a ruler at end of fingertips when arm is at 90 degrees. Fingers should not touch the ruler while reaching forward. The recorded measure is the distance forward that the fingers reach while the subject is in the most forward leaning position. When possible, ask the subject to use both arms when reaching to avoid rotation of the trunk.)

_____	4	able to reach forward confidently > 10" (25 cm)
_____	3	able to reach forward > 5" (12 cm)
___√___	2	able to reach forward > 2" (5 cm)
_____	1	reaches forward but needs supervision
_____	0	loses balance while trying/requires external support

9. PICK UP OBJECT FROM THE FLOOR FROM A STANDING POSITION

INSTRUCTIONS: Pick up the shoe/slipper that is placed in front of your feet.

_____	4	able to pick up slipper safely and easily
___√___	3	able to pick up slipper but needs supervision
_____	2	unable to pick up slipper but reaches 1" to 2" (2 to 5 cm) from slipper and keeps balance independently
_____	1	unable to pick up slipper and needs supervision while trying
_____	0	unable to try/needs assistance to keep from losing balance or falling

10. TURNING TO LOOK BEHIND OVER LEFT AND RIGHT SHOULDERS WHILE STANDING

INSTRUCTIONS: Turn to look directly behind you over your left shoulder. Repeat to the right. (Examiner may pick up an object behind the subject for him to look at to encourage a better twist turn.)

___√___	4	looks behind from both sides and shifts weight well
_____	3	looks behind one side only, other side shows less weight shift
_____	2	turns sideways only, but maintains balance
_____	1	needs supervision when turning
_____	0	needs assistance to keep from losing balance or falling

USING THE BERG FUNCTIONAL BALANCE SCALE
(continued)

Score (0-4)	Item	Activity

11. TURN 360 DEGREES

INSTRUCTIONS: Turn completely around in a full circle. Pause. Then turn a full circle in the other direction.

_____	4	able to turn 360 degrees safely in 4 seconds or less
_____	3	able to turn 360 degrees safely one side only in 4 seconds or less
___✓___	2	able to turn 360 degrees safely but slowly
_____	1	needs close supervision or verbal cueing
_____	0	needs assistance while turning

12. PLACING ALTERNATE FOOT ON STEP OR STOOL WHILE STANDING UNSUPPORTED

INSTRUCTIONS: Place each foot alternately on the step/stool. Continue until each foot has touched the step/stool four times.

_____	4	able to stand independently and safely complete 8 steps in 20 seconds
_____	3	able to stand independently and complete 8 steps > 20 seconds
_____	2	able to complete 4 steps without aid, with supervision
___✓___	1	able to complete > 2 steps, needs minimal assistance
_____	0	needs assistance to keep from falling/unable to try

13. STANDING UNSUPPORTED ONE FOOT IN FRONT

INSTRUCTIONS: Place one foot directly in front of the other. If you feel that you cannot place your foot directly in front, try to step far enough ahead that the heel of your forward foot is ahead of the toes of the other foot. (To score 3 points, the length of the step should exceed the length of the other foot and the width of the stance should approximate the subject's normal stride width.)

_____	4	able to place foot tandem independently and hold 30 seconds
_____	3	able to place foot ahead of other independently and hold 30 seconds
_____	2	able to take small step independently and hold 30 seconds
_____	1	needs help to step but can hold 15 seconds
___✓___	0	loses balance while stepping or standing

14. STANDING ON ONE LEG

INSTRUCTIONS: Stand on one leg as long as you can without holding on to the chair.

_____	4	able to lift leg independently and hold > 10 seconds
_____	3	able to lift leg independently and hold 5 to 10 seconds
_____	2	able to lift leg independently and hold 3 to 4 seconds
_____	1	tried to lift leg, unable to hold 3 seconds but remains standing independently
___✓___	0	unable to try or needs assistance to prevent fall

TOTAL
SCORE ___36___ / 56 (maximum)

Adapted with permission from Berg, K. et al. "Measuring Balance in the Elderly: Preliminary Development of an Instrument," *Physiotherapy of Canada* 41:304-311, 1989.

The Berg Functional Balance Scale consists of 14 tasks that incorporate sitting activities, transitional movements such as transfers, and static and dynamic standing activities, such as reaching and turning. The patient is graded on a scale of 0 to 4 for each of the tasks being evaluated. The maximum total score possible is 56. A score less than 45 out of 56 indicates an increased risk of falls.

This tool is relatively inexpensive and easy to use, taking approximately 15 to 20 minutes to complete and score in the clinical setting. Necessary equipment includes a stopwatch, two chairs, a ruler, and a stepstool. The evaluator needs no special training.

Denver Developmental Screening Test, revised (Denver II)

The Denver II, a 1990 revision of the Denver Developmental Screening test, is one of the most widely used tools for assessing a child's development. The tool can be used for any child from birth to age 6, and assesses a child's performance of age-appropriate activities compared to established norms for children of the same age. This assessment yields a score, which is expressed as the ratio of the "norm age" at which a child performs the skills to the child's developmental age. In other words, the tool provides objective information about how a child compares to his peer group in four major developmental areas.

The test consists of 125 tasks that address the areas of personal-social, fine motor-adaptive, language, and gross motor skills. The number of items varies by the child's age and time available for test administration. Each item tested is scored using one of the following: "P" for pass, "F" for fail, "N.O." for no opportunity, and

"R" for refusal. At least three items in each section need to be evaluated to identify relative risk and strengths.

When scoring each task evaluated on the Denver II, one of the following definitions is applied: *advanced performance, normal performance, caution* (indicating the child refuses to or can't perform at the 75th percentile), *delayed caution* (indicating the child refuses to or can't perform at the 90th percentile), and *no opportunity* (meaning the child hasn't had the opportunity to try a specific skill).

The results of the Denver II are interpreted as *normal, suspect,* or *untestable.* Children in the *suspect* or *untestable* categories should be rescreened to rule out such issues as illness, fatigue, and fear. If test results remain *suspect* or *untestable,* the child should be referred for further evaluation.

To administer the test, a special kit must be purchased. The examiner also needs special training in the procedure and interpretation of what is being observed. Otherwise, the results may be invalid.

The Denver II isn't indicated for diagnostic evaluation to quantify learning disability, language impairment, or emotional disturbance. However, results of this test may suggest the need for a more thorough assessment by an appropriate health care provider.

Functional independence measurement

Functional independence measurement forms were developed to serve as a database of functional outcomes for patients with a variety of diagnoses admitted to rehabilitation hospitals and subacute care settings. These interdisciplinary tools look at

MEASURING FUNCTIONAL INDEPENDENCE

Name _Richard Taber_   **Rater** _Thomas Baker_

Observation date _2/2/2000_

Self-care	Score
Feeding	6
Grooming	7
Bathing	6
Dressing: Upper body	7
Dressing: Lower body	3
Toileting	4
Sphincter control	
Bladder management	7
Bowel management	7
Mobility	
Transfer: Bed/chair↔wc	4
Toilet↔wc	3
Tub, shower	3
Locomotion	
Walking/Wheelchair	w 4
	c
Stairs	3

	Score
Communication	
Comprehension	7
Expression	7
Social cognition	
Social interaction	7
Problem solving	7
Memory	7
Total Score	99

FIM™ INSTRUMENT SCORING

7. Complete independence (Timely, safely)
6. Modified independence (Assistive device needed)
5. Supervision (Verbal cues)
4. Minimal assist (Subject 75%)
3. Moderate assist (Subject 50%)
2. Maximal assist (Subject 25%)
1. Total assist (Subject 0%)

FIM™ instrument. Copyright 1997 Uniform Data System for Medical Rehabilitation, a division of UB Foundation Activities, Inc. All rights reserved. Adapted with permission of UDSMR, February 2000.

activities addressed traditionally by physical therapy (ambulation and transfers); occupational therapy (dressing and grooming); speech therapy (language and swallowing ability); and nursing (bowel and bladder function).

The FIM™ assesses 18 specific activities that are divided into 6 major categories: self-care, sphincter control, mobility, locomotion, communication, and social cognition. Each activity is scored on a scale of 1 to 7, depending on the level of assistance required and assistive devices used by the patient. A score of 1 indicates total assistance is needed, while a score of 7 reflects complete independence. (See *Measuring functional independence*.)

The scores for the activities under mobility are derived from the Barthel index. Under locomotion, two specific criteria are evaluated when scoring: distance traveled and assistance required. The scorer must also indicate the means the patient uses to complete the activity, such as walking (with or without assistance) and the use of a wheelchair. For stair climbing, the scorer grades the number of stairs climbed and the level of assistance needed.

Functional reach

Functional reach is a single-task measure of standing balance. This tool was developed to identify elderly

MEASURING FUNCTIONAL REACH

Keeping a patient's frequently used items within "functional reach" — the distance that he can comfortably reach without straining — can help prevent falls. To determine a patient's functional reach:

● Have the patient stand upright with one shoulder about 6″ (15 cm) away from the wall and his face parallel to the wall.
● Put a piece of tape on the wall to mark the position of the front of the shoulder at the joint.
● With his arms outstretched from the shoulder and parallel to the floor, have the patient reach out as far as he can comfortably, while remaining balanced and not moving either foot.
● Have the patient make a fist while remaining in this position, and mark the wall again at that point.
● Measure the distance between the two marks to find the functional reach measure.

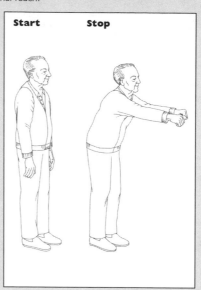

patients who might be at risk for falls. *Functional reach* is defined as the maximum forward distance a person can attain with a fixed base of support or as the distance a person can comfortably reach without straining.

The test is performed by asking the patient to stand upright with one shoulder approximately 6″ (15.2 cm) from a wall and his face parallel to the wall. A yardstick is placed at the level of the acromion process, which is the highest point of the shoulder. Next, the patient is asked to raise the arm to shoulder height parallel to the floor, with a fisted hand. Then he is asked to reach as far forward as possible without moving his feet or taking a step. The distance is marked and the measure of forward reach is

taken at the third metacarpal. (See *Measuring functional reach*.)

If appropriate, allow the patient to practice the test before data collection. The score of the functional reach measure is determined by taking the mean of three trials.

The functional reach measure is quick and easy to administer. Because it involves only one task, this tool provides valuable information for patients who may have impaired cognition and may not have the attention necessary for a more lengthy balance assessment.

Health Status Profile

The Health Status Profile is an assessment tool that identifies a relationship between how a patient views his health and his ability to perform usual activities. The Health Status Profile is used primarily as an initial screening tool, but it may be used again at the end of treatment and can be administered to anyone age 14 and older.

The test consists of 36 questions that are completed by the patient. The level of assessment in the test addresses both disability and functional limitations. Summary scores and scores within eight categories are obtained. (See *Completing the Health Status Profile,* pages 114 to 116.)

Mini-Mental Status Examination

The Mini–Mental Status Examination was developed as a screening tool to identify cognitive impairment in any patient. Performed quickly and easily, the examination addresses 5 major areas— orientation, registration, attention and calculation, recall, and language and motor skills. Each section of the test involves a related series of questions or commands. The patient receives one point for each correct answer. The patient's level of consciousness is also assessed along a continuum at the end of the test. (See *Performing the Mini–Mental Status examination,* pages 117 and 118.)

The test is administered by a clinician within the guidelines included with the test. The patient should be seated quietly in a well-lit room. The questions should be administered in the same order they appear on the form each time the test is given. The test takes approximately 10 minutes to administer, but it isn't a timed test. The maximum possible score is 30. Usually, a score less than 24 indicates cognitive impairment. A score less than 20 indicates dementia, delirium, schizophrenia, or affective disorder.

Motor Assessment Scale

The Motor Assessment Scale quantifies relevant motor skills and functional mobility during the acute recovery stage following a cerebrovascular accident. This tool quantifies both impairment and disability levels. However, the patient must be medically stable and able to follow two-step commands to be able to participate. Depending on the practice setting, this tool may be used repeatedly to monitor improvement or decline in the patient's status. (See *Using the motor assessment scale,* pages 119 to 121.)

The test consists of eight items that are scored using specific criteria based on the patient's best performance without any assistance from the examiner. Each item is scored from 1 to 6, with a score of 6 being the most functional. The maximum total score possible is 48. The last item, tonus, is a measure of tone and isn't included in the final score.

Oswestry Low Back Pain Disability Questionnaire

The Oswestry Low Back Pain Disability Questionnaire is a tool used to measure a patient's perception of his functional limitation related to the degree of lower back pain. The questionnaire consists of 10 sections that address pain intensity, personal care, lifting, walking, sitting, standing, sleeping, sex life, social life, and traveling. (See *Using the Oswestry questionnaire,* pages 122 and 123.)

Each section consists of six statements that are scored on a scale of 0 to 5 with 5 representing the greatest degree of disability. The patient indicates which single statement best de-
(Text continues on page 110.)

COMPLETING THE HEALTH STATUS PROFILE

Name _Paul Stevens_   **Date** _February 17, 2000_

INSTRUCTIONS: This survey asks for your views about your health. This information will help keep track of how you feel and how well you are able to do your
usual activities.

Answer every question by marking the answer as indicated. If you are unsure
about how to answer a question, please give the best answer you can.

1. In general, would you say your health is (circle one):
   Excellent 1   Very good 2   (Good   3)   Fair   4   Poor   5

2. Compared to one year ago, how would you rate your health in general now? (Circle
   one.)

   | Much better now than one year ago | 1 | (About the same as one year ago 3) | Much worse now than one year ago | 5 |
   | Somewhat better now than one year ago | 2 | Somewhat worse now than one year ago | 4 | |

3. The following items are about activities you might do during a typical day. Does your
   health now limit you in these activities? If so, how much? (Circle one number on each
   line.)

Activities	Yes, limited a lot	Yes, limited a little	No, not limited at all
a. Vigorous activities, such as running, lift ing heavy objects, participating in stren uous sports	1	②	3
b. Moderate activities, such as moving a table, pushing a vacuum cleaner, bowl- ing, or playing golf	1	2	③
c. Lifting or carrying groceries	1	2	③
d. Climbing several flights of stairs	1	2	③
e. Climbing one flight of stairs	1	2	③
f. Bending, kneeling, or stooping	1	②	3
g. Walking more than one mile	1	2	③
h. Walking several blocks	1	2	③
i. Walking one block	1	2	③
j. Bathing or dressing yourself	1	2	③

4. During the past 4 weeks, have you had any of the following problems with your work
   or other regular daily activities as a result of your physical health? (Circle one number
   on each line.)

	Yes	No
a. Cut down on the amount of time you spent on work or other activities	1	②
b. Accomplished less than you would like	1	②
c. Were limited in the kind of work or other activities	1	②
d. Had difficulty performing the work or other activities (for example, it took extra effort)	1	②

COMPLETING THE HEALTH STATUS PROFILE *(continued)*

5. During the past 4 weeks, have you had any of the following problems with your work or other regular daily activities as a result of any emotional problems (such as feeling depressed or anxious)? (Circle one number on each line.)

	Yes	No
a. Cut down the amount of time you spent on work or other activities	①	2
b. Accomplished less than you would like	①	2
c. Didn't do work or other activities as carefully as usual	①	2

6. During the past 4 weeks, to what extent has your physical health or emotional problems interfered with your normal social activities with family, friends, neighbors, or groups? (Circle one.)

Not at all	1	Slightly	2	Moderately	3
Quite a bit	4	Extremely	5		

7. How much bodily pain have you had during the past 4 weeks? (Circle one.)

None	1	Very mild	2	Mild	3
Moderate	4	Severe	5	Very severe	6

8. During the past 4 weeks, how much did pain interfere with your normal work (including both work outside the home and housework)? (Circle one.)

Not at all	1	A little bit	2	Moderately	3
Quite a bit	4	Extremely	5		

9. These questions are about how you feel and how things have been with you during the past 4 weeks. For each question, please give the one answer that comes closest to the way you have been feeling. How much of the time during the past 4 weeks (circle one number on each line):

	All of the time	Most of the time	A good bit of the time	Some of the time	A little of the time	None of the time
a. Did you feel full of pep?	1	2	3	④	5	6
b. Have you been a very nervous person?	1	2	3	4	⑤	6
c. Have you felt so down in the dumps that nothing could cheer you up?	1	2	3	④	5	6
d. Have you felt calm and peaceful?	1	2	3	4	⑤	6
e. Did you have a lot of energy?	1	2	3	④	5	6
f. Have you felt downhearted and blue?	1	2	3	4	⑤	6
g. Did you feel worn out?	1	2	③	4	5	6
h. Have you been a happy person?	1	2	3	④	5	6
i. Did you feel tired?	1	2	③	4	5	6

(continued)

COMPLETING THE HEALTH STATUS PROFILE (continued)

10. During the past 4 weeks, how much of the time has your physical health or emotional problems interfered with your social activities (like visiting with friends, relatives, etc.)? (Circle one.)

All of the time 1	(Some of the time 3)	None of the time 5
Most of the time 2	A little of the time 4	

11. How TRUE or FALSE is each of the following statements for you? (Circle one number on each line.)

	Definitely true	Mostly true	Don't know	Mostly false	Definitely false
a. I seem to get sick a little easier than other people.	1	2	3	(4)	5
b. I am as healthy as anybody I know.	1	(2)	3	4	5
c. I expect my health to get worse.	1	2	(3)	4	5
d. My health is excellent.	1	(2)	3	4	5

_____105_____ **Score**

scribes his current status. The questionnaire is scored by taking the percentage of the total value of the responses over a maximum score of 50. (If a patient doesn't score a particular section, the percentage is adjusted accordingly.)

The resulting percentage indicates the level of functional disability. Minimal disability is reflected as a percentage of 10% to 20%; moderate disability as 20% to 40%; severe disability as 40% to 60%; crippled as 60% to 80%; and bedridden (or, possibly, an inappropriate or exaggerated pain response) as 80% to 100%.

While the score may reflect how a patient is feeling on a day to day basis, the Oswestry questionnaire may not be as sensitive to improvements in function or lessening of pain over time as other measurement tools.

Rancho Los Amigos Cognitive Scale

The Rancho Los Amigos Cognitive Scale (RLACS) is a descriptive measurement tool developed for persons who have sustained traumatic brain injury. The RLACS is an eight-stage scale that categorizes behavioral and cognitive impairment along a continuum that reflects the spectrum of recovery from brain injury. The scale provides information about the general degree of impairment. When this scale is used, the examiner selects one of the eight stages that most

PERFORMING THE MINI–MENTAL STATUS EXAMINATION

Of the many assessment tools available for testing a patient's psychological condition, the Mini–Mental Status Examination offers a quick and simple way to quantify cognitive function and screen for cognitive loss. The examination tests the patient's orientation, registration, attention, calculation, recall, and language and motor skills. Each section of the test involves a related series of questions or commands. The patient receives one point for each correct answer; the total score provides a general idea of the patient's mental state.

To administer the examination, seat the patient in a quiet, well-lit room. Ask him to listen carefully and to answer each question as accurately as he can.

Don't time the test, but do score it right away by adding the number of correct responses. In the section on attention and calculation, include either items 14 to 18 or item 19, not both. The patient can receive a maximum total score of 30 points. Usually, a score below 24 indicates cognitive impairment, although this may not be an accurate cutoff for highly or poorly educated patients. A score below 20 usually appears in patients with delirium, dementia, schizophrenia, or affective disorder, and not in normal elderly people or in patients with neurosis or personality disorder.

Patient's name _Joseph Snead_

Date _February 12, 2000_

Orientation
Ask the patient for the date. Then ask for any missing information (year, month, day of the week). Ask if he knows what season it is. Ask him to name the hospital and the floor he's currently on. Finally, ask for the town or city, the county, and the state. Give a point for each correct answer (maximum score: 10).

1. Date ____ / ____
2. Year ____ / ____
3. Month ____ / ____
4. Day ____ / ____
5. Season ____ / ____
6. Hospital ____ / ____
7. Floor ____ 0 ____
8. Town or city ____ / ____
9. County ____ / ____
10. State ____ / ____

Registration
Tell the patient that you'd like to test his memory. Then say "ball," "flag," and "tree" clearly and slowly, taking about 1 second to say each word. After you've said all three words, ask him to repeat them. The first repetition determines the score (0 to 3), but keep saying the words (up to six trials) until he can repeat all three. If he doesn't eventually say all three, recall can't be meaningfully tested.

11. Ball ____ / ____
12. Flag ____ 0 ____
13. Tree ____ / ____
Number of trials ____ 2 ____

Attention and calculation
You may perform this section of the test in one of two ways. Begin by asking the patient to count backward from 100 by sevens. Stop after he has said 5 numbers (93, 86, 79, 72, 65). Score one point for each correct number.

Alternatively, if the patient can't or won't perform this task, ask him to spell "world" backward (D, L, R, O, W). Assign one point for each correctly placed letter. For example, DLROW=5, DLORW=3. Record how the patient spelled "world" backward.

14. 93 ____ / ____
15. 86 ____ / ____
16. 79 ____ / ____
17. 72 ____ 0 ____
18. 65 ____ 0 ____
19. Numbers of correctly spaced letters ____

Recall
Ask the patient to recall the three words you previously asked him to remember (in the registration section). Give one point for each correct answer.

20. Ball ____ / ____
21. Flag ____ 0 ____
22. Tree ____ 0 ____

(continued)

PERFORMING THE MINI-MENTAL STATUS EXAMINATION *(continued)*

Language and motor skills

This section of the assessment has six parts: naming, repetition, three-stage command, reading, writing, and copying.

Naming

Show the patient a wristwatch and ask, "What is this?" Repeat the question when holding a pencil. Give one point for each object named correctly.

23. Watch _____ / _____
24. Pencil _____ / _____

Repetition

Ask the patient to repeat "No ifs, ands, or buts." Allow only one try, and give one point for correct repetition.

25. Repetition _____ / _____

Three-stage command

Hand the patient a piece of blank paper and say, "Take the paper in your right hand, fold it in half, and put it on the floor." Score one point for each action performed correctly.

26. Takes in right hand _____ / _____
27. Folds in half _____ / _____
28. Places on floor _____ 0 _____

Reading

On a blank piece of paper, print "close your eyes" in letters large enough for the patient to see clearly. Ask him to read it and do what it says. Score one point only if he actually closes his eyes.

29. Closes eyes _____ / _____

Writing

Give the patient a blank piece of paper, and ask him to make up a sentence and write it. Evaluate whether the sentence contains a subject and a verb, and makes sense. Correct grammar and punctuation aren't necessary.

30. Writes sentence _____ / _____

Copying

On a clean piece of paper, draw intersecting pentagons, with each side about 1" long. Ask the patient to copy your drawing exactly as it appears. All 10 angles must be present and two must intersect to receive one point. Ignore tremor and rotation.

31. Draws pentagons _____ 0 _____

Total score _____ 22 _____

Adapted with permission from Folstein, M.F., et al. "Mini-Mental State: A Practical Method for Grading the Cognitive State of Patients for the Clinician," *Journal of Psychiatric Research* 12(3):189-198, November 1975.

closely reflects the patient's current status. (See *Assessing cognitive function,* page 124.)

The RLACS is used in rehabilitation settings and may be reused to track the patient's status. Additional specific information about an individual's cognitive deficits requires neuropsychological testing.

Six-Minute Walk Test

The Six-Minute Walk Test aims to quantify functional exercise capacity

USING THE MOTOR ASSESSMENT SCALE

Scoring Sheet

Name _Ken Cole._   **Date** _1/17/2000_   **Total Score** _16_

1. Supine to side-lying onto intact side   Score _3_

1. Pulls himself into side-lying position. (Starting position must be supine, not knee-flexed. Patient pulls himself into side-lying position with intact arm, moves affected leg with intact leg.)

2. Actively moves leg across and lower half of body follows. (Starting position as above. Arm is left behind.)

3. Arm is lifted across body with other arm. Leg is moved actively and body follows in a block. (Starting position as above.)

4. Moves arm across body actively and the rest of the body moves as a block. (Starting position as above.)

5. Moves arm and leg and rolls to side but overbalances. (Starting position as above. Shoulder protracts and arm flexes forward.)

6. Rolls to side in 3 seconds. (Starting position as above. Must not use hands.)

2. Supine to sitting over side of bed   Score _3_

1. Side-lying position, lifts head sideways but can't sit up. (Patient assisted to side-lying position.)

2. Side-lying position to sitting over side of bed. (Therapist assists patient with movement. Patient controls head position throughout.)

3. Side-lying position to sitting over side of bed. (Therapist gives stand-by help [see instructions] by assisting legs over side of bed.)

4. Side-lying position to sitting over side of bed. (With no stand-by help.)

5. Supine to sitting over side of bed. (With no stand-by help.)

6. Supine to sitting over side of bed within 10 seconds. (With no stand-by help.)

3. Balanced sitting   Score _4_

1. Sits only with support. (Therapist should assist patient into sitting.)

2. Sits unsupported for 10 seconds. (Without holding on, knees and feet together, feet can be supported on the floor.)

3. Sits unsupported with weight well forward and evenly distributed. (Weight should be well forward at the hips, head and thoracic spine extended, weight evenly distributed on both sides.)

4. Sits unsupported, turns head and trunk to look behind. (Feet supported and together on the floor. Do not allow legs to abduct or feet to move. Have hands resting on thighs, do not allow hands to move onto plinth.)

5. Sits unsupported, reaches forward to touch the floor, and returns to starting position. (Feet supported on floor. Do not allow patient to hold on. Do not allow legs and feet to move, support affected arm if necessary. Hand must touch floor at least 10 cm [4 in] in front of feet.)

6. Sits on stool unsupported, reaches sideways to touch floor, and returns to starting position. (Feet supported on floor. Do not allow patient to hold on. Do not allow legs and feet to move, support affected arm if necessary. Patient must reach sideways and not forward.)

(continued)

4. Sitting to standing   Score _2_

1. Gets to standing with help from therapist. (Any method.)

2. Gets to standing with stand-by help. (Weight unevenly distributed, uses hands for support.)

3. Gets to standing. (Do not allow uneven weight distribution or help from hands.)

4. Gets to standing and stands for 5 seconds with hips and knees extended. (Do not allow uneven weight distribution.)

5. Sitting to standing to sitting with no stand-by help. (Do not allow uneven weight distribution. Full extension of hips and knees.)

6. Sitting to standing to sitting with no stand-by help three times in 10 seconds. (Do not allow uneven weight distribution.)

5. Walking   Score _2_

1. Stands on affected leg and steps forward with the other leg. (Weight bearing hip must be extended. Therapist may give stand-by help.)

2. Walks with stand-by help from one person.

3. Walks 3 m (10 ft) alone or uses an aid but no stand-by help.

4. Walks 4 m (13 ft) with no aid in 15 seconds.

5. Walks 10 m (33 ft) with no aid, turns around, picks up a small sandbag from the floor, and walks back in 25 seconds. (May use either hand.)

6. Walks up and down four steps with or without an aid but without holding on to the rail three times in 35 seconds.

6. Upper-arm function   Score _1_

1. Lying, protract shoulder girdle with arm in elevation. (Therapist places arm in position and supports it with elbow in extension.)

2. Lying, hold extended arm in elevation for 2 seconds. (Therapist should place arm in position and patient must maintain position with external rotation. Elbow must be held within 20 degrees of full extension.)

3. Flexion and extension of the elbow to take palm to forehead with arm as in #2. (Therapist may assist supination of forearm.)

4. Sitting, hold extended arm in forward flexion at 90 degrees to body for 2 seconds. (Therapist should place arm in position and patient must maintain position with some external rotation and elbow extension. Do not allow excess shoulder elevation.)

5. Sitting, patient lifts arm to above position, holds it there for 10 seconds, and then lowers it. (Patient must maintain position with external rotation. Do not allow pronation.)

6. Standing, hand against wall. Maintain arm position while turning body toward wall. (Have arm abducted to 90 degrees with palm flat against wall.)

USING THE MOTOR ASSESSMENT SCALE *(continued)*

7. Hand movements Score __/__

1. Sitting, extension of wrist. (Therapist should have patient sitting at table with forearm resting on table. Therapist places cylindrical objects in palm of patient's hand. Patient is asked to lift object off table by extending the wrist. Do not allow elbow flexion.)

2. Sitting, radial deviation of the wrist. (Therapist should place forearm in midpronation-supination, fingers around a cylindrical object. Patient is asked to lift object off table. Do not allow elbow flexion or pronation.)

3. Sitting, elbow into side, pronation and supination. (Elbow unsupported and at a right angle. Three-quarter range is acceptable.)

4. Reach forward, pick up a large ball of 14 cm (5 in) diameter with both hands and put it down. (Ball should be on table so far in front of the patient that he has to extend arms fully to reach it. Shoulders must be protracted, elbows extended, wrist neutral or extended. Palms should be in contact with the ball.)

5. Pick up polystyrene cup from table and put it on table across other side of body. (Do not show alteration in shape of cup.)

6. Continuous opposition of the thumb with each finger more than 14 times in 10 seconds. (Each finger in turn taps thumb, starting with index finger. Do not allow thumb to slide from one finger to the other, or to go backwards.)

8. Advanced hand activities Score __O__

1. Picking up the top of a pen and putting it down again. (Patient stretches arm forward, picks up pen top, releases it on table close to body.)

2. Picking up one jellybean from a cup and placing it in another cup. (Teacup contains eight jellybeans. Both cups must be at arms length. Left hand takes jellybean from cup on right and releases it in cup on left.)

3. Drawing horizontal lines to stop at vertical line 10 times in 20 seconds. (At least 5 lines must touch and stop at the vertical line.)

4. Holding a pencil, making rapid consecutive dots on a sheet of paper. (Patient must make at least 2 dots per second for 5 seconds. Patient picks a pencil up and positions it without assistance. Patient must make a dot and not a stroke.)

5. Taking a dessert spoon of liquid to the mouth. (Do not allow head to lower towards spoon. Do not allow liquid to spill.)

6. Holding a comb and combing hair to back of head.

9. General tonus *Not used on overall score*

Adapted with permission from Carr, J.H. et al. "Investigation of a New Motor Assessment Scale for Stroke Patients, " *Physical Therapy* 65:175-180, 1985.

in persons with chronic disability. This assessment tool has been used to quantify functional status in patients with a variety of conditions, including heart failure, chronic lung disease, lung transplantation, and total hip replacement. It may be used on admission and at discharge as well as at specific intervals determined by the physical therapist to evaluate improvement or decline in the patient's status.

When administering this test, the patient is asked to ambulate at a preferred, comfortable speed. He may use assistive devices but may not receive physical assistance. He may stop for rest periods as needed. The test scores

USING THE OSWESTRY QUESTIONNAIRE

Name _David Doan_   **Date** _3/21/2000_

INSTRUCTIONS: Mark in each section only the one box that applies to you. We realize that you may consider that two of the statements in any one section relate to you, but please just mark the box which most closely describes your problem.

Section 1 — Pain Intensity
- [ ] I can tolerate the pain I have without having to use pain killers.
- [ ] The pain is bad, but I manage without taking pain killers.
- [x] Pain killers give complete relief from pain.
- [ ] Pain killers give moderate relief from pain.
- [ ] Pain killers give very little relief from pain.
- [ ] Pain killers have no effect on the pain and I do not use them.

Section 2 — Personal Care (Washing, Dressing, etc.)
- [ ] I can look after myself normally without pain.
- [x] I can look after myself normally, but it causes extra pain.
- [ ] It is painful to look after myself and I am slow and careful.
- [ ] I need some help but manage most of my personal care.
- [ ] I need help everyday in most aspects of my self-care.
- [ ] I do not get dressed and I wash with difficulty and stay in bed.

Section 3 — Lifting
- [ ] I can lift heavy weights without extra pain.
- [ ] I can lift heavy weight but it gives extra pain.
- [ ] Pain prevents me from lifting heavy weights off the floor, but I can manage if they are conveniently positioned (e.g., on a table).
- [ ] Pain prevents me from lifting heavy weights but I can manage light to medium weights if they are conveniently positioned.
- [x] I can lift only very light weights.
- [ ] I cannot lift or carry anything at all.

Section 4 — Walking
- [ ] Pain does not prevent me from walking any distance.
- [ ] Pain prevents me from walking more than 1 mile.

- [ ] Pain prevents me from walking more than ½ mile.
- [x] Pain prevents me from walking more than ½ mile.
- [ ] I can only walk using a stick or crutches.
- [ ] I am in bed most of the time and have to crawl to the toilet.

Section 5 — Sitting
- [ ] I can sit in any chair as long as I like.
- [ ] I can only sit in my favorite chair as long as I like.
- [ ] Pain prevents me from sitting more than 1 hour.
- [x] Pain prevents me from sitting more than ½ hour.
- [ ] Pain prevents me from sitting more than 10 minutes.
- [ ] Pain prevents me from sitting at all.

Section 6 — Standing
- [ ] I can stand as long as I want without extra pain.
- [x] I can stand as long as I want, but it gives me extra pain.
- [ ] Pain prevents me from standing for more than 1 hour.
- [ ] Pain prevents me from standing for more than 30 minutes.
- [ ] Pain prevents me from standing for more than 10 minutes.
- [ ] Pain prevents me from standing at all.

Section 7 — Sleeping
- [ ] Pain does not prevent me from sleeping well.
- [x] I can sleep well only by using tablets.
- [ ] Even when I take tablets I have less than 6 hours of sleep.
- [ ] Even when I take tablets I have less than 4 hours of sleep.
- [ ] Even when I take tablets I have less than 2 hours of sleep.
- [ ] Pain prevents me from sleeping at all.

USING THE OSWESTRY QUESTIONNAIRE *(continued)*

Section 8 — Sex Life
- ☐ My sex life is normal and causes no extra pain.
- ☐ My sex life is normal but causes some extra pain.
- ☐ My sex life is nearly normal but is very painful.
- ☑ My sex life is severely restricted by pain.
- ☐ My sex life is nearly absent because of pain.
- ☐ Pain prevents any sex life at all.

Section 9 — Social Life
- ☐ My social life is normal and causes no extra pain.
- ☐ My social life is normal but increases the degree of pain.
- ☐ Pain has no significant effect on my social life apart from limiting my more energetic interests (e.g., dancing, etc.)
- ☑ Pain has restricted my social life and I do not go out as often.
- ☐ Pain has restricted my social life to my home.
- ☐ I have no social life because of pain.

Section 10 — Travelling
- ☐ I can travel anywhere without extra pain.
- ☐ I can travel anywhere, but it gives me extra pain.
- ☐ Pain is bad, but I manage journeys over 2 hours.
- ☑ Pain restricts me to journeys of less than 1 hour.
- ☐ Pain restricts me to short necessary journeys of less than 30 minutes.
- ☐ Pain prevents me from travelling except to the doctor or hospital.

Adapted with permission from Fairbanks, S.C. et al. "The Oswestry Low Back Pain Disability Questionnaire," *Physiotherapy* 66:271-273, 1980.

the distance traveled during the timed interval.

Timed Up and Go

The Timed Up and Go is a multistep functional performance measure to assess basic mobility, primarily in frail, elderly patients. This test evolved from another "get-up-and-go" measurement tool that scored performance on a numerical scale of 1 to 5. Timed Up and Go measures the time required for a patient to rise from a standard chair, walk 3 m (10″), turn around, return, and sit down. The patient must be able to transfer and ambulate without physical assistance but may use an assistive device to complete the activity safely.

Persons who are independent in functional mobility typically complete the multistep task in less than 10 seconds; 20 seconds is the cutoff time for independent functional ability. Patients who need more than 30 seconds to complete the activity are likely to have impaired mobility and be at increased risk for falls.

Tinetti Performance Oriented Mobility Assessment

The Tinetti Performance Oriented Mobility Assessment (POMA) was developed as a screening tool to identify older adults who may be at risk for falls and frailty. The POMA assesses two areas: gait and balance. The balance portion of the assessment consists of eight functional tasks. The gait portion measures specific gait parameters during ambulation. (See *Tinetti balance and gait evaluation,* pages 125 and 126.)

Each item in the balance and gait subtests is scored on a scale of 0 to 2 based on objective criteria for the performance of each task. The subtests may be performed in isolation. Assistive devices may be used during as-

ASSESSING COGNITIVE FUNCTION

The Rancho Los Amigos Cognitive Scale is a tool widely used to classify brain-injured patients according to their behavior. This tool, shown below, describes the phases of recovery from coma to dependent functioning on a scale of I (unresponsive) to VIII (purposeful, appropriate, alert, and oriented). This chart is useful when assessing patients who have experienced posttraumatic amnesia.

Level	Response	Characteristics
I	None	Patient is unresponsive to any stimulus.
II	Generalized	Patient makes limited, inconsistent, nonpurposeful responses, often to pain only.
III	Localized	Patient can localize and withdraw from painful stimuli, can make purposeful responses and focus on presented objects, and may follow simple commands, but inconsistently and in a delayed manner.
IV	Confused and agitated	Patient is alert but agitated, confused, disoriented, and aggressive. He can't perform self-care and has no awareness of present events. Bizarre behavior is likely; agitation appears related to internal confusion.
V	Confused and inappropriate	Patient is alert and responds to commands, but is easily distracted and can't concentrate on tasks or learn new information. He becomes agitated in response to external stimuli, and his behavior and speech are inappropriate. His memory is severely impaired and he can't carry over learning from one situation to another.
VI	Confused and appropriate	Patient has some awareness of self and others but is inconsistently oriented. He can follow simple directions consistently with cuing and can relearn some old skills, such as activities of daily living, but continues to have serious memory problems (especially with short-term memory).
VII	Automatic and appropriate	Patient is consistently oriented with little or no confusion, but frequently appears robotlike when performing daily routines. His awareness of self and his interaction with his environment increase, but he lacks insight, judgment, problem-solving skills, and the ability to plan realistically.
VIII	Purposeful and appropriate	Patient is alert and oriented, recalls and integrates past events, learns new activities, and performs activities of daily living independently; however, deficits in stress tolerance, judgment, and abstract reasoning persist. He may function in society at a reduced level.

Adapted with permission from Rancho Los Amigos Hospital Professional Staff Association.

sessment. The maximum combined total score possible on the POMA is 28: 16 points from the balance portion and 12 from the gait portion. Patients scoring between 19 and 24 are thought to be at moderate risk for falls. A score less than 19 indicates a high risk of falls.

TINETTI BALANCE AND GAIT EVALUATION

This tool can be used to evaluate how successfully a patient remains at rest or moves about in ordinary activities. It takes 5 to 15 minutes to administer. To prepare, you'll need an armless upholstered chair, a walking space (such as a large room or a hallway), and any of the patient's walking aids (such as a cane or walker).

Observe the patient during each of the maneuvers listed below and select the number that best describes his performance. The maximum score is 28; the lowest is 0. The higher the score, the better the patient's gait and balance. You can assess any deterioration in his condition by periodically repeating the evaluation and comparing later scores to the baseline score.

Balance
INSTRUCTIONS: Seat the patient in a hard, armless chair and test the following maneuvers.

1. Sitting balance
   0 = Leans or slides in chair
   1 = Steady, safe

2. Arising
   0 = Unable without help
   1 = Able but uses arm to help
   2 = Able without use of arms

3. Attempts to arise
   0 = Unable without help
   1 = Able but requires more than one attempt
   2 = Able to arise with one attempt

4. Immediate standing balance (first 5 seconds)
   0 = Unsteady (staggers, moves feet, marked trunk sway)
   1 = Steady but uses walker or cane or grabs other object for support
   2 = Steady without walker, cane, or other support

5. Standing balance
   0 = Unsteady
   1 = Steady but wide stance (medial heels more than 4" apart) or uses walker, cane, or other support
   2 = Narrow stance without support

6. Nudge (Patient at maximum position with feet as close together as possible. Examiner pushes lightly on patient's sternum with palm of hand three times.)
   0 = Begins to fall
   1 = Staggers, grabs, but catches self
   2 = Steady

7. Eyes closed (at maximum position, as in number 6)
   0 = Unsteady
   1 = Steady

8. Turn 360 degrees
   0 = Discontinuous steps
   1 = Continuous steps
   0 = Unsteady (grabs, staggers)
   1 = Steady

9. Sit down
   0 = Unsafe (misjudged distance, falls into chair)
   1 = Uses arms or not a smooth motion
   2 = Safe, smooth motion

BALANCE SCORE _11_ /16

(continued)

TINETTI BALANCE AND GAIT EVALUATION *(continued)*

Gait

INSTRUCTIONS: Patient stands with examiner. He then walks down hallway or across room, first at his usual pace, then back at a rapid but safe pace (using usual walking aid, such as walker or cane).

10. Initiation of gait (immediately after told to go)
  0 = Any hesitancy or multiple attempts to start
  ① = No hesitancy

11. Step length and height (right-foot swing)
  0 = Does not pass left stance foot with step
  ① = Passes left stance foot
  0 = Right foot does not clear floor completely with step
  ① = Right foot completely clears floor

12. Step length and height (left-foot swing)
  0 = Does not pass right stance foot with step
  ① = Passes right stance foot
  0 = Left foot does not clear floor completely with step
  ① = Left foot completely clears floor

13. Step symmetry
  0 = Right and left step length not equal (estimate)
  ① = Right and left step length appear equal

14. Step continuity
  0 = Stopping or discontinuity between steps
  ① = Steps appear continuous

15. Path (Estimated in relation to floor tiles 12" wide. Observe excursion of one foot over about 10' of course.)
  0 = Marked deviation
  ① = Mild to moderate deviation or uses a walking aid
  2 = Straight without walking aid

16. Trunk
  0 = Marked sway or uses walking aid
  ① = No sway but flexes knees or back or spreads arms out while walking
  2 = No sway, no flexion, no use of arms, and no walking aid

17. Walk stance
  ① = Heels apart
  1 = Heels almost touching while walking

___9___ /12 **GAIT SCORE**

___20___ /28 **TOTAL MOBILITY SCORE (BALANCE AND GAIT)**

Adapted with permission from Galindo, D.J., et al. "Gait Training and Falls in the Elderly," *Journal of Gerontological Nursing* 21(6):15-16, June 1995.

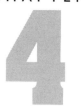

CHAPTER

4

Diagnostic tests

Findings and implications

Common diagnostic tests   128

Common diagnostic tests

Arthroscopy

Arthroscopy is the visual examination of the interior of a joint, most often the knee, using a specially designed fiber-optic endoscope. With about 98% diagnostic accuracy, it may prove to be the definitive diagnostic procedure for evaluating patient with suspected or confirmed joint disease.

Unlike radiographic studies, arthroscopy permits concurrent surgery or biopsy using a technique called triangulation, in which instruments are passed through a separate cannula. Thus, arthroscopy provides a safe, convenient alternative to open surgery (arthrotomy) and separate biopsy. Although arthroscopy is commonly performed under a local anesthetic, it may also be performed under a spinal or general anesthetic, especially when surgery is anticipated.

Purpose

- To detect and diagnose meniscal, patellar, condylar, extrasynovial, and synovial diseases
- To monitor the progression of disease
- To perform joint surgery
- To monitor the effectiveness of therapy

Normal findings

The knee is a typical diarthrodial joint surrounded by muscles, ligaments, cartilage, and tendons and lined with synovial membrane. (See *Understanding knee arthroscopy.*)

In children, menisci are smooth and opaque, with thick outer edges attached to the joint capsule and their inner edges lying snugly against the condylar surfaces, unattached. Articular cartilage appears smooth and white; ligaments and tendons appear cablelike and silvery. The synovium is smooth and marked by a fine vascular network. Degenerative changes begin during adolescence.

Implications of results

Arthroscopy can reveal meniscal diseases and injuries, such as a torn medial or lateral meniscus; patellar diseases and injuries, such as chondromalacia, dislocations, subluxations, fractures, osteochondritis dissecans, loose bodies, and parapatellar synovitis condylar disease such as degenerative articular cartilage; extrasynovial diseases and injuries, such as torn anterior cruciate or tibial collateral ligaments, Baker's cyst, and ganglionic cyst; and synovial diseases, such as synovitis, rheumatoid and degenerative arthritis, and foreign bodies associated with gout, pseudogout, and osteochondromatosis.

Depending on test findings, appropriate treatment or surgery can follow arthroscopy. If arthroscopic surgery can't be performed, arthrotomy is the procedure of choice.

Interfering factors

- Failure to use the arthroscope properly can result in an incomplete examination of the joint.

Bone densitometry

Bone densitometry quantifies bone mass. This noninvasive procedure, also known as dual energy X-ray absorptiometry (DEXA), uses an X-ray tube to measure bone mineral density while exposing the patient to only minimal radiation. The images are analyzed by computer to determine bone mineral status. The computer calculates the size and thickness of

UNDERSTANDING KNEE ARTHROSCOPY

Arthroscopic techniques vary, depending on the surgeon and the type of arthroscope used. In most cases, as much blood as possible is drained from the leg by wrapping it in an elastic bandage and elevating the leg or by instilling a mixture of lidocaine with epinephrine and sterile normal saline solution into the patient's knee to distend the knee and help reduce bleeding. Then the joint is anesthetized, a small incision is made, and a cannula is passed through the incision and positioned in the joint cavity with the patient's knee flexed about 40 degrees. The examiner moves the knee into various degrees of flexion, extension, and rotation to obtain different arthroscopic views of the joint space. Photographs may also be taken if needed for further study.

Some possible arthroscopic views are shown here. Counterclockwise from the top, you'll see a normal patellofemoral joint, showing smooth joint surfaces; the articular surface of the patella, showing chondromalacia; and a tear in the anterior cruciate ligament.

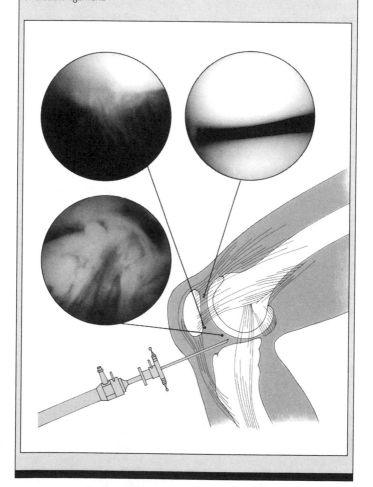

the bone as well as its volumetric density to determine its potential resistance to mechanical stress.

This test can scan the lumbar spine and the proximal femur, two sites at high risk for fractures. It's precise enough to scan three lumbar vertebrae and the introchanteric area of the hip. Scanning the distal forearm is also useful because research has shown a high correlation between its bone mineral density and that of the spine and femur.

This test may be done in the radiology department of a hospital, a doctor's office, or a clinic. It's usually performed by a technician or a nurse.

Purpose

• To determine bone mineral density
• To identify people at risk for osteoporosis
• To evaluate a patient's clinical response to therapy aimed at reducing the rate of bone loss

Normal findings

Results of the scan are analyzed by a computer program according to the patient's age, sex, and height. Rate of bone loss can be tracked over time.

Implications of results

The value and reliability of bone densitometry as a predictor of fractures are under investigation. Experts disagree about the scanning site and whether bone loss occurs as a general phenomenon or occurs first in the spine. Also, large-scale studies are being conducted to establish an "at-risk" level of bone density to help predict fractures.

Interfering factors

• The accuracy of the test may be influenced by osteoarthritis, fractures,

the size of the region scanned, and fatty tissue distribution.

Chest radiography

In chest radiography (commonly known as chest X-ray), X-ray beams penetrate the chest and react on specially sensitized film. Because normal pulmonary tissue is radiolucent, such abnormalities as infiltrates, foreign bodies, fluids, and tumors appear as densities on the film. A chest X-ray is most useful when compared with the patient's previous films because it allows the radiologist to detect changes.

Although chest radiography was once performed routinely as a cancer screening test, the associated expense and exposure to radiation have caused many authorities to question its usefulness for this purpose. The American Cancer Society recommends sputum culture instead — even for patients at high risk.

Purpose

• To detect pulmonary disorders, such as pneumonia, atelectasis, pneumothorax, bullae, and tumors
• To detect cardiac disease and mediastinal abnormalities such as tumors
• To determine the correct placement of pulmonary artery catheters, endotracheal tubes, and chest tubes
• To determine the location of objects, such as coins and broken central lines, that were swallowed or aspirated
• To gauge lesion location and size
• To help assess pulmonary status
• To evaluate the response to therapy

Normal findings

For an explanation of normal and abnormal findings, see *Clinical implications of chest X-ray findings*.

CLINICAL IMPLICATIONS OF CHEST X-RAY FINDINGS

Anatomic structure and normal appearance	Abnormality	Implications
Trachea Visible midline in the anterior mediastinal cavity; translucent tubelike appearance	• Deviation from midline	• Tension pneumothorax, atelectasis, pleural effusion, consolidation, mediastinal lymph nodes; in children, enlarged thymus
	• Narrowing, with hourglass appearance and deviation to one side	• Substernal thyroid
Heart Visible in the anterior left mediastinal cavity; solid appearance due to blood contents; edges may be clear in contrast with the surrounding air density of the lung	• Shift	• Atelectasis, pneumothorax
	• Hypertrophy of right side of the heart	• Cor pulmonale, heart failure
	• Cardiac borders obscured by stringy densities	• Cystic fibrosis
Aortic knob Visible as water density; formed by the aortic arch	• Solid densities, possibly indicating calcifications	• Atherosclerosis
	• Tortuous shape	• Atherosclerosis
Mediastinum (mediastinal shadow) Visible as the space between the lungs; shadowy appearance that widens at the hila of the lungs	• Deviation to nondiseased side; deviation to diseased side by traction	• Pleural effusion or tumor, fibrosis, collapsed lung
	• Gross widening	• Neoplasms of the esophagus, bronchi, lungs, thyroid, thymus, peripheral nerves, or lymphoid tissue; aortic aneurysm; mediastinitis; cor pulmonale
Ribs Visible as the thoracic cavity encasement	• Break or misalignment	• Fractured sternum or ribs
	• Widening of intercostal spaces	• Emphysema
Spine Visible midline in the posterior chest; straight, bony structure	• Spinal curvature • Break or misalignment	• Scoliosis, kyphosis • Fractures
Clavicles Visible in the upper thorax; intact and equidistant in properly centered X-ray films	• Break or misalignment	• Fractures

(continued)

CLINICAL IMPLICATIONS OF CHEST X-RAY FINDINGS (continued)

Anatomic structure and normal appearance	Abnormality	Implications
Hila (lung roots) Visible above the heart, where pulmonary vessels, bronchi, and lymph nodes join the lungs; appear as small, white, bilateral densities	• Shift to one side • Accentuated shadows	• Atelectasis • Pneumothorax, emphysema, pulmonary abscess, tumor, enlarged lymph nodes
Mainstem bronchus Visible as part of the hila; translucent, tubelike appearance	• Spherical or oval density	• Bronchogenic cyst
Bronchi Usually not visible	• Visible	• Bronchial pneumonia
Lung fields Usually not visible throughout, except for the blood vessels	• Visible • Irregular, patchy densities	• Atelectasis • Resolving pneumonia, infiltrates, silicosis, fibrosis, metastatic neoplasm
Hemidiaphragm Rounded, visible; right side ⅜" to ¾" (1 to 2 cm) higher than left	• Elevation of diaphragm (difference in elevation can be measured on inspiration and expiration to detect movement) • Flattening of diaphragm • Unilateral elevation of either side • Unilateral elevation of left side only	• Active tuberculosis, pneumonia, pleurisy, acute bronchitis, active disease of abdominal viscera, bilateral phrenic nerve involvement, atelectasis • Asthma, emphysema • Possibly unilateral phrenic nerve paresis • Perforated ulcer (rare), gas distention of stomach, splenic flexure of colon, free air in abdomen

Implications of results

For accurate diagnosis, radiography findings must be correlated with additional radiologic and pulmonary tests and physical assessment findings. Pulmonary hyperinflation with a low diaphragm and generalized increased radiolucency may suggest emphysema but may also appear in a healthy person's X-rays.

Interfering factors

• Portable chest X-rays taken in the anteroposterior position may show larger cardiac shadowing than other X-rays because the distance from the anterior structures to the beam is shorter.
• Portable chest X-rays — primarily those taken to detect atelectasis, pneumonia, pneumothorax, and me-

diastinal shift or to evaluate treatment—may be less reliable than stationary X-rays.

• Films taken with the patient in a supine position won't show fluid levels. (However, decubitus views can demonstrate fluid levels.)

• Because chest X-ray findings vary with the patient's age and sex, these factors should be considered when the films are evaluated.

• The patient's inability to take a full inspiration may interfere with X-ray results.

• Under- or over-exposure of the films may result in poor quality X-rays.

Computed tomography of the spine

Computed tomography (CT) scans of the spine provide detailed, high-resolution images in the cross-sectional, longitudinal, sagittal, and lateral planes. In this procedure, multiple X-ray beams from a computerized body scanner are directed at the spine from different angles. They pass through the body and strike radiation detectors, producing electrical impulses. A computer converts these impulses into digital information, which is displayed as a three-dimensional image on a video monitor. Digitized images are stored as a permanent record, which allows reexamination without repeating the procedure.

Two variations of spinal CT scanning further expand the procedure's diagnostic capabilities. Contrast-enhanced CT scanning accentuates spinal vasculature and highlights even subtle differences in tissue density. Air CT scanning, which involves removing a small amount of cerebrospinal fluid (CSF) and injecting air via lumbar puncture, intensifies the contrast between the subarachnoid space and surrounding tissue.

Purpose

• To diagnose spinal lesions and abnormalities
• To monitor the effects of spinal surgery or therapy

Normal findings

In the CT image, spinal tissue appears black, white, or gray, depending on its density. Vertebrae, the densest tissues, are white. Soft tissues appear in shades of gray. CSF is black.

Implications of results

By highlighting areas of altered density and depicting structural malformation, CT scanning can reveal all types of spinal lesions and abnormalities. It's particularly useful in detecting and localizing tumors, which appear as masses of varying density. Measuring this density and noting the configuration and location relative to the spinal cord can often identify the type of tumor. For example, a neurinoma (schwannoma) appears as a spherical mass dorsal to the cord; a darker, wider mass lying more laterally or ventrally to the cord may be a meningioma.

CT scanning also reveals degenerative processes and structural changes in detail. Herniated nucleus pulposus appears as an obvious herniation of disk material with unilateral or bilateral nerve root compression; if the herniation is midline, spinal cord compression will be evident. Cervical spondylosis appears as cervical cord compression due to bony hypertrophy of the cervical spine. Lumbar stenosis appears as hypertrophy of the lumbar vertebrae, causing cord compression by decreasing space within the spinal column.

Facet disorders appear as soft-tissue changes, bony overgrowth, and spurring of the vertebrae, resulting in nerve root compression.

Fluid-filled arachnoidal and other paraspinal cysts appear as dark masses displacing the spinal cord. Vascular malformations, evident after contrast enhancement, appear as masses or clusters, usually on the dorsal aspect of the spinal cord. Congenital spinal malformations, such as meningocele, myelocele, and spina bifida, show as abnormally large, dark gaps between the white vertebrae.

Interfering factors

• Excessive movement by the patient during the scanning procedure may create artifacts, making the images difficult to interpret.
• Failure to remove metal objects from the scanning field may cause unclear images.

Doppler ultrasonography

Doppler ultrasonography is a noninvasive test that evaluates blood flow in the major veins and arteries of the arms and legs and in the extracranial cerebrovascular system. Developed as an alternative to arteriography and venography, Doppler ultrasonography is safer and less costly and requires a shorter test period than invasive tests. Although this test is 95% accurate in detecting arteriovenous disease that impairs blood flow by at least 50%, it may fail to detect mild arteriosclerotic plaques and smaller thrombi, and it usually fails to detect major calf vein thrombosis.

In Doppler ultrasonography, a handheld transducer directs high-frequency sound waves to the artery or vein being tested. The sound waves strike moving red blood cells and are reflected back to the transducer at frequencies that correspond to the velocity of blood flow through the vessel. The transducer then amplifies the sound waves to permit direct listening and graphic recording of blood flow. (See *How the Doppler probe works*.)

The measurement of systolic pressure during this test helps detect the presence, location, and extent of peripheral arterial occlusive disease. Normally, venous blood flow fluctuates with respiration, so observing changes in sound-wave frequency during respiration helps detect venous occlusive disease. Compression maneuvers can also help detect occlusion of the veins as well as occlusion or stenosis of carotid arteries.

Pulse volume recorder testing may be performed along with Doppler ultrasonography to yield a quantitative recording of changes in blood volume or flow in an extremity or organ.

Purpose

• To aid diagnosis of venous insufficiency and superficial and deep vein thromboses (popliteal, femoral, iliac)
• To aid diagnosis of peripheral artery disease and arterial occlusion
• To monitor patients who have had arterial reconstruction and bypass grafts
• To detect abnormalities of carotid artery blood flow associated with such conditions as aortic stenosis
• To evaluate possible arterial trauma

Normal findings

Arterial waveforms of the arms and legs are multiphasic, with a prominent systolic component and one or more diastolic sounds. The ankle-arm pressure index — the ratio between ankle systolic pressure and brachial systolic pressure — is nor-

HOW THE DOPPLER PROBE WORKS

The Doppler ultrasonic probe directs high-frequency sound waves through layers of tissue. When these waves strike red blood cells (RBCs) moving through the bloodstream, their frequency changes in proportion to the flow velocity of the RBCs. Recording these waves permits the detection of arterial and venous obstruction but not a quantitative measurement of blood flow.

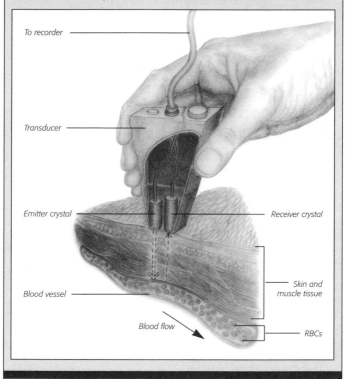

mally equal to or greater than 1. (The ankle-arm pressure index is also known as the arterial ischemia index, the ankle-brachial index, and the pedal-brachial index.) Proximal thigh pressure is normally 20 to 30 mm Hg higher than arm pressure, but pressure measurements at adjacent sites are similar. In the arms, pressure readings should remain unchanged despite postural changes.

Venous blood flow velocity is normally phasic with respiration and is of a lower pitch than arterial flow. Distal compression or release of prox-

imal limb compression increases blood flow velocity. In the legs, abdominal compression eliminates respiratory variations, but release increases blood flow; Valsalva's maneuver also interrupts venous flow velocity.

In cerebrovascular testing, a strong velocity signal is present. In the common carotid artery, blood flow velocity increases during diastole, due to low peripheral vascular resistance of the brain. The direction of periorbital arterial flow is normally anterograde out of the orbit.

Implications of results

Arterial stenosis or occlusion diminishes the blood flow velocity signal, with no diastolic sound and a less prominent systolic component distal to the lesion. At the lesion, the signal is high-pitched and, occasionally, turbulent. If complete occlusion is present and collateral circulation hasn't taken over, the velocity signal may be absent.

A pressure gradient exceeding 20 to 30 mm Hg at adjacent sites of measurement in the leg may indicate occlusive disease. Specifically, low proximal thigh pressure signifies common femoral or aortoiliac occlusive disease. An abnormal gradient between the proximal thigh and the above- or below-knee cuffs indicates superficial femoral or popliteal artery occlusive disease; an abnormal gradient between the below-knee and ankle cuffs indicates tibiofibular disease. Abnormal gradients of arm and forearm pressure readings may indicate brachial artery occlusion.

An abnormal ankle-arm pressure index is directly proportional to the degree of circulatory impairment: mild ischemia, 1 to 0.75; claudication, 0.75 to 0.50; pain at rest, 0.50 to 0.25; and pregangrene, 0.25 to 0.

Venous blood flow velocity that is unchanged by respirations, doesn't increase in response to compression or Valsalva's maneuver, or is absent indicates venous thrombosis. In chronic venous insufficiency and varicose veins, the flow velocity signal may be reversed. Confirmation of results may require venography.

The inability to identify Doppler signals during cerebrovascular examination indicates total arterial occlusion. Reversed periorbital arterial flow indicates significant arterial occlusive disease of the extracranial internal carotid artery; in addition, the audible signal may take on the acoustic characteristics of a normal peripheral artery. Stenosis of the internal carotid artery causes turbulent signals. Collateral circulation can be assessed by compression maneuvers.

Oculoplethysmography, carotid phonoangiography, or carotid imaging may further evaluate cerebrovascular disease. Retrograde blood velocity in the vertebral artery may indicate subclavian steal syndrome. Weak velocity signal on comparison of contralateral vertebral arteries may indicate diffuse vertebral artery disease.

Interfering factors

• Failure of the patient to remain still during this test may invalidate results.

Electrocardiography

Electrocardiography (ECG), the most commonly used test for evaluating cardiac status, graphically records the electrical current (electrical potential) generated by the heart. This current radiates from the heart in all directions and, on reaching the skin, is measured by electrodes connected to an amplifier and strip chart recorder.

ECG tracings normally consist of three identifiable waveforms: the P wave, the QRS complex, and the T wave. The P wave depicts atrial depolarization; the QRS complex, ventricular depolarization; and the T wave, ventricular repolarization. Although the ECG records only about 50 to 100 of the more than 100,000 cardiac cycles that occur in 24 hours, it's useful for detecting the presence and location of myocardial infarction (MI), ischemia, conduction delays, chamber enlargement, arrhythmias, and myocardial necrosis.

New, computerized ECG machines routinely use electrodes with small tabs that peel off a sheet and adhere to the patient's skin. The leads coming from the ECG machine are clearly marked (LA, RA, LL, RL, V_1 through V_6) and are applied to the electrodes with alligator clamps. In a standard 12-lead ECG, 10 electrodes (4 limb, 6 chest) record the heart's electrical potential from 12 different views or leads: the standard bipolar limb leads (I, II, III), the augmented unipolar limb leads (aV_F, aV_L, and aV_R), and the precordial, or chest, leads (V_1 through V_6). The entire ECG tracing is displayed on a screen so that abnormalities (loose leads or artifacts) can be corrected before printing; then it's printed on one sheet of paper. The electrode tabs can remain on the patient's chest, arms, and legs to provide continuous lead placements for serial ECG studies.

Purpose

• To help identify primary conduction abnormalities, cardiac arrhythmias, cardiac hypertrophy, pericarditis, electrolyte imbalance, myocardial ischemia, and the site and extent of an MI
• To monitor recovery from an MI
• To evaluate the effectiveness of cardiac medication, such as digitalis glycosides, antiarrhythmics, antihypertensives, and vasodilators
• To observe pacemaker performance
• To determine the effectiveness of thrombolytic therapy and the resolution of ST-segment depression or elevation and T-wave changes

Normal findings

The lead II waveform, known as the rhythm strip, depicts the heart's rhythm more clearly than any other waveform. (See *Normal ECG waveforms,* page 138.) In lead II, the normal P wave doesn't exceed 2.5 mm (0.25 mV) in height or last longer than 0. 11 second. The PR interval,

which includes the P wave and the PR segment, persists for 0.12 to 0.2 second for cardiac rates over 60 beats/minute. The QT interval varies with the cardiac rate and lasts 0.4 to 0.52 second for rates above 60; the voltage of the R wave in leads V_1 through V_6 doesn't exceed 27 mm. The total QRS interval lasts 0.06 to 0.1 second. ST-segment data is also useful for assessing myocardial ischemia.

Implications of results

An abnormal ECG may show MI, right or left ventricular hypertrophy, arrhythmias, right or left bundle-branch block, ischemia, conduction defects, pericarditis, electrolyte abnormalities such as hypokalemia, or the effects of cardioactive drugs such as digoxin Sometimes an ECG may reveal abnormal waveforms only during episodes of angina or during exercise. (See chapter 5, Understanding rhythm strips, for more information.)

Interfering factors

• Mechanical difficulties, such as ECG machine malfunction, electrode patches that don't adhere well (for example, from diaphoresis), or electromagnetic interference, can produce artifacts.
• Improper placement of electrodes, patient movement or muscle tremor, strenuous exercise before the test, or reactions to medication can produce inaccurate test results.

Electromyography

Electromyography (EMG) is the recording of the electrical activity of selected skeletal muscle groups at rest and during voluntary contraction. In this test, a needle electrode is inserted percutaneously into a muscle. The

NORMAL ECG WAVEFORMS

Because each lead takes a different view of heart activity, it generates its own characteristic tracing. The traces shown here represent each of the 12 leads. Leads aV_R, V_1, V_2, and V_3 normally show strong negative deflections below the baseline. Negative deflections indicate that the electrical current is flowing away from the positive electrode; positive deflections indicate that the current is flowing toward the positive electrode.

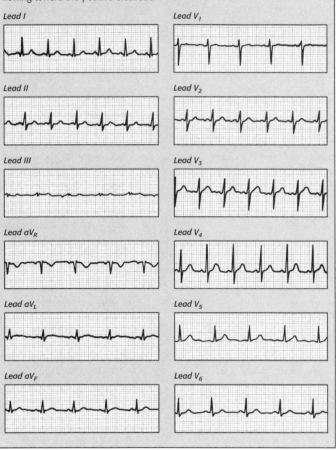

Lead I

Lead II

Lead III

Lead aV_R

Lead aV_L

Lead aV_F

Lead V_1

Lead V_2

Lead V_3

Lead V_4

Lead V_5

Lead V_6

electrical discharge (or motor unit potential) of the muscle is then displayed and measured on an oscilloscope screen. Although a separate procedure, *nerve conduction time* (distance between point of stimulation and recorded response divided by time between stimulus and detected response) is often measured simulta-

neously. EMG is a useful diagnostic technique for evaluating muscle disorders.

Purpose

• To help differentiate between primary muscle disorders, such as muscular dystrophies, and those that are secondary

• To help determine diseases characterized by central neuronal degeneration such as amyotrophic lateral sclerosis (ALS)

• To help diagnose neuromuscular disorders such as myasthenia gravis

Normal findings

At rest, a normal muscle exhibits minimal electrical activity. During voluntary contraction, however, electrical activity increases markedly. A sustained contraction, or one of increasing strength, produces a rapid "train" of motor unit potentials that can be heard over the audioamplifier as a crescendo of sounds, similar to the sound of an outboard motor.

At the same time, the oscilloscope screen displays a sequence of waveforms that vary in amplitude (height) and frequency. Waveforms that are close together indicate a high frequency; waveforms that are far apart signify a low frequency.

Implications of results

In primary muscle disease, such as muscular dystrophy, motor unit potentials are short (low amplitude), with frequent, irregular discharges. In such disorders as ALS and peripheral nerve disorders, motor unit potentials are isolated and irregular but show increased amplitude and duration. In myasthenia gravis, motor unit potentials may be normal initially, but they diminish in amplitude progressively with continuing contractions. The interpreter makes a distinction between waveforms that indicate a muscle disorder and those that indicate denervation.

Findings must be correlated with the patient's history, clinical features, and the results of other neurodiagnostic tests.

Interfering factors

• The patient's inability to comply with instructions during the test may invalidate results.

• Drugs that affect myoneural junctions, such as cholinergics, anticholinergics, and skeletal muscle relaxants, interfere with test results.

Exercise electrocardiography

Exercise electrocardiography (ECG), commonly known as a stress test, evaluates heart action during physical stress — when the demand for oxygen increases — and, thus, provides important diagnostic information that can't be obtained from a resting ECG alone.

In this test, ECG and blood pressure readings are taken while the patient walks on a treadmill or pedals a stationary bicycle, and his response to a constant or increasing workload is observed. Unless complications develop, the test continues until the patient reaches the target heart rate (determined by an established protocol) or experiences chest pain or fatigue. A patient who recently had a myocardial infarction (MI) or coronary artery surgery may walk the treadmill at a slow pace to determine his activity tolerance before being discharged from the hospital.

The risk of MI during exercise ECG is less than 1 in 500; the risk of death, less than 1 in 10,000.

Purpose

• To help diagnose the cause of chest pain or other possible cardiac pain

• To determine the functional capacity of the heart after surgery or MI

• To screen for asymptomatic coronary artery disease (CAD), particularly in men over age 35

• To help set limitations for an exercise program
• To identify cardiac arrhythmias that develop during physical exercise
• To evaluate the effectiveness of antiarrhythmic or antianginal therapy

Normal findings

In a normal exercise ECG, the P wave, QRS complex, T wave, and ST segment change slightly; a slight ST-segment depression occurs in some patients, especially women. The heart rate rises in direct proportion to the workload and metabolic oxygen demand; systolic blood pressure also rises as workload increases. The endurance levels attained should be appropriate to the patient's age and the exercise protocol.

Implications of results

Although criteria for judging test results vary, two findings strongly suggest an abnormality: a flat or downsloping ST-segment depression of 1 mm or more for at least 0.08 second after the junction of the QRS complex and ST segment (J point) and a markedly depressed J point, with an upsloping but depressed ST segment of 1.5 mm below the baseline 0.08 second after the J point. T-wave inversion also signifies ischemia. Initial ST-segment depression on the resting ECG must be further depressed by 1 mm during exercise to be considered abnormal.

Hypotension resulting from exercise, ST-segment depression of 3 mm or more, downsloping ST segments, and ischemic ST segments appearing within the first 3 minutes of exercise and lasting 8 minutes into the posttest recovery period may indicate multivessel or left main coronary artery disease. ST-segment elevation may indicate dyskinetic left ventricular wall motion or severe transmural ischemia.

The predictive value of this test for CAD varies with the patient's history and gender; however, false-negative and false-positive test results are common. To detect CAD accurately, thallium imaging and stress testing, exercise multiple-gated acquisition scanning, or coronary angiography may be necessary.

Interfering factors

• The patient's failure to observe pretest restrictions hinders the heart's ability to respond to stress.
• Use of beta-adrenergic blockers may make test results difficult to interpret.
• Inability to exercise to the target heart rate because of fatigue or failure to cooperate interferes with accurate testing.
• Wolff-Parkinson-White syndrome (anomalous atrioventricular excitation), electrolyte imbalance, or the use of a digitalis glycoside may cause false-positive results.
• Conditions that cause left ventricular hypertrophy, such as congenital abnormalities and hypertension, may interfere with testing for ischemia.

Fasting plasma glucose

Commonly used to screen for diabetes mellitus, the fasting plasma glucose test (also known as the fasting blood sugar test) measures plasma glucose levels following a 12- to 14-hour fast.

In the fasting state, plasma glucose levels decrease, stimulating the release of the hormone glucagon. Glucagon then acts to raise plasma glucose by accelerating glycogenolysis, stimulating gluconeogenesis, and inhibiting glycogen synthesis. Normally, the secretion of insulin checks this rise in glucose levels. In diabetes, however, absence or deficiency of insulin allows persistently high glucose levels.

Purpose

• To screen for diabetes mellitus
• To monitor drug or diet therapy in patients with diabetes mellitus

Reference values

The normal range for fasting plasma glucose varies according to the laboratory procedure. Generally, normal values after a 12- to 14-hour fast are 70 to 100 mg of "true glucose" per deciliter of blood when measured by the glucose oxidase and hexokinase methods.

Implications of results

A fasting plasma glucose level greater than or equal to 126 mg/dl or more obtained on two or more occasions confirms diabetes mellitus. However, a borderline or transiently elevated level requires the 2-hour postprandial plasma glucose test or the oral glucose tolerance test to confirm the diagnosis.

Although increased fasting plasma glucose levels most commonly occur with diabetes, they can also result from pancreatitis, recent acute illness (such as myocardial infarction), Cushing's syndrome, acromegaly, and pheochromocytoma. Hyperglycemia may also stem from hyperlipoproteinemia (especially type III, IV, or V), chronic hepatic disease, nephrotic syndrome, brain tumor, sepsis, or gastrectomy with dumping syndrome and is typical in eclampsia, anoxia, and seizure disorders.

Depressed plasma glucose levels can result from hyperinsulinism, insulinoma, von Gierke's disease, functional or reactive hypoglycemia,

myxedema, adrenal insufficiency, congenital adrenal hyperplasia, hypopituitarism, malabsorption syndrome, and some cases of hepatic insufficiency.

Interfering factors

• False-positive findings may be caused by acetaminophen when the glucose oxidase or hexokinase method is used. Other drugs known to elevate plasma glucose levels are chlorthalidone, thiazide diuretics, furosemide, triamterene, oral contraceptives (estrogen-progestin combination), benzodiazepines, phenytoin, phenothiazines, lithium, epinephrine, arginine, phenolphthalein, dextrothyroxine, diazoxide, large doses of nicotinic acid, corticosteroids, and recent I.V. glucose infusions. Ethacrynic acid may also cause hyperglycemia, but large doses can produce hypoglycemia in patients with uremia.
• Decreased plasma glucose levels may be caused by beta-adrenergic blockers, ethanol, clofibrate, insulin, oral antidiabetic agents, and monoamine oxidase inhibitors.
• Failure to observe dietary restrictions may elevate plasma glucose levels.
• Recent illness, infection, or pregnancy can elevate plasma glucose levels; strenuous exercise can depress them.
• Glycolysis caused by failure to refrigerate the sample or send it to the laboratory immediately can result in false-negative results.

Hematocrit

Hematocrit (HCT), a common, reliable test, may be done by itself or as part of a complete blood count. This test measures the percentage by volume of packed red blood cells (RBCs) in a whole blood sample. For exam-

NORMAL HEMATOCRIT VALUES BY AGE

Age	Hematocrit values (%)
Newborn	55 to 68
1 week	47 to 65
1 month	37 to 49
3 months	30 to 36
1 year	29 to 41
10 years	36 to 40
Adult male	42 to 54
Adult female	38 to 46

ple, an HCT of 40% means that a 100-ml sample contains 40 ml of packed RBCs. This packing is achieved by centrifugation of anticoagulated whole blood in a capillary tube, so that RBCs are tightly packed without hemolysis.

Most commonly, HCT is measured electronically, producing results 3% lower than when HCT is measured manually. (Manual measurement traps plasma in the column of packed RBCs.) Test results may be used to calculate two erythrocyte indices: mean corpuscular volume and mean corpuscular hemoglobin concentration.

Purpose

• To aid diagnosis of abnormal states of hydration, polycythemia, and anemia
• To aid in calculating RBC indices

Reference values

Hematocrit values vary, depending on the patient's sex and age, type of sample, and the laboratory performing the test. (See *Normal hematocrit values by age.*)

Implications of results

Low HCT suggests anemia, hemodilution, or massive blood loss; high HCT indicates polycythemia or hemoconcentration due to blood loss and dehydration.

Interfering factors

• Failure to use the proper anticoagulant in the collection tube, fill the tube appropriately, or adequately mix the sample and the anticoagulant may alter test results.
• Hemolysis due to rough handling of the sample may affect test results.
• Tourniquet constriction for longer than 1 minute causes hemoconcentration and typically raises HCT by 2.5% to 5%.
• Taking the blood sample from the same arm that is being used for I.V. infusion causes hemodilution.

Lower-limb venography

Venography, the radiographic examination of a vein, is commonly used to assess the condition of the deep leg veins after injection of a contrast medium. It's the definitive test for deep vein thrombosis (DVT), an acute condition marked by inflammation and thrombus formation in the deep veins of the legs. Such thrombi usually develop in valve pockets — venous junctions or sinuses of the calf muscle — then travel to the deep calf veins. If untreated, they may occlude the popliteal, femoral, and iliac vein systems, which may lead to pulmonary embolism, a potentially lethal complication. Predisposing factors to DVT include vein wall injury, prolonged bed rest, coagulation abnormalities, surgery, childbirth, and the use of oral contraceptives.

Venography shouldn't be used for routine screening because it exposes the patient to relatively high doses of radiation and can cause complications, such as phlebitis, local tissue damage and, occasionally, DVT itself. It's also expensive and isn't easily repeated. A combination of three noninvasive tests — Doppler ultrasonography, impedance plethysmography, and ^{125}I fibrinogen scanning — provides an acceptable, though less accurate, alternative to venography. Radionuclide tests, such as the ^{125}I fibrinogen scan, are also used to detect DVT in a patient who is too ill for venography or is hypersensitive to the contrast medium.

Purpose

• To confirm diagnosis of DVT
• To distinguish clot formation from venous obstruction (such as a large tumor of the pelvis impinging on the venous system)
• To evaluate congenital venous abnormalities
• To assess deep vein valvular competence (especially helpful in identifying underlying causes of leg edema)
• To locate a suitable vein for arterial bypass grafting

Normal findings

A normal venogram shows steady opacification of the superficial and deep vasculature with no filling defects.

Implications of results

A venogram that shows consistent filling defects on repeat views, abrupt termination of a column of contrast material, unfilled major deep veins, or diversion of flow (through collaterals, for example) is diagnostic of DVT. (See *Abnormal venograms*, page 144.)

Interfering factors

• If the patient places weight on the leg being tested, the contrast medium may fail to fill the leg veins.
• Movement of the leg being tested, excessive tourniquet constriction, insufficient injection of contrast medium, and delay between injection and radiography affect the accuracy of test results.

Myelography

Myelography combines fluoroscopy and radiography to evaluate the spinal subarachnoid space after injection of a contrast medium. Because the contrast medium is heavier than cerebrospinal fluid (CSF), it will flow through the subarachnoid space to the dependent area when the patient, lying prone on a fluoroscopic table, is tilted up or down. The fluoroscope allows visualization of the flow of the contrast medium and the outline of the subarachnoid space. X-rays are taken for a permanent record.

Myelography can help locate a spinal lesion, a ruptured disk, spinal stenosis, or an abscess. Sometimes it's

ABNORMAL VENOGRAMS

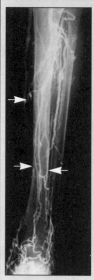

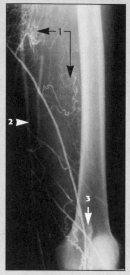

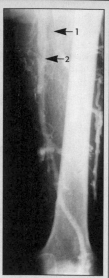

This venogram of the calf shows incompetent veins (arrows).

This venogram of the thigh shows the development of collateral veins (1), filling of some superficial veins (2), and obstruction of the popliteal vein (3).

This venogram of the thigh shows a filling defect due to a thrombus (1) and backflow from a blockage of the iliac veins (2).

performed to confirm the need for surgery; in such cases, a neurosurgeon may stand by. If this test confirms a spinal tumor, the patient may be taken directly to the operating room. Immediate surgery may also be necessary when the contrast medium causes a total block of the subarachnoid space.

Purpose

• To demonstrate lesions that partially or totally block the flow of CSF in the subarachnoid space, such as tumors and herniated intervertebral disks
• To help detect arachnoiditis, spinal nerve root injury, or tumors in the posterior fossa of the skull

Normal findings

The contrast medium should flow freely through the subarachnoid space, showing no obstruction or structural abnormalities.

Implications of results

This test can identify and localize lesions within or surrounding the spinal cord or subarachnoid space. Common extradural lesions include herniated intervertebral disks and metastatic tumors. Common lesions within the subarachnoid space include neurofibromas and meningiomas; lesions within the spinal cord include ependymomas and astrocytomas. This test may also detect syringomyelia, a congenital abnormality marked by fluid-filled cavities in the spinal cord and widening of the cord itself. Myelography may also detect arachnoiditis, spinal nerve root injury, and tumors in the posterior fossa of the skull. Test results must be correlated with the patient's history and clinical status.

Interfering factors

• Incorrect needle placement or the patient's failure to cooperate may alter results.

Partial thromboplastin time

The partial thromboplastin time (PTT) test evaluates all the clotting factors of the intrinsic pathway — except platelets — by measuring the time required for formation of a fibrin clot after the addition of calcium and phospholipid emulsion to a plasma sample. Because most congenital coagulation deficiencies occur in the intrinsic pathway, the PTT test is valuable in preoperative screening for bleeding tendencies. It's also the test of choice for monitoring heparin therapy.

Purpose

• To screen for deficiencies of the clotting factors in the intrinsic pathways
• To monitor the patient's response to heparin therapy

Reference values

Normally, a fibrin clot forms 25 to 36 seconds after addition of reagents. For a patient on anticoagulant therapy, check with the doctor to find out the desirable values for the therapy being delivered.

Implications of results

Prolonged PTT may indicate a deficiency of certain plasma clotting factors, the presence of heparin, or the presence of fibrin split products, plasmin, or circulating anticoagulants that are antibodies to specific clotting factors.

Interfering factors

• Failure to use the proper anticoagulant, fill the collection tube completely, or mix the sample and the anticoagulant adequately may affect the accuracy of test results.
• Hemolysis due to rough handling of the sample or excessive probing at the venipuncture site may alter test results.
• Failure to send the sample to the laboratory immediately or to place it on ice may cause spurious test results.

Prothrombin time

Prothrombin time (PT), commonly known as "pro time," measures the time required for a fibrin clot to form in a citrated plasma sample after addition of calcium ions and tissue thromboplastin (factor III). It's an excellent screening procedure for the overall evaluation of extrinsic coagulation factors V, VII, and X, and of prothrombin and fibrinogen. PT is the test of choice for monitoring oral anticoagulant therapy.

Purpose

• To evaluate the extrinsic coagulation system
• To monitor response to oral anticoagulant therapy

INTERNATIONAL NORMALIZED RATIO

The International Normalized Ratio (INR) system is generally viewed as the best means of standardizing measurement of prothrombin time (PT) to monitor oral anticoagulant therapy. However, the INR should never be used to screen patients for coagulopathies — because PT testing is performed using different thromboplastin reagents and different instruments, each laboratory may have different "normal values."

Many types of thromboplastin are used in PT testing (rabbit brain, human brain, recombinant). Each type of reagent has a different sensitivity. The greater the reagent's sensitivity, the longer the PT will be. For example, when using the same patient plasma, a sensitive thromboplastin will result in a PT of approximately 30 seconds, but a less sensitive thromboplastin will result in a PT of approximately 20 seconds.

The INR helps to standardize oral anticoagulant therapy so that a patient's therapy outcomes can be easily evaluated by various institutions that may use different instruments and thromboplastin reagents. Recent guidelines for patients receiving warfarin therapy recommend an INR of 2.0 to 3.0, except for those with mechanical prosthetic heart valves. For these patients, an INR of 2.5 to 3.5 is suggested.

Reference values

Normally, PT ranges from 10 to 14 seconds. In a patient receiving warfarin therapy, PT is usually maintained between 1½ and 2 times the normal control value. (See *International Normalized Ratio.*)

Implications of results

Prolonged PT may indicate hepatic disease or deficiencies in fibrinogen; prothrombin; factors V, VII, or X (specific assays can pinpoint such deficiencies); or vitamin K. It may also result from ongoing oral anticoagulant therapy. Prolonged PT that exceeds 2½ times the control value is commonly associated with abnormal bleeding.

Prolonged PT can result from the overuse of alcohol or from the use of adrenocorticotropic hormone, anabolic steroids, cholestyramine resin, I.V. heparin (within 5 hours of collection), indomethacin, mefenamic acid, methimazole, oxyphenbuta-

zone, phenylbutazone, phenytoin, propylthiouracil, quinidine, quinine, thyroid hormones, or vitamin A.

Prolonged or shortened PT can follow ingestion of antibiotics, barbiturates, hydroxyzine, sulfonamides, salicylates (more than 1 g/day prolongs PT), mineral oil, or clofibrate.

Interfering factors

• Hemolysis may interfere with the accuracy of test results.
• Failure to mix the sample and anticoagulant adequately or send the sample to the laboratory promptly may alter test results.
• Fibrin or fibrin split products in the sample or plasma fibrinogen levels less than 100 mg/dl can prolong PT.
• Falsely prolonged results may occur if the collection tube isn't filled to capacity with blood; this results in too much anticoagulant for the blood sample.
• Shortened PT can result from the use of antihistamines, chloral hydrate, corticosteroids, digitalis glyco-

sides, diuretics, glutethimide, griseo-fulvin, estrogen-progestin combina-tions, pyrazinamide, vitamin K, or xanthines (caffeine, theophylline).

Pulmonary function

Pulmonary function tests (including volume, capacity, and flow rate tests) are a series of measurements that evaluate ventilatory function through spirometric measurements; they're performed on patients with suspected pulmonary dysfunction. Of the seven tests that are performed to determine volume, tidal volume (V_T) and expi-ratory reserve volume (ERV) are di-rect spirographic measurements; minute volume (MV), carbon dioxide (CO_2) response, inspiratory reserve volume (IRV), and residual volume (RV) are calculated from the results of other pulmonary function tests; and thoracic gas volume (TGV) is calculated from body plethysmog-raphy.

Of the pulmonary capacity tests, vital capacity (VC), inspiratory capac-ity (IC), functional residual capacity (FRC), total lung capacity (TLC), and forced expiratory flow (FEF) may be measured directly or calculated from the results of other tests. Forced vital capacity (FVC), flow-volume curve, forced expiratory volume (FEV), peak expiratory flow rate (PEFR), and maximal voluntary ven-tilation (MVV) are direct spirographic measurements. The diffusing capaci-ty for carbon monoxide (DLCO) is calculated from the amount of car-bon monoxide exhaled.

Purpose

• To determine the cause of dyspnea

• To assess the effectiveness of a spe-cific therapeutic regimen
• To determine whether a functional abnormality is obstructive or restric-tive
• To measure pulmonary dysfunction
• To evaluate the patient before surgery

Reference values

Normal values are predicted for each patient based on age, height, weight, and sex and are expressed as percent-ages:
• V_T: 5 to 7 mg/kg of body weight
• *ERV:* 25% of VC
• *IC:* 75% of VC
• FEV_1: 83% of VC (after 1 second)
• FEV_2: 94% of VC (after 2 seconds)
• FEV_3: 97% of VC (after 3 seconds).
  Values such as these can be calcu-lated at bedside with a portable spirometer. Results are usually con-sidered abnormal if they're less than 80% of these values.

Implications of results

For information on the implications of test results, see *Interpreting pul-monary function tests,* pages 148 to 150.

Interfering factors

• Lack of patient cooperation, hypox-ia, and metabolic disturbances can make testing difficult or impossible.
• Pregnancy or gastric distention may displace lung volume.
• A narcotic analgesic or sedative can decrease inspiratory and expiratory forces.
• Bronchodilators may temporarily improve pulmonary function.

(Text continues on page 150.)

INTERPRETING PULMONARY FUNCTION TESTS

Test	Method of calculation	Implications
Tidal volume (V_T): amount of air inhaled or exhaled during normal breathing	Determine the spirographic measurement for 10 breaths and divide by 10.	Decreased V_T may indicate restrictive disease and requires further testing, such as full pulmonary function studies and chest radiography.
Minute volume (MV): total amount of air expired per minute	Multiply V_T by the respiration rate.	Normal MV can occur in emphysema; decreased MV may indicate other diseases such as pulmonary edema. Increased MV can occur with acidosis, increased CO_2, decreased partial pressure of arterial oxygen, exercise, and low compliance states.
Carbon dioxide (CO_2) response: increase or decrease in MV after breathing various CO_2 concentrations	Plot changes in MV against increasing inspired CO_2 concentrations.	Reduced CO_2 response may occur in emphysema, myxedema, obesity, hypoventilation syndrome, and sleep apnea.
Inspiratory reserve volume (IRV): amount of air inspired after normal inspiration	Subtract V_T from inspiratory capacity (IC).	Abnormal IRV alone doesn't indicate respiratory dysfunction; IRV decreases during normal exercise.
Expiratory reserve volume (ERV): amount of air exhaled after normal expiration	Determine by direct spirographic measurement.	ERV varies, even in healthy people, but usually decreases in obese people.
Residual volume (RV): amount of air remaining in the lungs after forced expiration	Subtract ERV from FRC.	RV greater than 35% of TLC after maximal expiratory effort may indicate obstructive disease.
Vital capacity (VC): total volume of air that can be exhaled after maximum inspiration	Determine by direct spirographic measurement or add V_T, IRV, and ERV.	Normal or increased VC with decreased flow rates may indicate any condition that reduces functional pulmonary tissue such as pulmonary edema. Decreased VC with normal or increased flow rates may indicate decreased respiratory effort resulting from neuromuscular disease, drug overdose, or head injury; decreased thoracic expansion; or limited movement of diaphragm.
Inspiratory capacity (IC): amount of air that can be inhaled after normal expiration	Determine by direct spirographic measurement or add IRV and V_T.	Decreased IC indicates restrictive disease.

INTERPRETING PULMONARY FUNCTION TESTS (continued)

Test	Method of calculation	Implications
Thoracic gas volume (TGV): total volume of gas in lungs from both ventilated and nonventilated airways	Determine using body plethysmography.	Increased TGV indicates air trapping, which may result from obstructive disease.
Functional residual capacity (FRC): amount of air remaining in lungs after normal expiration	Determine using nitrogen washout, helium dilution technique, or add ERV and RV.	Increased FRC indicates overdistention of lungs, which may result from obstructive pulmonary disease.
Total lung capacity (TLC): total volume of lungs when maximally inflated	Add V_T, IRV, ERV, and RV; FRC and IC; or VC and RV.	Low TLC indicates restrictive disease; high TLC indicates overdistended lungs caused by obstructive disease.
Forced vital capacity (FVC): measurement of the amount of air exhaled forcefully and quickly after maximum inspiration	Determine by direct spirographic measurement (expressed as a percentage of the total volume of gas exhaled).	Decreased FVC indicates flow resistance in respiratory system from obstructive disease such as chronic bronchitis or from restrictive disease such as pulmonary fibrosis.
Flow-volume curve (also called flow-volume loop): greatest rate of flow (Vmax) during FVC maneuvers versus lung volume change	Determine by direct spirographic measurement at 1-second intervals, calculated from flow rates (expressed in liters/second) and lung volume changes (expressed in liters) during maximal inspiratory and expiratory maneuvers.	Decreased flow rates at all volumes during expiration indicate an obstructive disease of the small airways such as emphysema. A plateau of expiratory flow near TLC, a plateau of inspiratory flow at mid-VC, and a square wave pattern through most of VC indicate obstructive disease of large airways. Normal or increased peak expiratory flow, decreased flow with decreasing lung volume, and markedly decreased VC indicate restrictive disease.
Forced expiratory volume (FEV): volume of air expired in the 1st, 2nd, or 3rd second of FVC maneuver	Determine by direct spirographic measurement (expressed as a percentage of FVC).	Decreased FEV_1 and increased FEV_2 and FEV_3 may indicate obstructive disease; decreased or normal FEV_1 may indicate restrictive disease.
Forced expiratory flow (FEF): average rate of flow during middle half of FVC	Calculate from the flow rate and the time needed for expiration of middle 50% of FVC.	Low FEF (25% to 75%) indicates obstructive disease of the small and medium-sized airways.

(continued)

INTERPRETING PULMONARY FUNCTION TESTS *(continued)*

Test	Method of calculation	Implications
Peak expiratory flow rate (PEFR): Vmax during forced expiration	Calculate from flow-volume curve or by direct spirographic measurement using a pneumotachometer or electronic tachometer with a transducer to convert flow to electrical output display.	Decreased PEFR may indicate a mechanical problem, such as upper airway obstruction, or obstructive disease. PEFR is usually normal in restrictive disease but decreases in severe cases. Because PEFR is effort-dependent, it's also low in a person who has poor expiratory effort or doesn't understand the procedure.
Maximal voluntary ventilation (MVV) (also called maximum breathing capacity [MBC]): greatest volume of air breathed per unit of time	Determine by direct spirographic measurement.	Decreased MVV may indicate obstructive disease; normal or decreased MVV may indicate restrictive disease such as myasthenia gravis.
Diffusing capacity for carbon monoxide (DCO): milliliters of carbon monoxide diffused per minute across the alveolocapillary membrane	Calculate from analysis of the amount of carbon monoxide exhaled compared with the amount inhaled.	Decreased DCO because of thickened alveolocapillary membrane occurs in interstitial pulmonary diseases, such as pulmonary fibrosis, asbestosis, and sarcoidosis; it's reduced in emphysema because of the loss of the alveolocapillary membrane.

Radiopharmaceutical myocardial perfusion imaging

This imaging test (also known as chemical stress imaging) is an alternative method of assessing coronary vessel function for patients who can't tolerate exercise or treadmill electrocardiography (ECG). The drugs used to chemically stress the patient include adenosine, dobutamine, and dipyridamole. Infusion of the selected drug I.V. simulates the effects of exercise by increasing blood flow in the coronary arteries. Next, a radiopharmaceutical is injected I.V. to allow imaging, which assists in evaluating the cardiac vessels' response to the drug-induced stress. Both resting and stress images are obtained to evaluate coronary perfusion.

Purpose

• To assess the presence and degree of coronary artery disease (CAD)
• To evaluate therapeutic procedures, such as bypass surgery and coronary angioplasty

Normal findings

Imaging should reveal characteristic distribution of the radiopharmaceutical throughout the left ventricle with no visible defects.

Implications of results

Cold spots are usually due to CAD but may result from myocardial fibrosis, attenuation due to soft tissue (for example, breast and diaphragm), or coronary spasm. The absence of cold spots in the presence of CAD may result from insignificant obstruction, single-vessel disease, or collateral circulation.

Interfering factors

• Cold spots may result from artifacts, such as implants and electrodes.

• The absence of cold spots in the presence of CAD may result from delayed imaging.

Technetium Tc 99m pyrophosphate scanning

Technetium Tc 99m pyrophosphate scanning is used to detect recent myocardial infarction (MI) and to determine its extent. In this test, an I.V. tracer isotope (technetium Tc 99m pyrophosphate) is injected into a vein. The isotope accumulates in damaged myocardial tissue, possibly by combining with calcium in the damaged myocardial cells, where it forms a hot spot on a scan made with a scintillation camera. Such hot spots first appear within 12 hours of infarction, are most apparent after 48 to 72 hours, and usually disappear after 1 week. Hot spots that persist longer than 1 week usually suggest ongoing myocardial damage.

This test is most useful for confirming recent MI when serum enzyme tests are unreliable or when patients suffer from obscure cardiac pain (postoperative cardiac patients) or have equivocal electrocardio-grams, as in left bundle branch block or old myocardial scars.

Purpose

• To confirm recent MI
• To define the size and location of recent MI
• To assess the prognosis after acute MI

Normal findings

A normal technetium scan shows no isotope in the myocardium.

Implications of results

The isotope is absorbed by the sternum and ribs, and their activity is compared with the heart's; 2+, 3+, and 4+ activity (equal to or greater than bone) indicate a positive myocardial scan. The technetium scan can reveal areas of isotope accumulation, or hot spots, in damaged myocardium, particularly 48 to 72 hours after the onset of acute MI. However, hot spots are apparent as early as 12 hours after acute MI. In most patients with MI, hot spots disappear after 1 week. They may persist for several months if necrosis continues in the area of infarction.

Knowing where the infarct is makes it possible to anticipate complications and to plan patient care. About 25% of patients with unstable angina pectoris show hot spots due to subclinical myocardial necrosis and may require coronary arteriography and bypass grafting.

Interfering factors

• In about 10% of patients who undergo this test, isotope accumulation may result from ventricular aneurysm associated with dystrophic calcification, pulmonary neoplasm, recent cardioversion, or valvular heart disease associated with severe calcification.

Thallium imaging

Thallium imaging (also known as cold spot myocardial imaging and thallium scintigraphy) evaluates myocardial blood flow after I.V. injection of the radioisotope thallium-201. Because thallium, the physiologic analogue of potassium, concentrates in healthy myocardial tissue but not in necrotic or ischemic tissue, areas of the heart with normal blood supply and intact cells absorb it rapidly. Areas with poor blood flow and ischemic cells fail to absorb the isotope and appear as cold spots on a scan.

This test is performed in a resting state or after stress. Resting imaging can detect acute myocardial infarction (MI) within the first few hours of symptoms but doesn't distinguish between old and new infarcts. Stress imaging is performed on the patient after he has exercised on a treadmill to the point that he experiences angina or rate-limiting fatigue. It can assess known or suspected coronary artery disease (CAD) and can evaluate the effectiveness of antianginal therapy or balloon angioplasty and the patency of grafts after coronary artery bypass surgery. Complications of stress testing include arrhythmias, angina pectoris, and MI.

Purpose

• To assess myocardial scarring and perfusion
• To demonstrate the location and extent of acute or chronic MI, including transmural and postoperative infarction (resting imaging)
• To diagnose CAD (stress imaging)
• To evaluate the patency of grafts after coronary artery bypass surgery

• To evaluate the effectiveness of antianginal therapy or balloon angioplasty (stress imaging)

Normal findings

Thallium imaging should show normal distribution of the isotope throughout the left ventricle with no defects (cold spots).

Implications of results

Persistent defects indicate MI; transient defects (those that disappear after a 3- to 6-hour rest) indicate ischemia due to CAD. After coronary artery bypass surgery, improved regional perfusion suggests patency of the graft. Increased perfusion after ingestion of antianginal drugs can show that the drugs relieve ischemia. Improved perfusion after balloon angioplasty suggests increased coronary flow.

Interfering factors

• Cold spots may result from sarcoidosis, myocardial fibrosis, cardiac contusion, coronary spasm, or attenuation due to soft tissue and artifacts, such as breast tissue, the diaphragm, implants, and electrodes.
• The absence of cold spots in the presence of CAD may result from an insignificant obstruction, inadequate stress, delayed imaging, single-vessel disease (particularly the right or left circumflex coronary arteries), or collateral circulation.

Total hemoglobin

This test, usually performed as part of a complete blood count, measures the grams of hemoglobin (Hb) found in 100 ml of whole blood. Hemoglobin concentration correlates closely with the red blood cell (RBC) count

NORMAL HEMOGLOBIN VALUES BY AGE

Age	Hemoglobin value (g/dl)
Newborn	17 to 22
1 week	15 to 20
1 month	11 to 15
Children	11 to 13
Adult male	14 to 18
Adult female	12 to 16
Middle-aged adult male	12.4 to 14.9
Middle-aged adult female	11.7 to 13.8

and affects the Hb-RBC ratio (mean corpuscular hemoglobin [MCH] and mean corpuscular hemoglobin concentration [MCHC]). In the laboratory, hemoglobin is chemically converted to pigmented compounds and is measured by spectrophotometry or colorimetry.

Purpose

• To measure the severity of anemia or polycythemia and monitor the response to therapy
• To supply figures for calculating MCH and MCHC

Reference values

Hemoglobin concentration varies, depending on the patient's age and sex and the type of blood sample drawn. (See *Normal hemoglobin values by age*.)

Implications of results

Low hemoglobin concentration may indicate anemia, recent hemorrhage, or hemodilution caused by fluid retention. Elevated hemoglobin suggests hemoconcentration caused by polycythemia or dehydration.

Interfering factors

• Failure to use the proper anticoagulant in the collection tube or to adequately mix the sample and anticoagulant may affect the test results.
• Hemolysis due to rough handling of the sample may adversely affect the test results.
• Prolonged tourniquet constriction may cause hemoconcentration.
• Very high white blood cell counts, hyperlipidemia, or RBCs that are resistant to lysis will falsely elevate hemoglobin values.

Wound culture

A wound culture involves the microscopic analysis of a lesion specimen to confirm infection. Wound cultures may be aerobic (for detection of organisms that usually require oxygen to grow and typically appear in a superficial wound) or anaerobic (for organisms that need little or no oxygen and appear in areas of poor tissue perfusion, such as postoperative wounds, ulcers, and compound fractures). Indications for wound culture include fever as well as inflammation and drainage in damaged tissue.

Purpose

• To identify an infectious microbe in a wound

Normal findings

No pathogenic organisms should be present in a clean wound.

Implications of results

The most common aerobic pathogens in wounds are *Staphylococcus aureus,* group A beta-hemolytic streptococci, *Proteus, Escherichia coli* and other Enterobacteriaceae, and some *Pseudomonas* species. The most common anaerobic pathogens are some *Clostridium* and *Bacteroides* species.

Interfering factors

• Failure to report recent or current antimicrobial therapy may cause false-negative results.
• Poor collection techniques, such as exposing a specimen to oxygen, may contaminate or invalidate the specimen.
• Failure to use the proper transport media may cause the specimen to dry up and the bacteria to die, affecting the accuracy of test results.

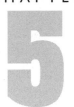

CHAPTER

5

Understanding rhythm strips

Tracing cardiac function

Normal ECG 156

Sinus arrhythmias 159

Atrial arrhythmias 163

Junctional arrhythmias 167

Ventricular arrhythmias 169

Atrioventricular blocks 175

Normal ECG

How to read any ECG: An 8-step guide

An electrocardiogram (ECG) waveform has three basic elements: a P wave, a QRS complex, and a T wave. These are joined by five other useful diagnostic elements: the PR interval, the U wave, the ST segment, the J point, and the QT interval. The diagram below shows how they're related.

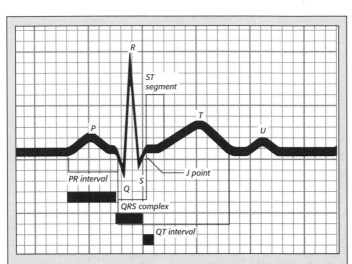

The following 8-step guide will enable you to read any ECG.

Step 1: Evaluate the P wave
Observe the P wave's size, shape, and location in the waveform. If the P wave consistently precedes the QRS complex, the electrical impulse is being initiated by the sinoatrial node, as it should be.

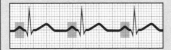

Step 2: Evaluate the atrial rhythm
The P wave should occur at regular intervals with only small variations that are associated with respiration. Using a pair of calipers, you can easi-ly measure the interval between P waves (the P-P interval). Compare the P-P intervals in several ECG cycles. Make sure the calipers are set at the same point — at the beginning of the wave or on its peak. Instead of lifting the calipers, rotate one of its legs to the next P wave, to ensure accurate measurements.

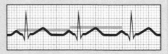

Step 3: Determine the atrial rate
To determine the atrial rate quickly, count the number of P waves in two 3-second segments. Multiply this number by 10.

For a more accurate determination, count the number of small squares between two P waves using either the apex of the wave or the initial upstroke of the wave. Each small square equals 0.04 second; 1,500 squares equal 1 minute (0.04 × 1,500 = 60 seconds). So, divide 1,500 by the number of squares you counted between the P waves. This gives you the atrial rate — the number of contractions per minute.

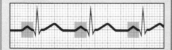

Step 4: Calculate duration of the PR interval

Count the number of small squares between the beginning of the P wave and the beginning of the QRS complex. Multiply the number of squares by 0.04 second. The normal interval is between 0.12 and 0.2 second, or between 3 and 5 small squares wide. A wider interval indicates delayed conduction of the impulse through the atrioventricular (AV) node to the ventricles. A short PR interval indicates that the impulse originated in an area other than the sinoatrial (SA) node.

Step 5: Evaluate the ventricular rhythm

Use the calipers to measure the R-R intervals. Remember to place the calipers on the same point of the QRS complex. If the R-R intervals remain consistent, the ventricular rhythm is regular.

Step 6: Determine the ventricular rate

To determine the ventricular rate, use the same formula as in Step 3. In this case, however, count the number of small squares between two R waves to do the calculation. Also check that the QRS complex is shaped appropriately for the lead you're monitoring.

Step 7: Calculate the duration of the QRS complex

Count the number of squares between the beginning and the end of the QRS complex and multiply by 0.04 second. A normal QRS complex is less than 0.12 second, or less than 3 small squares wide. Some references specify 0.06 to 0.1 second as the normal duration for the QRS complex.

Step 8: Calculate the duration of the QT interval

Count the number of squares from the beginning of the QRS complex to the end of the T wave. Multiply this number by 0.04 second. The normal range is 0.36 to 0.44 second, or 9 to 11 small squares wide.

Normal sinus rhythm

When the heart functions normally, the sinoatrial (SA) node acts as the primary pacemaker, initiating the electrical impulses that set the rhythm for cardiac contractions. The SA node assumes this role because its automatic firing rate exceeds that of the heart's other pacemakers, allowing cells to depolarize spontaneously. Two factors account for increased automaticity. First, during the resting phase of the depolarization-repolarization cycle, SA node cells have the least negative charge. Second, depolarization actually begins during the resting phase.

Based on an electrical disturbance's location, arrhythmias can be classified as sinus, atrial, junctional, or ventricular arrhythmias or atrioventricular (AV) blocks. Functional

disturbances in the SA node produce sinus arrhythmias. Enhanced automaticity of atrial tissue or reentry may produce atrial arrhythmias, the most common arrhythmias.

Junctional arrhythmias originate in the area around the AV node and the bundle of His. These arrhythmias usually result from a suppressed higher pacemaker or blocked impulses at the AV node.

Ventricular arrhythmias originate in ventricular tissue below the bifurcation of the bundle of His. These rhythms may result from reentry or enhanced automaticity or after depolarization.

An AV block results from an abnormal interruption or delay of atrial impulse conduction to the ventricles. It may be partial or total and may occur in the AV node, the bundle of His, or the Purkinje system.

Characteristics and interpretation

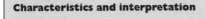
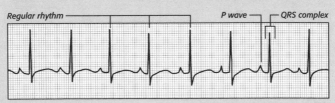

Regular rhythm ———— P wave —— ┌ QRS complex

Lead II

Atrial rhythm: regular
Ventricular rhythm: regular
Atrial rate: 60 to 100 beats/minute (80 beats/minute shown)
Ventricular rate: 60 to 100 beats/minute (80 beats/minute shown)
P wave: normally shaped (All P waves have similar size and shape; a P wave precedes each QRS complex.)
PR interval: within normal limits (0.12 to 0.2 second) and constant (0.20-second duration shown)

QRS complex: within normal limits of 0.06 to 0.1 second (All QRS complexes have the same configuration. Duration of 0.12 second is shown.)
T wave: normally shaped, upright and rounded (A T wave follows each QRS complex.)
QT interval: within normal limits of 0.36 to 0.44 second and constant (0.44-second duration shown)

Sinus arrhythmias

Sinus arrhythmia

In this type of arrhythmia, the heart rate stays within normal limits but the rhythm is irregular and corresponds to the respiratory cycle and variations of vagal tone. During inspiration, an increased volume of blood returns to the heart, reducing vagal tone and increasing sinus rate. During expiration, venous return decreases, vagal tone increases, and sinus rate slows.

Conditions unrelated to respiration may also produce sinus arrhythmia. These conditions include an inferior wall myocardial infarction, digitalis toxicity, and increased intracranial pressure.

Sinus arrhythmia is easily recognized in elderly, pediatric, and sedated patients. The patient's pulse rate increases with inspiration and decreases with expiration. Usually, the patient will be asymptomatic.

Intervention

Treatment isn't usually necessary, unless the patient is symptomatic or the sinus arrhythmia stems from an underlying cause. When the patient is symptomatic, atropine may be administered if the heart rate falls below 40 beats/minute.

Characteristics and interpretation

Cyclic, irregular rhythm

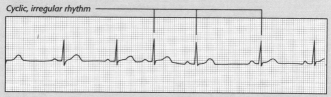

Lead II

Atrial rhythm: irregular, corresponding to the respiratory cycle
Ventricular rhythm: irregular, corresponding to the respiratory cycle
Atrial rate: within normal limits; varies with respiration (60 beats/minute shown)
Ventricular rate: within normal limits; varies with respiration (60 beats/minute shown)
P wave: normal size and configuration (A P wave precedes each QRS complex.)

PR interval: within normal limits and constant (0.16-second duration shown)
QRS complex: normal duration and configuration (0.06-second duration shown)
T wave: normal size and configuration
QT interval: within normal limits (0.36-second duration shown)
Other: phasic slowing and quickening of the rhythm

Sinus bradycardia

Characterized by a sinus rate of less than 60 beats/minute, sinus bradycardia usually occurs as the normal response to a reduced demand for blood flow. It's common among athletes, whose well-conditioned hearts can maintain stroke volume with reduced effort. It may also be caused by drugs, such as digitalis glycosides, calcium channel blockers, and beta-adrenergic blockers.

Sinus bradycardia may occur after an inferior wall myocardial infarction involving the right coronary artery, which provides the blood supply to the sinoatrial node. The rhythm may develop during sleep and in patients with elevated intracranial pressure. It may also result from vagal stimulation caused by vomiting or defecating. Pathologic sinus bradycardia may occur with sick sinus syndrome.

The patient with sinus bradycardia will be asymptomatic if he's able to compensate for the drop in heart rate by increasing stroke volume. If not, he may have signs and symptoms of decreased cardiac output, such as hypotension, syncope, confusion, and blurred vision.

Intervention

If the patient is asymptomatic, treatment isn't necessary. If he has signs and symptoms, treatment aims to identify and correct the underlying cause. The heart rate may be increased with such drugs as atropine or isoproterenol (Isuprel). A temporary or permanent pacemaker may be inserted if the bradycardia persists.

Characteristics and interpretation

Regular rhythm with rate less than 60 beats/minute

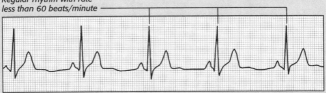

Lead II

Atrial rhythm: regular
Ventricular rhythm: regular
Atrial rate: less than 60 beats/minute (50 beats/minute shown)
Ventricular rate: less than 60 beats/minute (50 beats/minute shown)
P wave: normal size and configuration (A P wave precedes each QRS complex.)

PR interval: within normal limits and constant (0.14-second duration shown)
QRS complex: normal duration and configuration (0.08-second duration shown)
T wave: normal size and configuration
QT interval: within normal limits (0.4-second duration shown)

Sinus tachycardia

A normal response to cellular demands for increased oxygen delivery and blood flow commonly produces sinus tachycardia. Conditions causing such a demand include heart failure, shock, anemia, exercise, fever, hypoxia, pain, and stress. Drugs that stimulate the beta-receptors in the heart will also cause sinus tachycardia. These include isoproterenol (Isuprel), aminophylline (Aminophyllin), and inotropic agents such as dobutamine. Alcohol, caffeine, and nicotine may also produce sinus tachycardia.

An elevated heart rate increases myocardial oxygen demands. If the patient can't meet these demands (for example, because of coronary artery disease), ischemia and further myocardial damage may occur. If tachycardia exceeds 140 beats/minute for longer than 30 minutes, ECG may show ST-segment and T-wave changes, indicating ischemia.

Intervention

Treatment focuses on finding the primary cause. If it's high catecholamine levels, a beta-adrenergic blocker may slow the heart rate. After myocardial infarction, persistent sinus tachycardia may precede heart failure or cardiogenic shock.

Characteristics and interpretation

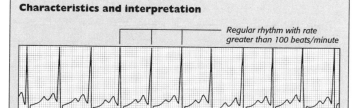

Regular rhythm with rate greater than 100 beats/minute

Lead II

Atrial rhythm: regular
Ventricular rhythm: regular
Atrial rate: 100 to 160 beats/minute (110 beats/minute shown)
Ventricular rate: 100 to 160 beats/minute (110 beats/minute shown)
P wave: normal size and configuration (A P wave precedes each QRS complex. As the sinus rate reaches roughly 150 beats/minute, the P wave merges with the preceding T wave and may be difficult to identify. Examine the descending slope of the preceding T wave closely for notches, indicating the presence of the P wave; normal P wave shown.)
PR interval: within normal limits and constant (0.16-second duration shown)
QRS complex: normal duration and configuration (0.1-second duration shown)
T wave: normal size and configuration
QT interval: within normal limits and constant (0.36-second duration shown)
Other: gradual onset and cessation

Sinus arrest

Failure of the sinoatrial node to generate an impulse interrupts the sinus rhythm, producing sinus pause when one or two beats are dropped and sinus arrest when three or more beats are dropped. Such failure may result from an acute inferior wall myocardial infarction, increased vagal tone, or use of certain drugs, such as digitalis glycosides, calcium channel blockers, and beta-adrenergic blockers. The arrhythmia may also be linked to sick sinus syndrome.

The patient will have an irregular pulse rate associated with the sinus rhythm pauses. If the pauses are infrequent, the patient will be asymptomatic. If they occur frequently and last for several seconds, the patient may have signs of decreased cardiac output.

Intervention

For the symptomatic patient, treatment focuses on maintaining cardiac output and discovering the cause of the sinus arrest. If indicated, atropine may be given or a temporary or permanent pacemaker may be inserted.

Characteristics and interpretation

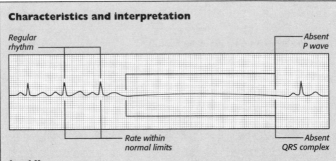

Regular rhythm

Absent P wave

Rate within normal limits

Absent QRS complex

Lead II

Atrial rhythm: regular, except for the missing complex
Ventricular rhythm: regular, except for the missing complex
Atrial rate: within normal limits but varies because of the pauses (94 beats/minute shown)
Ventricular rate: within normal limits but varies because of pauses (94 beats/minute shown)
P wave: normal size and configuration (A P wave precedes each QRS complex but is absent during a pause.)

PR interval: within normal limits and constant when P wave is present; immeasurable when P wave is absent (0.2-second duration shown on all complexes surrounding the arrest)
QRS complex: normal duration and configuration; QRS complex absent during a pause (0.08-second duration shown)
T wave: normal size and configuration; absent during a pause
QT interval: within normal limits and constant; immeasurable during a pause (0.4-second interval shown)

Atrial arrhythmias

Premature atrial contractions

An irritable focus in the atria that supersedes the sinoatrial node as the pacemaker for one or two beats can cause premature atrial contractions (PACs). Although PACs commonly occur in normal hearts, they're also associated with ischemic and valvular heart disease. In an inferior wall myocardial infarction (MI), PACs may indicate a concomitant right atrial infarct. In an anterior wall MI, PACs are an early sign of left-sided heart failure. They also may warn of a more severe atrial arrhythmia, such as atrial flutter and atrial fibrillation.

Possible causes include digitalis toxicity, hyperthyroidism, elevated catecholamine levels, acute respiratory failure, and chronic obstructive pulmonary disease.

Intervention

Symptomatic patients may be treated with propranolol (Inderal) and disopyramide (Norpace).

Characteristics and interpretation

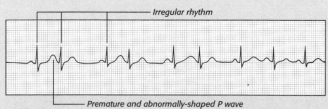

Irregular rhythm

Premature and abnormally-shaped P wave

Lead II

Atrial rhythm: irregular; incomplete compensatory pause follows PAC; underlying rhythm possibly regular
Ventricular rhythm: irregular; incomplete compensatory pause follows PAC; underlying rhythm possibly regular
Atrial rate: varies with underlying rhythm (90 beats/minute shown)
Ventricular rate: varies with underlying rhythm (90 beats/minute shown)
P wave: premature and abnormally shaped; possibly lost in previous T wave (Varying configurations indicate multiform PACs.)

PR interval: usually normal and constant but may be shortened or slightly prolonged, depending on the origin of the ectopic focus (0.16-second duration shown)
QRS complex: usually normal and constant duration and configuration. (0.08-second duration shown)
T wave: usually normal configuration; may be distorted if P wave is hidden in previous T wave
QT interval: usually normal and constant (0.36-second duration shown)
Other: possible occurrence in bigeminy or couplets

Atrial tachycardia

In this arrhythmia, the atrial rhythm is ectopic and the atrial rate is rapid, shortening diastole. This results in a loss of atrial kick, reduced cardiac output, reduced coronary perfusion, and ischemic myocardial changes.

Although atrial tachycardia occurs in healthy patients, it's usually associated with high catecholamine levels, digitalis toxicity, myocardial infarction, cardiomyopathy, hyperthyroidism, hypertension, and valvular heart disease. Three types of atrial tachycardia exist: atrial tachycardia with block, multifocal atrial tachycardia, and paroxysmal atrial tachycardia.

Intervention

If the patient is symptomatic, prepare for immediate cardioversion. If the patient is stable, the doctor may perform carotid sinus massage (if no bruits are present) or order drug therapy, such as adenosine (Adenocard), verapamil (Calan), digoxin (Lanoxin), beta-adrenergic blockers, or diltiazem (Cardizem). If these measures fail, cardioversion may be necessary.

Characteristics and interpretation

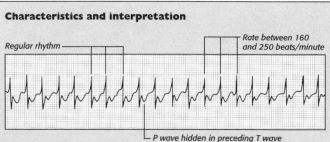

Regular rhythm

Rate between 160 and 250 beats/minute

P wave hidden in preceding T wave

Lead II

Atrial rhythm: regular
Ventricular rhythm: regular
Atrial rate: three or more successive ectopic atrial beats at a rate of 160 to 250 beats/minute (210 beats/minute shown)
Ventricular rate: varies with atrioventricular (AV) conduction ratio (210 beats/minute shown)
P wave: 1:1 ratio with QRS complex, though often indiscernible due to rapid rate; possibly hidden in previous ST segment or T wave
PR interval: may be immeasurable if P wave can't be distinguished from preceding T wave (If P wave is present, PR interval is short when conduction through the AV node is 1:1. On this strip, the PR interval isn't discernible.)
QRS complex: usually normal unless aberrant intraventricular conduction is present (0.1-second duration shown)
T wave: may be normal or inverted if ischemia is present (inverted T waves shown)
QT interval: usually normal but may be shorter due to rapid rate (0.2-second duration shown)
Other: ST-segment and T-wave changes if tachyarrhythmia persists longer than 30 minutes

Atrial flutter

Characterized by an atrial rate of 300 beats/minute or more, atrial flutter results from multiple reentry circuits within the atrial tissue. Causes include conditions that enlarge atrial tissue and elevate atrial pressures, such as myocardial infarction, increased catecholamine levels, hyperthyroidism, and digitalis toxicity. A ventricular rate of 300 beats/minute suggests the presence of an anomalous pathway.

If the patient's pulse rate is normal, he usually has no symptoms. If his pulse rate is high, he'll probably have signs and symptoms of decreased cardiac output, such as hypotension and syncope.

Intervention

The doctor may perform vagal stimulation to slow the ventricular response and demonstrate the presence of flutter waves. This is contraindicated if carotid bruit is present. If the patient is symptomatic, prepare for immediate cardioversion.

Drugs that may be ordered to slow atrioventricular conduction include calcium channel blockers (diltiazem, verapamil) and beta-adrenergic blockers (esmolol, metoprolol). Digoxin may be ordered, but some experts question its use for urgent treatment. After the rate slows, if conversion to a normal rhythm hasn't occurred, procainamide (Pronestyl) or quinidine (Quinidex) may be ordered.

Characteristics and interpretation

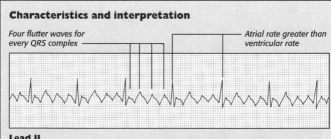

Four flutter waves for every QRS complex

Atrial rate greater than ventricular rate

Lead II

Atrial rhythm: regular
Ventricular rhythm: regular or irregular, depending on the conduction ratio (regular rhythm shown)
Atrial rate: 300 to 350 beats/minute (300 beats/minute shown)
Ventricular rate: variable (70 beats/minute shown)
P wave: atrial activity seen as flutter waves, often with a saw-toothed appearance

PR interval: not measurable
QRS complex: usually normal, but possibly distorted by the underlying flutter waves (0.1-second, normal duration shown)
T wave: not identifiable
QT interval: not measurable

Atrial fibrillation

Defined as chaotic, asynchronous electrical activity in the atrial tissue, atrial fibrillation results from impulses in many reentry pathways. These impulses cause the atria to quiver instead of contract regularly. With this arrhythmia, blood may pool in the left atrial appendage and form thrombi that can be ejected into the systemic circulation. An associated rapid ventricular rate can decrease cardiac output.

Possible causes include valvular disorders, hypertension, coronary artery disease, myocardial infarction, and the use of certain drugs, such as aminophylline (Aminophyllin) and digitalis glycosides.

Intervention

If the patient is symptomatic, synchronized cardioversion should be used immediately. Vagal stimulation may be used to slow the ventricular response, but it won't convert the arrhythmia.

Drugs that may be ordered to slow atrioventricular conduction include calcium channel blockers (diltiazem) and beta-adrenergic blockers (metoprolol). Digoxin may be ordered if the patient is stable. After the rate slows, if conversion to a normal sinus rhythm hasn't occurred, amiodarone (Cordarone), procainamide (Pronestyl) or quinidine (Quinidex) may be ordered. If atrial fibrillation is of several days' duration, anticoagulant therapy is recommended before pharmacologic or electrical conversion. If atrial fibrillation is of recent onset, ibutilide (Corvert) may be used to convert the rhythm.

Characteristics and interpretation

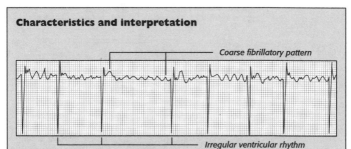

Coarse fibrillatory pattern

Irregular ventricular rhythm

Lead II

Atrial rhythm: grossly irregular
Ventricular rhythm: grossly irregular
Atrial rate: greater than 400 beats/minute
Ventricular rate: 60 to 150 beats/minute, depending on treatment (80 beats/minute shown)
P wave: absent; erratic baseline fibrillatory waves (f waves) in place (When the f waves are pronounced, the arrhythmia is called coarse atrial

fibrillation. When the f waves aren't pronounced, the arrhythmia is known as fine atrial fibrillation. On this strip, the f waves are pronounced.)
PR interval: indiscernible
QRS complex: duration usually within normal limits, with aberrant intraventricular conduction (0.08-second duration shown)
T wave: indiscernible
QT interval: not measurable

Junctional arrhythmias

Junctional rhythm

This arrhythmia occurs in the atrioventricular junctional tissue, producing retrograde depolarization of the atrial tissue and antegrade depolarization of the ventricular tissue. It results from conditions that depress sinoatrial node function, such as an inferior wall myocardial infarction (MI), digitalis toxicity, and vagal stimulation. The arrhythmia may also stem from an increased automaticity of the junctional tissue, which can be brought about by digitalis toxicity or ischemia associated with an inferior wall MI.

A junctional rhythm with a ventricular rate of 60 to 100 beats/minute is known as an accelerated junctional rhythm. If the ventricular rate exceeds 100 beats/minute, the arrhythmia is called junctional tachycardia.

Intervention

Treatment aims to identify and manage the arrhythmia's primary cause. If the patient is symptomatic, treatment may include atropine to increase the sinus or junctional rate. Alternatively, the doctor may insert a pacemaker to maintain an effective heart rate.

Characteristics and interpretation

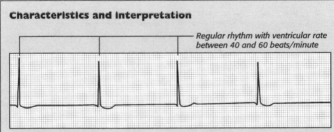

Regular rhythm with ventricular rate between 40 and 60 beats/minute

Lead II

Atrial rhythm: regular
Ventricular rhythm: regular
Atrial rate: if discernible, 40 to 60 beats/minute (On this strip, the rate isn't discernible.)
Ventricular rate: 40 to 60 beats/minute (40 beats/minute shown)
P wave: usually inverted; may precede, follow, or fall within the QRS complex or may be absent (On this strip, the P wave is absent.)

PR interval: less than 0.12 second and constant if the P wave precedes the QRS complex, otherwise not measurable (On this strip, it can't be measured.)
QRS complex: duration normal; configuration usually normal (0.08-second duration shown)
T wave: usually normal configuration
QT interval: usually normal (0.32-second duration shown)

Premature junctional contractions

A junctional beat that occurs before the next normal sinus beat in a rhythm is called a premature junctional contraction (PJC). Ectopic beats, PJCs commonly result from increased automaticity in the bundle of His or the surrounding junctional tissue. This interrupts the underlying rhythm. The patient may complain of palpitations if PJCs are frequent.

PJCs most commonly result from digitalis toxicity. Their other causes include ischemia associated with an inferior wall myocardial infarction, excessive caffeine ingestion, and excessive levels of amphetamines.

Intervention

In most cases, treatment is directed at the underlying cause.

Characteristics and interpretation

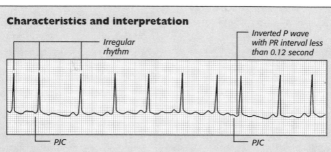

Irregular rhythm

Inverted P wave with PR interval less than 0.12 second

PJC   PJC

Lead II

Atrial rhythm: irregular with PJC, but underlying rhythm may be regular
Ventricular rhythm: irregular with PJC, but underlying rhythm may be regular
Atrial rate: follows the underlying rhythm (100 beats/minute shown)
Ventricular rate: follows the underlying rhythm (100 beats/minute shown)
P wave: usually inverted; may precede, follow, or fall within the QRS complex or may be absent (On this strip, it precedes the QRS complex.)

PR interval: less than 0.12 second on the PJC if P wave precedes the QRS complex, otherwise not measurable (0.14-second, constant duration shown on the underlying rhythm, 0.06-second duration shown on the PJC)
QRS complex: normal duration and configuration (0.06-second duration shown)
T wave: usually normal configuration
QT interval: usually within normal limits (0.3-second duration shown)

Ventricular arrhythmias

Premature ventricular contractions

Among the most common arrhythmias, premature ventricular contractions (PVCs) occur in both healthy and diseased hearts. These ectopic beats may occur singly or in clusters of two or more. They also occur in bigeminy, trigeminy, or quadrageminy.

PVCs may result from the use of digitalis glycosides and sympathomimetic drugs or from electrolyte imbalances, such as hypokalemia and hypocalcemia. They may also result from exercise or ingestion of caffeine, tobacco, or alcohol. The arrhythmia may also result from hypoxia, myocardial infarction, and myocardial irritation by pacemaker electrodes.

When you detect PVCs, you must determine whether they appear in a pattern that indicates danger. Paired PVCs, for instance, can produce ventricular tachycardia because the second PVC usually meets refractory tissue. A salvo, three or more PVCs in a row, is considered a run of ventricular tachycardia. Multiform PVCs look different from one another and arise from different ventricular sites; alternatively, they may arise from the same site but be abnormally conducted. In R-on-T phenomenon, the PVC occurs so early that it falls on the T wave of the preceding beat. Because the cells haven't fully depolarized, ventricular tachycardia or fibrillation can result.

When palpating the peripheral pulse in a patient with PVCs, you may feel a longer than normal pause immediately after the PVC, depending on how early in the cardiac cycle the beat occurs. The earlier the beat, the shorter the diastolic filling time and the lower the stroke volume. Some patients complain of palpitations with frequent PVCs.

Intervention

If the PVCs are thought to result from a serious cardiac problem, lidocaine (Xylocaine) or other antiarrhythmics, such as procainamide (Pronestyl) and quinidine (Quinidex, Quinora), may be given to suppress ventricular irritability. When a patient's PVCs are thought to result from a noncardiac problem, treatment aims at correcting the underlying cause — correcting an acid-base or electrolyte disturbance, discontinuing an antiarrhythmic, treating hypothermia, or correcting high catecholamine levels.

(continued)

Characteristics and interpretation

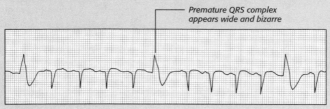

Premature QRS complex appears wide and bizarre

Lead II

Atrial rhythm: irregular during PVC; underlying rhythm may be regular
Ventricular rhythm: irregular during PVC; underlying rhythm may be regular
Atrial rate: follows underlying rhythm (120 beats/minute shown)
Ventricular rate: follows underlying rhythm (120 beats/minute)
P wave: atrial activity independent of the PVC (If retrograde atrial depolarization exists, a retrograde P wave will distort the ST segment of the PVC. On this strip, no P wave appears before the PVC but one occurs with each QRS complex.)
PR interval: determined by underlying rhythm, not associated with the PVC

(0.12-second, constant duration shown)
QRS complex: occurs earlier than expected with duration that exceeds 0.12 second and a complex of bizarre configuration; possibly normal underlying rhythm (0.08-second duration shown in the normal beats; bizarre and 0.12-second duration shown in the PVC)
T wave: occurs in the direction opposite the QRS complex; normal in the underlying complexes
QT interval: not usually measured in the PVC but may be within normal limits in the underlying rhythm (0.28-second duration shown in the underlying rhythm)

Ventricular tachycardia

This life-threatening arrhythmia develops when three or more premature ventricular contractions occur in a row and the rate exceeds 100 beats/minute. It may result from enhanced automaticity or reentry within the Purkinje system. The rapid ventricular rate reduces ventricular filling time and, because atrial kick is lost, cardiac output drops.

Ventricular tachycardia usually results from acute myocardial infarction, coronary artery disease, valvular heart disease, heart failure, or cardiomyopathy. The arrhythmia can also stem from an electrolyte imbalance or from toxic levels of such drugs as a digitalis glycoside, procainamide (Pronestyl), or quinidine (Quinidex). You may detect two variations of this arrhythmia: R-on-T phenomenon and torsades de pointes.

Intervention

This rhythm often degenerates into ventricular fibrillation and cardiovascular collapse, requiring immediate cardiopulmonary resuscitation and defibrillation. If the patient is symptomatic, prepare for immediate cardioversion, followed by antiarrhythmic therapy. Lidocaine (Xylocaine) is usually administered immediately. If it proves ineffective, procainamide (Pronestyl) or bretylium (Bretylol) is used.

Characteristics and interpretation

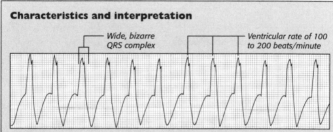

Wide, bizarre QRS complex

Ventricular rate of 100 to 200 beats/minute

Lead II

Atrial rhythm: independent P waves possibly discernible with slower ventricular rates (On this strip, the P waves aren't visible.)
Ventricular rhythm: usually regular, but may be slightly irregular (On this strip, it's regular.)
Atrial rate: can't be determined
Ventricular rate: usually 100 to 200 beats/minute (120 beats/minute shown)

P wave: usually absent; may be obscured by the QRS complex; possible presence of retrograde P waves
PR interval: not measurable
QRS complex: duration greater than 0.12 second; bizarre appearance, usually with increased amplitude (0.16-second duration shown)
T wave: opposite the terminal forces of the QRS complex
QT interval: not measurable

Ventricular fibrillation

Defined as chaotic, asynchronous electrical activity within the ventricular tissue, ventricular fibrillation results in death if the rhythm isn't stopped immediately. Conditions leading to ventricular fibrillation include myocardial ischemia, hypokalemia, cocaine toxicity, hypoxia, hypothermia, severe acidosis, and severe alkalosis.

Patients with myocardial infarctions have the greatest risk of ventricular fibrillation during the initial 2 hours after the onset of chest pain. Those who experience ventricular fibrillation will have a reduced risk of recurrence as healing progresses and scar tissue forms.

In ventricular fibrillation, a lack of cardiac output results in a loss of consciousness, pulselessness, and respiratory arrest. Coarse fibrillatory waves may initially be seen on the electrocardiogram strip. As acidosis develops, the waves become fine and progress to asystole unless defibrillation restores cardiac rhythm.

Intervention

Perform cardiopulmonary resuscitation until the patient can receive defibrillation. Administer epinephrine if the initial defibrillation series is unsuccessful. Other drugs that may be used include lidocaine (Xylocaine), bretylium (Bretylate), and procainamide (Pronestyl). Magnesium sulfate may be used for torsades de pointes or refractory ventricular fibrillation.

Characteristics and interpretation

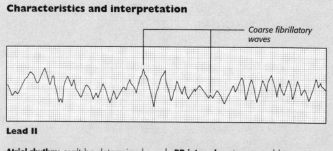

Coarse fibrillatory waves

Lead II

Atrial rhythm: can't be determined
Ventricular rhythm: irregular
Atrial rate: can't be determined
Ventricular rate: can't be determined
P wave: indiscernible

PR interval: not measurable
QRS complex: replaced with fibrillatory waves; duration can't be determined
T wave: can't be determined
QT interval: not measurable

Idioventricular rhythm

This life-threatening arrhythmia acts as a safety mechanism when all potential pacemakers above the ventricles fail to discharge or when a block prevents supraventricular impulses from reaching the ventricles.

The slow ventricular rate and loss of atrial kick associated with this arrhythmia will markedly reduce the patient's cardiac output. In turn, this will cause hypotension, confusion, vertigo, and syncope.

Intervention

Treatment aims to identify and manage the primary problem that triggered this safety mechanism.

Atropine may be given to increase the patient's atrial rate. A pacemaker may also be inserted to increase the heart rate and improve cardiac output.

Characteristics and interpretation

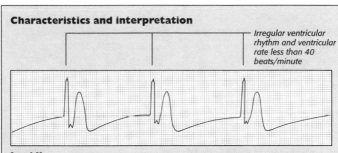

Irregular ventricular rhythm and ventricular rate less than 40 beats/minute

Lead II

Atrial rhythm: unable to be determined

Ventricular rhythm: usually regular, except with isolated escape beats (On this strip, the rhythm is irregular.)

Atrial rate: unable to be determined

Ventricular rate: less than 40 beats/minute (30 beats/minute shown)

P wave: absent

PR interval: usually not measurable

QRS complex: duration greater than 0.12 second; wide complex with bizarre configuration (0.2-second, bizarre complex shown)

T wave: directed opposite terminal forces of QRS complex

QT interval: usually greater than 0.44 second (0.46-second duration shown)

Accelerated idioventricular rhythm

When the pacemaker cells above the ventricles fail to generate an impulse or when a block prevents supraventricular impulses from reaching the ventricles, life-threatening idioventricular rhythms result. When the rate of an idioventricular rhythm ranges from 40 to 100 beats/minute, it's considered accelerated idioventricular rhythm, denoting a rate greater than the inherent pacemaker.

In this rhythm, the cells of the His-Purkinje system operate as pacemaker cells. The characteristic waveform results from an area of enhanced automaticity within the ventricles, which may be associated with myocardial infarction, digitalis toxicity, or metabolic imbalances. In addition, the arrhythmia commonly occurs during myocardial reperfusion following thrombolytic therapy.

The patient may or may not be symptomatic, depending on his heart rate and ability to compensate for the loss of the atrial kick. If symptomatic, he may experience signs and symptoms of decreased cardiac output, including hypotension, confusion, syncope, and blurred vision.

Intervention

An asymptomatic patient needs no treatment. For a symptomatic patient, treatment focuses on maintaining cardiac output and identifying the cause of the arrhythmia. The patient may require an atrial pacemaker to enhance cardiac output.

ALERT Accelerated idioventricular rhythm protects the heart from ventricular standstill and never should be treated with lidocaine (Xylocaine) or other antiarrhythmic agents.

Characteristics and interpretation

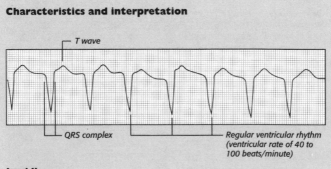

T wave

QRS complex

Regular ventricular rhythm (ventricular rate of 40 to 100 beats/minute)

Lead II

Atrial rhythm: can't be determined
Ventricular rhythm: usually regular
Atrial rate: can't be determined
Ventricular rate: 40 to 100 beats/minute
P wave: absent
PR interval: can't be measured

QRS complex: duration greater than 0.12 second; wide and bizarre configuration
T wave: deflection usually opposite that of QRS complex
QT interval: within normal limits or possibly prolonged

Atrioventricular blocks

First-degree atrioventricular block

Defined as delayed conduction velocity through the atrioventricular (AV) node or His-Purkinje system, first-degree AV block is associated with an inferior wall myocardial infarction and the effects of digitalis glycosides or amiodarone (Cordarone). The arrhythmia is also associated with chronic degeneration of the conduction system.

Usually, patients with first-degree AV block are asymptomatic.

Intervention

Management of first-degree AV block includes identifying and treating the underlying cause as well as monitoring the patient for signs of progressive AV block.

Characteristics and interpretation

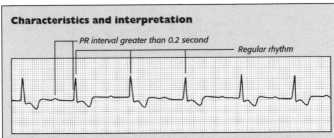

PR interval greater than 0.2 second

Regular rhythm

Lead II

Atrial rhythm: regular
Ventricular rhythm: regular
Atrial rate: usually within normal limits (60 beats/minute shown)
Ventricular rate: usually within normal limits (60 beats/minute shown)
P wave: normal size and configuration (One P wave precedes each QRS complex.)

PR interval: greater than 0.20 second and constant (0.32-second duration shown)
QRS complex: usually normal duration and configuration (0.08-second duration and normal configuration shown)
T wave: normal size and configuration
QT interval: usually within normal limits (0.32-second duration shown)

Type I second-degree atrioventricular block

In Type I (Wenckebach or Mobitz type I) second-degree atrioventricular (AV) block, diseased AV node tissues conduct impulses to the ventricles increasingly later until one of the atrial impulses fails to be conducted or is blocked. Type I block most commonly occurs at the level of the AV node and is caused by an inferior wall myocardial infarction, vagal stimulation, or digitalis toxicity.

The arrhythmia usually doesn't cause symptoms. However, a patient may have signs and symptoms of decreased cardiac output, such as hypotension, confusion, and syncope. These effects occur especially if the patient's ventricular rate is slow.

Intervention

If the patient is asymptomatic, no intervention is required other than monitoring the electrocardiogram frequently to see if a more serious form of AV block develops.

If the patient is symptomatic, the doctor may order atropine to increase the rate and stop the decremental conduction through the AV node. Occasionally, the doctor may insert a temporary pacemaker to maintain effective cardiac output.

Characteristics and interpretation

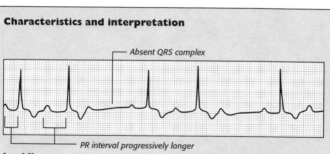

— Absent QRS complex

— PR interval progressively longer

Lead II

Atrial rhythm: regular
Ventricular rhythm: irregular
Atrial rate: determined by the underlying rhythm (80 beats/minute shown)
Ventricular rate: slower than the atrial rate (50 beats/minute shown)
P wave: normal size and configuration
PR interval: progressively prolonged with each beat until a P wave appears without a QRS complex

QRS complex: normal duration and configuration; periodically absent. (0.08-second duration shown)
T wave: normal size and configuration
QT interval: usually within normal limits (0.46-second and constant duration shown)
Other: usually distinguished by a pattern of group beating, referred to as the footprints of Wenckebach

Type II second-degree atrioventricular block

Produced by a conduction disturbance in the His-Purkinje system, a Type II (Mobitz type II) second-degree atrioventricular (AV) block causes an intermittent absence of conduction. In this life-threatening arrhythmia, two or more atrial impulses are conducted to the ventricles with constant PR intervals; suddenly, without warning, the atrial impulse is blocked. This type of block occurs in an anterior wall myocardial infarction (MI), severe coronary artery disease, and chronic degeneration of the conduction system.

Intervention

If the patient is hypotensive, treatment aims at increasing his heart rate to improve cardiac output. Because the conduction block occurs in the His-Purkinje system, drugs that act directly on the myocardium usually prove more effective than those that increase the atrial rate. As a result, dopamine (Intropin), instead of atropine, may be ordered to increase the ventricular rate.

If the patient has an anterior wall MI, the doctor will immediately insert a temporary pacemaker to prevent ventricular asystole. For long-term management, the patient will usually need a permanent pacemaker.

Characteristics and interpretation

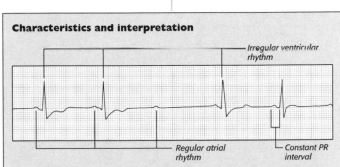

Irregular ventricular rhythm

Regular atrial rhythm

Constant PR interval

Lead II

Atrial rhythm: regular
Ventricular rhythm: regular or irregular
Atrial rate: usually within normal limits (60 beats/minute shown)
Ventricular rate: may be within normal limits but less than the atrial rate (40 beats/minute shown)
P wave: normal size and configuration (Not all P waves will be followed by a QRS complex.)

PR interval: constant and commonly within normal limits for all conducted beats
QRS complex: usually greater than 0.16 second due to the presence of a preexisting bundle branch heart block (0.12-second complex shown)
T wave: usually normal size and configuration
QT interval: usually within normal limits (0.44-second duration shown)

Third-degree atrio-ventricular block

Also called complete heart block, third-degree atrioventricular (AV) block is a life-threatening arrhythmia that occurs when all supraventricular impulses are prevented from reaching the ventricles. If this type of block originates at the AV node, a junctional escape rhythm occurs; if it originates below the AV node, an idioventricular escape rhythm occurs.

Third-degree AV block involving the AV node may result from an inferior wall myocardial infarction (MI) or drug toxicity (digitalis glycosides, beta-adrenergic blockers, calcium channel blockers). Third-degree AV block below the AV node may result from an anterior wall MI or chronic degeneration of the conduction system.

Intervention

If cardiac output isn't adequate or the patient's condition is deteriorating, the doctor will order therapy to improve the ventricular rhythm. Initially, atropine may be ordered to increase the ventricular rate and improve cardiac output until a pacemaker is available.

Characteristics and interpretation

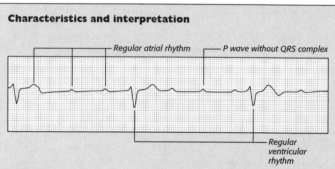

Regular atrial rhythm — P wave without QRS complex

Regular ventricular rhythm

Lead II

Atrial rhythm: usually regular
Ventricular rhythm: usually regular
Atrial rate: usually within normal limits (90 beats/minute shown)
Ventricular rate: slow (30 beats/minute shown)
P wave: normal size and configuration
PR interval: not measurable because the atria and ventricles beat independently of each other
QRS complex: determined by the site of the escape rhythm (With a junctional escape rhythm, the duration and configuration are normal; with an idioventricular escape rhythm, the duration is greater than 0.12 second and the complex is distorted. In the complex shown, duration is 0.16 second, configuration is abnormal, and the complex is distorted.)
T wave: normal size and configuration
QT interval: may or may not be within normal limits (0.56-second interval shown)

Common disorders

Responding to patient needs

Musculoskeletal disorders

Achilles tendon contracture

This condition is a shortening of the Achilles tendon (tendo calcaneus or heel cord) that causes foot pain and strain, with limited ankle dorsiflexion.

Causes

Achilles tendon contracture may reflect a congenital structural anomaly or a muscular reaction to chronic poor posture, especially in women who wear high-heeled shoes or joggers who land on the balls of their feet instead of their heels. Other causes include paralytic conditions of the legs, such as poliomyelitis or cerebral palsy.

Signs and symptoms

Sharp, spasmodic pain during dorsiflexion of the foot characterizes the reflex type of Achilles tendon contracture. In footdrop (fixed equinus), contracture of the flexor foot muscle prevents placing the heel on the ground.

Diagnostic tests

Physical examination and patient history suggest Achilles tendon contracture. A simple test confirms the condition: While the patient keeps his knee flexed, the examiner places the foot in dorsiflexion; gradual knee extension forces the foot into plantar flexion.

Treatment

Achilles tendon contracture is treated conservatively by raising the inside heel of the shoe in the reflex type; gradually lowering the heels of shoes (sudden lowering can aggravate the problem) and stretching exercises, if the cause is high heels; or using support braces or casting to prevent footdrop in a paralyzed patient. Alternative therapy includes using wedged plaster casts or stretching the tendon by manipulation. Analgesics may be given to relieve pain.

With fixed footdrop, treatment may include surgery (Z-tenotomy), although this procedure may weaken the tendon. Z-tenotomy allows further stretching by cutting the tendon. After surgery, a short leg cast maintains the foot in 90-degree dorsiflexion for 6 weeks. Some surgeons allow partial weight bearing on a walking cast after 2 weeks.

Physical therapy considerations

After surgery to lengthen the Achilles tendon, follow these therapy guidelines:
• Elevate the casted foot to decrease venous pressure and edema by raising the foot of the bed or supporting the foot with pillows.
• Prepare the patient for ambulation by having him dangle his foot over the side of the bed for short periods (5 to 15 minutes) before he gets out of bed, allowing for gradual increase of venous pressure.
• Assist the patient in walking (usually within 24 hours of surgery), using crutches and a non-weight-bearing or touch-down gait.
• To prevent Achilles tendon contracture in paralyzed patients, apply support braces, universal splints, casts, or high-topped sneakers. Make sure the weight of the sheets doesn't keep paralyzed feet in plantar flexion.

Teaching points

• Make sure the patient understands how much exercise and walking are recommended after discharge.

• For patients who aren't paralyzed, teach good foot care, and urge them to seek immediate medical care for foot problems.

• Warn women against wearing high heels constantly, and suggest regular weight-bearing exercises to promote dorsiflexion.

Carpal tunnel syndrome

The most common nerve entrapment syndrome, carpal tunnel syndrome results from repetitive compression of the median nerve where it passes through the carpal tunnel at the wrist, along with blood vessels and flexor tendons, to the fingers and thumb. The resulting compression neuropathy causes sensory and motor changes in the median distribution of the hand.

Carpal tunnel syndrome usually occurs in women between the ages of 30 and 60 and poses a serious occupational health problem. Assembly-line workers and packers, secretary-typists, and persons who repeatedly use poorly designed tools are most likely to develop this disorder. Any strenuous use of the hands — sustained grasping, twisting, or flexing — aggravates this condition.

Causes

The carpal tunnel is formed by the carpal bones and the transverse carpal ligament. (See *The carpal tunnel*.) Inflammation or fibrosis of the tendon sheaths that pass through the carpal tunnel often causes edema and compression of the median nerve.

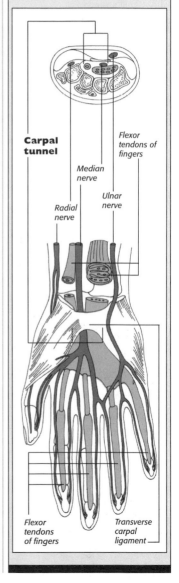

THE CARPAL TUNNEL

The carpal tunnel is clearly visible in this palmar view and cross section of a right hand. Note the median nerve, flexor tendons of fingers, and the blood vessels passing through the tunnel on their way from the forearm to the hand.

Carpal tunnel

Flexor tendons of fingers

Median nerve

Ulnar nerve

Radial nerve

Flexor tendons of fingers

Transverse carpal ligament

Many conditions can cause the contents or structure of the carpal tunnel to swell and press the median nerve against the transverse carpal ligament. Such conditions include rheumatoid arthritis, flexor tenosynovitis (often associated with rheumatic disease), nerve compression, pregnancy, renal failure, menopause, diabetes mellitus, acromegaly, edema following Colles' fracture, hypothyroidism, amyloidosis, myxedema, benign tumors, tuberculosis, and other granulomatous diseases. Another source of damage to the median nerve is dislocation or acute sprain of the wrist.

Signs and symptoms

The patient with carpal tunnel syndrome usually complains of weakness, pain, burning, numbness, or tingling in one or both hands. This paresthesia affects the thumb, forefinger, middle finger, and half of the fourth finger. The patient is unable to clench his hand into a fist. The nails may be atrophic, and the skin, dry and shiny.

Because of vasodilation and venous stasis, symptoms are often worse at night and in the morning. The pain may spread to the forearm and, in severe cases, as far as the shoulder. The patient can usually relieve such pain by shaking his hands vigorously or dangling his arms at his side.

Diagnostic tests

Physical examination reveals decreased sensation to light touch or pinpricks in the affected fingers. Thenar muscle atrophy occurs in about half of all cases of carpal tunnel syndrome. The patient exhibits a positive Tinel's sign (tingling over the median nerve on light percussion) and also responds positively to Phalen's wrist-flexion test (holding the forearms vertically and allowing both hands to drop into complete flexion at the wrists for 1 minute reproduces symptoms of carpal tunnel syndrome).

A compression test supports this diagnosis: A blood pressure cuff inflated above systolic pressure on the forearm for 1 to 2 minutes provokes pain and paresthesia along the distribution of the median nerve.

Electromyography detects a median nerve motor conduction delay of more than 5 milliseconds. Other laboratory tests may identify underlying disease.

Treatment

Conservative treatment is the first approach, including resting the hands by splinting the wrist in neutral extension for 1 to 2 weeks. If a definite link is established between the patient's occupation and the development of carpal tunnel syndrome, he may have to seek other work. Effective treatment may also require correction of an underlying disorder.

When conservative treatment fails, the only alternative is surgical decompression of the nerve by resecting the entire transverse carpal tunnel ligament or by using endoscopic surgical techniques. Neurolysis (freeing of the nerve fibers) may also be necessary.

Physical therapy considerations

• Long-term treatment considerations include maintaining the length of the flexor tendons and muscles through stretching exercises, conditioning intrinsics and flexors of the wrist to increase endurance to ensure return to work without reoccurrence, and modalities as indicated.

Teaching points

• Advise the patient who is about to be discharged to exercise his hands regularly. If the arm is in a sling, tell him to remove the sling several times a day to do exercises for his elbow and shoulder.

• Suggest occupational counseling for the patient who must change jobs because of carpal tunnel syndrome.

• For the patient who can't change jobs, suggest an ergonomic assessment of the work environment to prevent further problems.

• Teach the patient how to apply a splint. Tell him not to make it too tight. Show him how to remove the splint for his exercises.

• Teach him how to perform gentle range-of-motion exercises, which should be done daily. Make sure he knows how to do them before he's discharged.

Clubfoot

The most common congenital disorder of the lower extremities, clubfoot, or talipes, is marked primarily by a deformed talus and shortened Achilles tendon, which give the foot a characteristic clublike appearance. In talipes equinovarus, the foot points downward (equinus) and turns inward (varus), while the front of the foot curls toward the heel (forefoot adduction). (See *Recognizing clubfoot,* page 184.)

Clubfoot occurs in approximately 1 per 1,000 live births, usually occurs bilaterally, and is twice as common in boys as in girls. It may be associated with other birth defects, such as myelomeningocele, spina bifida, and arthrogryposis. Clubfoot is correctable with prompt treatment.

Causes

A combination of genetic and environmental factors in utero appears to cause clubfoot. Heredity is a definite factor in some cases, although the mechanism of transmission is undetermined. If a child is born with clubfoot, his sibling has a 1 in 35 chance of being born with the same anomaly; children of a parent with clubfoot have 1 chance in 10.

In children without a family history of clubfoot, this anomaly seems linked to arrested development during the 9th and 10th weeks of embryonic life, when the feet are formed. Researchers also suspect muscle abnormalities, leading to variations in length and tendon insertions, as possible causes of clubfoot.

Signs and symptoms

Talipes equinovarus varies in severity. Deformity may be so extreme that the toes touch the inside of the ankle, or it may be only vaguely apparent. In every case, the talus is deformed, the Achilles tendon shortened, and the calcaneus somewhat shortened and flattened. Depending on the degree of the varus deformity, the calf muscles are shortened and underdeveloped, with soft-tissue contractures at the site of the deformity. The foot is tight in its deformed position and resists manual efforts to push it back into normal position.

Clubfoot is painless, except in older, arthritic patients. In older children, clubfoot may be secondary to paralysis, poliomyelitis, or cerebral palsy, in which case treatment must include management of the underlying disease.

Diagnostic tests

An early diagnosis of clubfoot is usually no problem because the deformi-

RECOGNIZING CLUBFOOT

Clubfoot may have various names, depending on the orientation of the deformity, as shown in the illustrations.

Talipes equinus

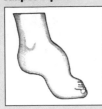

Talipes calcaneus

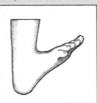

Talipes cavus

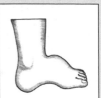

Talipes varus

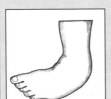

Talipes equinovarus

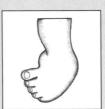

Talipes calcaneovarus

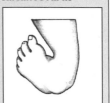

Talipes valgus

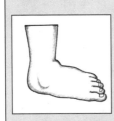

Talipes calcaneovalgus

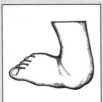

Talipes equinovalgus

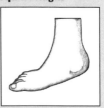

ty is obvious. In subtle deformity, however, true clubfoot must be distinguished from apparent clubfoot (metatarsus varus or pigeon toe).

Apparent clubfoot results when a fetus maintains a position in utero that gives his feet a clubfoot appearance at birth. This can usually be corrected manually.

Another form of apparent clubfoot is inversion of the feet, resulting from the peroneal type of progressive muscular atrophy and progressive muscular dystrophy. In true clubfoot, X-rays show superimposition of the talus and the calcaneus and a ladderlike appearance of the metatarsals.

Treatment

Appropriate treatment for clubfoot is administered in three stages:
• correcting the deformity
• maintaining the correction until the foot regains normal muscle balance

• observing the foot closely for several years to prevent the deformity from recurring.

In newborns, corrective treatment for true clubfoot should begin at once. An infant's foot contains large amounts of cartilage; the muscles, ligaments, and tendons are supple. The ideal time to begin treatment is during the first few days and weeks of life, when the foot is most malleable.

Sequential correction

Clubfoot deformities are usually corrected in sequential order: forefoot adduction first, then varus (or inversion), then equinus (or plantar flexion). Trying to correct all three deformities at once only results in a misshapen, rocker-bottomed foot.

Forefoot adduction is corrected by uncurling the front of the foot away from the heel (forefoot abduction); the varus deformity is corrected by turning the foot so the sole faces outward (eversion); and equinus is corrected by casting the foot with the toes pointing up (dorsiflexion). This last correction may have to be supplemented with a subcutaneous tenotomy of the Achilles tendon and posterior capsulotomy of the ankle joint.

Treatment methods

Several therapeutic methods have been tested and found effective in correcting clubfoot. The first is simple manipulation and casting, whereby the foot is gently manipulated into a partially corrected position and then held there in a cast for several days or weeks. (The skin should be painted with a nonirritating adhesive liquid beforehand to prevent the cast from slipping.)

After cast removal, the foot is manipulated into an even better position and casted again. This procedure is repeated as many times as necessary. In some cases, the shape of the cast can be transformed through a series of wedging maneuvers, instead of changing the cast each time.

After correction of clubfoot, proper foot alignment is maintained through exercise, night splints, and orthopedic shoes. With manipulating and casting, correction usually takes about 3 months. The Denis Browne splint — a device that consists of two padded, metal footplates connected by a flat, horizontal bar — is sometimes used as a follow-up measure to help promote bilateral correction and strengthen the foot muscles.

Resistant clubfoot may require surgery. Older children, for example, with recurrent or neglected clubfoot usually need surgery, such as tenotomy, tendon transfer, stripping of the plantar fascia, or capsulotomy. In severe cases, bone surgery (wedge resections, osteotomy, or astragalectomy) may be appropriate. After surgery, a cast is applied to preserve the correction. Whenever clubfoot is severe enough to require surgery, it's rarely totally correctable. However, surgery can usually ameliorate the deformity.

Physical therapy considerations

• Look for any exaggerated attitudes in an infant's feet. Make sure you can recognize the difference between true clubfoot and apparent clubfoot.
• Don't use excessive force in trying to manipulate a clubfoot. An apparent clubfoot moves easily.

Teaching points

• Stress to parents the importance of prompt treatment. Make sure they understand that clubfoot demands immediate therapy and orthopedic supervision until growth is completed.
• Explain to the older child and his parents that surgery can improve clubfoot with good function, but can't totally correct it; the affected

calf muscle will remain slightly underdeveloped.

• Emphasize the need for long-term orthopedic care to maintain correction, including range-of-motion exercises to increase triplanar motion of the ankle joint, strengthening exercises of the gastrocnemius-soleus complex, weight-bearing activities to encourage proper alignment, and ankle stabilizers.

• Teach the parents the prescribed exercises that their child can do at home.

• Urge the parents to make sure their child wears corrective shoes as ordered and the splints during naps and at night.

• Make sure parents understand that treatment for clubfoot continues during the entire growth period. Correcting this defect permanently takes time and patience.

Developmental hip dysplasia

Developmental hip dysplasia, an abnormality of the hip joint present from birth, is the most common disorder affecting hip joints of children under age 3. Developmental hip dysplasia can be unilateral or bilateral. This abnormality occurs in three forms of varying severity: *unstable hip dysplasia,* in which the hip is positioned normally but can be dislocated by manipulation; *subluxation, or incomplete dislocation,* in which the femoral head rides on the edge of the acetabulum; and *complete dislocation,* in which the femoral head is totally outside the acetabulum. (See *Complete dysplasia of the hip.*) Developmental hip subluxation or dislocation can cause abnormal acetabular development and permanent disability. About 85% of affected infants are females.

Causes

Experts are unsure what causes developmental hip dysplasia; however, it is known that dislocation is 10 times more common after breech delivery (malpositioning in utero) than after cephalic delivery. The condition is also more common among large neonates and among twins.

Signs and symptoms

Clinical effects of hip dysplasia vary with age. In newborns, dysplasia produces no gross deformity or pain. However, in complete dysplasia, the hip rides above the acetabulum, causing the level of the knees to be uneven. As the child grows older and begins to walk, the abduction on the dislocated side is limited. Uncorrected bilateral dysplasia may cause him to sway from side to side, a condition known as "duck waddle"; unilateral dysplasia may produce a limp. If corrective treatment isn't begun until after age 2, developmental hip dysplasia may cause degenerative hip changes, lordosis, joint malformation, and soft-tissue damage.

Diagnostic tests

Several observations during physical examination of the relaxed child strongly suggest developmental hip dysplasia. First, place the child on his back, and inspect the folds of skin over his thighs. Usually, a child in this position has an equal number of thigh folds on each side, but a child with subluxation or dislocation may have an extra fold on the affected side (which is also apparent when the child lies prone). Next, with the child lying prone, check for alignment of the buttock fold. In a child with dysplasia, the buttock fold on the affected side is higher. In addition, abduction of the affected hip is restricted.

A positive Ortolani's or Trendelenburg's sign confirms developmental hip dysplasia. To test for Ortolani's sign, place the infant on his back, with his hip flexed and in abduction. Abduct the hip while pressing the femur downward. This will dislocate the hip. Then, abduct the hip while moving the femur upward. If you hear a click or feel a jerk (produced by the femoral head moving over the acetabular rim), this indicates subluxation in an infant younger than 1 month; this sign indicates subluxation or complete dislocation in an older infant.

To elicit Trendelenburg's sign, have the child rest his weight on the side of the dislocation and lift his other knee. His pelvis drops on the normal side because of weak abductor muscles in the affected hip. However, when the child stands with his weight on the normal side and lifts the other knee, the pelvis remains horizontal.

X-rays show the location of the femur head and a shallow acetabulum; they can also monitor the progress of the disease or treatment. Sonography and magnetic resonance imaging may also be used to assess reduction.

Treatment

The earlier the infant receives treatment, the better his chances are for normal development. Treatment varies with the patient's age. In infants younger than 3 months, treatment includes *gentle* manipulation to reduce the dislocation, followed by holding the hips in a flexed and abducted position with a splint-brace or harness to maintain the reduction. The infant must wear this apparatus continuously for 2 to 3 months and then use a night splint for another month, so the joint capsule can tighten and stabilize in correct alignment.

COMPLETE DYSPLASIA OF THE HIP

In complete dislocation, the femoral head is totally displaced outside the acetabulum (see arrow).

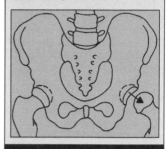

If treatment doesn't begin until after age 3 months, it may include bilateral skin traction (in infants) or skeletal traction (in children who have started walking) in an attempt to reduce the dislocation by gradually abducting the hips. Bryant's traction or divarication traction is used to treat developmental hip dysplasia. Both extremities are placed in traction, even if only one is affected. This helps to maintain immobilization. This type of traction is used in children who are younger than age 3 and weigh less than 35 lb (16 kg). The length of treatment is 2 to 3 weeks.

If traction fails, gentle closed reduction under a general anesthetic can further abduct the hips; the child is then placed in a spica cast for 4 to 6 months. If closed treatment fails, open reduction, followed by immobilization in a spica cast for an average of 6 months or osteotomy may be considered.

In the child ages 2 to 5, treatment is difficult and includes skeletal traction and subcutaneous adductor tenotomy. Treatment started after age 5 rarely restores satisfactory hip function.

Physical therapy considerations

If treatment requires a spica cast:
• When transferring the child immediately after casting, use your palms to avoid making dents in the cast. Such dents predispose the patient to pressure ulcers. Remember that the cast needs 24 to 48 hours to dry naturally. Don't use heat to make it dry faster because heat also makes it more fragile.
• Turn the child every 2 hours during the day and every 4 hours at night. Check color, sensation, and motion of the infant's legs and feet. Be sure to examine all his toes. Notify the doctor of dusky, cool, or numb toes.
• Maintain skin integrity and check circulation at least every 2 hours.
• Shine a flashlight under the cast every 4 hours to check for objects and crumbs.
• Check the cast daily for odors, which may herald infection. Record the child's temperature daily.
• If the child complains of itching, he may benefit from diphenhydramine. Alternately, you may try aiming a hair dryer set on cool at the cast edges to relieve itching. Don't scratch or probe under the cast. Investigate any persistent itching.
• Provide adequate stimuli to promote growth and development. If the child's hips are abducted in a froglike position, tell parents that he may be able to fit on a tricycle that the parent can push (if the child is unable to pedal) or an electric child's car. Encourage parents to let the child sit at a table by seating him on pillows on a chair, to put him on the floor for short periods of play, and to let him play with other children his age.
After cast removal:
• Perform passive range-of-motion exercises to maintain joint integrity.
• Perform massage for edema control.

• Initiate strengthening exercises with emphasis on abductors, gluteus, and lateral rotators.
• Initiate cardiac conditioning.
• Encourage joint mobilization to decrease capsular restriction.

Teaching points
• Listen sympathetically to the parents' expressions of anxiety and fear. Explain possible causes of developmental hip dislocation, and give reassurance that early, prompt treatment will probably result in complete correction.
• During the child's first few days in a cast or splint-brace, encourage his parents to stay with him as much as possible to calm and reassure him because restricted movement will make him irritable.
• Assure parents that the child will adjust to this restriction and return to normal sleeping, eating, and playing behavior in a few days.
• Teach parents how to correctly splint or brace the hips, as ordered.
• Instruct them to remove braces and splints while bathing the infant but to replace them immediately afterward. Stress good hygiene; parents should bathe and change the child frequently and wash his perineum with warm water and soap at each diaper change.
• Stress the need for frequent check-ups.
For the child in a spica cast:
• Tell the parents to watch for signs that the child is outgrowing the cast (cyanosis, cool extremities, pain).
• Tell them that treatment may be prolonged and requires patience.
• If the child is in Bryant's traction, inform the parents that they may care for him at home by learning traction application and maintenance.
• Teach the parents how to maintain the child's skin integrity.
• Encourage the parents to cuddle and hold their child and encourage

his interaction with siblings and friends.

• If necessary, refer the child and parents to a child life specialist to ensure continued developmental progress.

Epicondylitis

Also known as tennis elbow or epitrochlear bursitis, epicondylitis is inflammation of the forearm extensor supinator tendon fibers at their common attachment to the lateral humeral epicondyle, which produces acute or subacute pain.

Causes

Epicondylitis probably begins as a partial tear and is common among tennis players or people whose activities require a forceful grasp, wrist extension against resistance, or frequent rotation of the forearm. Untreated epicondylitis may become disabling.

Signs and symptoms

The patient's initial symptom is elbow pain that gradually worsens and often radiates to the forearm and back of the hand whenever he grasps an object or twists his elbow.

Other associated signs and symptoms include tenderness over the involved lateral or medial epicondyle or over the head of the radius and a weak grasp. In rare instances, epicondylitis may cause local heat, swelling, or restricted range of motion (ROM).

Diagnostic tests

Because X-rays are almost always negative, diagnosis typically depends on clinical signs and symptoms and a patient history of playing tennis or engaging in similar activities. The pain can be reproduced by wrist extension and supination with lateral involvement, or by flexion and pronation with medial epicondyle involvement.

Treatment

The aim of treatment is to relieve pain, usually by local injection of corticosteroid and a local anesthetic and by systemic anti-inflammatory therapy with aspirin or indomethacin.

Supportive measures

Supportive treatment includes an immobilizing splint from the distal forearm to the elbow, which generally relieves pain in 2 to 3 weeks; heat therapy, such as warm compresses, short-wave diathermy, and ultrasound (alone or in combination with diathermy); and physical therapy, such as manipulation and massage to detach the tendon from the chronically inflamed periosteum.

A "tennis elbow strap" benefits many patients. This strap, which is wrapped snugly around the forearm approximately 1″ (2.5 cm) below the epicondyle, helps relieve the strain on affected forearm muscles and tendons.

If these measures prove ineffective, surgery to release the tendon at the epicondyle may be necessary.

Physical therapy considerations

• Assess the patient's level of pain, ROM, and sensory function. Monitor heat therapy to prevent burns.
• Remove the elbow support daily, and gently move the arm to prevent stiffness and contracture.
• Provide physical therapy for specific strengthening exercises to build the endurance of the damaged muscle and prevent reinjury.

Teaching points

• Instruct the patient to rest the elbow until inflammation subsides.

• Teach him the prescribed exercise program that he'll need to follow. For example, he may stretch his arm and flex his wrist to the maximum, then press the back of his hand against a wall until he can feel a pull in his forearm, and hold this position for 1 minute.

• Advise the patient to warm up for 15 to 20 minutes before beginning any sports activity.

• Suggest that he assess the equipment or have it assessed for proper size and weight. The playing field may also need to be reevaluated.

• Urge him to wear an elastic support or splint during any activity that stresses the forearm or elbow.

Herniated disk

Also called a ruptured or slipped disk or a herniated nucleus pulposus, a herniated disk occurs when all or part of the nucleus pulposus — the soft, gelatinous, central portion of an intervertebral disk — is forced through the disk's weakened or torn outer ring (annulus fibrosus).

When this happens, the extruded disk may impinge on spinal nerve roots as they exit from the spinal canal or on the spinal cord itself, resulting in back pain and other signs of nerve root irritation. Herniated disks usually occur in adults (mostly men) under age 45.

Causes

Herniated disks may result from severe trauma or strain or may be related to intervertebral joint degeneration. In older patients, whose disks have begun to degenerate, minor trauma may cause herniation. About 90% of herniated disks occur in the lumbar and lumbosacral regions, 8% occur in the cervical area, and 1% to 2% in the thoracic area.

Patients with a congenitally small lumbar spinal canal or with osteophyte formation along the vertebrae may be more susceptible to nerve root compression with a herniated disk and more likely to have neurologic symptoms.

Signs and symptoms

The overriding symptom of lumbar herniated disk is severe low back pain, which radiates to the buttocks, legs, and feet, usually unilaterally. When herniation follows trauma, the pain may begin suddenly, subside in a few days, and then recur at shorter intervals and with progressive intensity.

Sciatic pain follows, beginning as a dull pain in the buttocks. Valsalva's maneuver, coughing, sneezing, or bending intensifies the pain, which is often accompanied by muscle spasms. A herniated disk may also cause sensory and motor loss in the area innervated by the compressed spinal nerve root and, in later stages, weakness and atrophy of leg muscles.

Diagnostic tests

Obtaining a careful patient history is vital because the mechanisms that intensify disk pain are diagnostically significant. The following test results support the diagnosis:

• The straight-leg-raising test and its variants are perhaps the best tests for diagnosing a herniated disk. For this test, the patient lies in a supine position while the examiner places one hand on the patient's ilium, to stabilize the pelvis, and the other hand under the ankle, and then slowly raises the patient's leg. The test is positive only if the patient complains of posterior leg (sciatic) pain, not back pain.

• In the Lesègue test, the patient lies flat while the thigh and knee are flexed to a 90-degree angle. Resistance and pain, as well as loss of ankle or knee-jerk reflex, indicate spinal root compression.

• X-rays of the spine are essential to rule out other abnormalities but may not diagnose a herniated disk because a marked disk prolapse can be present despite a normal X-ray.

• Peripheral vascular status check — including posterior tibial and dorsalis pedis pulses, and the skin temperature of extremities — helps rule out ischemic disease, another cause of leg pain or numbness.

Aside from the physical examination and X-rays, myelography, a computed tomography scan, and magnetic resonance imaging provide the most specific diagnostic information, showing spinal canal compression by herniated disk material.

Treatment

Initial treatment is conservative and consists of several weeks of bed rest (possibly with pelvic traction), heat applications, an exercise program, and medication. If neurologic impairment progresses rapidly, surgery may be necessary.

Drug therapy

Aspirin reduces inflammation and edema at the site of injury; rarely, corticosteroids, such as dexamethasone, may be prescribed for the same purpose. Muscle relaxants, especially diazepam or methocarbamol, also may be beneficial.

Surgery

A herniated disk that fails to respond to conservative treatment may necessitate surgery. The most common procedure, laminectomy, involves excision of a portion of the lamina and removal of the protruding disk (nucleus pulposus).

If laminectomy doesn't alleviate pain and disability, a spinal fusion may be necessary to overcome segmental instability. Laminectomy and spinal fusion are sometimes performed concurrently to stabilize the spine.

Other treatments

Chemonucleolysis — injection of the enzyme chymopapain into the herniated disk to dissolve the nucleus pulposus — is a possible alternative to laminectomy. Microdiskectomy can also be used to remove fragments of nucleus pulposus.

Physical therapy considerations

• Herniated disk requires supportive care, careful patient teaching, and strong emotional support to help the patient cope with the discomfort and frustration of chronic low back pain.

Nonoperative considerations

• Conservative measures to decrease mechanical forces acting on the impaired disk involve exercises to increase strength and ROM.

• Functional (cervical) lumbar stabilization with musculus multifidus strengthening is the treatment of choice to maintain proper, pain-free positioning of the spine.

• McKenzie extension or Williams flexion exercises may be appropriate depending on the anatomy or location of the herniation.

Postoperative considerations

• Clarify the doctor's order for the type of exercise prescribed for the patient. Common options include stretching, strengthening, and cardiovascular exercises, many of which the patient can also do in water.

• Avoid trunk extension exercises for spinal fusion patients. Exercising without a brace requires the doctor's permission.

• Avoid painful end-range exercises on patients who have undergone a diskectomy.

• After a laminectomy or diskectomy, maintain normal ROM of lower extremities with flexibility training. Continue a strengthening program, such as one of those previously listed under nonoperative considerations.

• After spinal fusion, traction is contraindicated for 6 months. Continue strengthening and stretching exercises, such as those mentioned previously under nonoperative considerations.

• In manual therapy, include myofascial release, muscle energy technique, joint mobilization, trigger points, massage, strain-counterstrain, craniosacral technique, and neural tension.

• When performing work simulation, don't exceed prescribed weight limits. Assess the patient's work environment ergonomically. Include body mechanics during static and dynamic postures and conditioning.

Teaching point

• Teach the patient proper body mechanics, lifting techniques, and posture and compensatory strategies.

Muscular dystrophy

Muscular dystrophy is actually a group of congenital disorders characterized by progressive symmetrical wasting of skeletal muscles without neural or sensory defects. Paradoxically, these wasted muscles tend to enlarge because of connective tissue and fat deposits, giving an erroneous impression of muscle strength.

Four main types of muscular dystrophy occur: Duchenne's (pseudohypertrophic) muscular dystrophy, which accounts for 50% of all cases; Becker's (benign pseudohypertrophic) muscular dystrophy; facioscapulohumeral (Landouzy-Dejerine) dystrophy; and limb-girdle dystrophy.

The prognosis varies. Duchenne's muscular dystrophy generally strikes during early childhood and usually results in death by age 20. Patients with Becker's muscular dystrophy live into their 40s. Facioscapulohumeral and limb-girdle dystrophies usually don't shorten life expectancy.

Causes

Muscular dystrophy is caused by various genetic mechanisms. Duchenne's and Becker's muscular dystrophies are X-linked recessive disorders. They result from defects in the gene coding for the muscle protein dystrophin. The defect can be mapped genetically to the Xp2l locus.

Duchenne's and Becker's muscular dystrophies affect males almost exclusively. The incidence of Duchenne's muscular dystrophy in males is 13 to 33 per 100,000. Becker's muscular dystrophy occurs in about 1 to 3 males per 100,000.

Facioscapulohumeral dystrophy is an autosomal dominant disorder. Limb-girdle dystrophy may be inherited in several ways, but it's usually an autosomal recessive trait. These two types affect both sexes about equally.

Signs and symptoms

Although the four types of muscular dystrophy cause progressive muscular deterioration, the degree of severity and the age of onset vary.

Duchenne's muscular dystrophy

Duchenne's muscular dystrophy begins insidiously, between ages 3 and 5. At first it affects leg and pelvic muscles, eventually spreading to the involuntary muscles. Muscle weakness produces a waddling gait, toe-walking, and lordosis. A protuberant abdomen and exaggerated lordosis are secondary to weak pelvic muscles.

Children with this disorder have difficulty climbing stairs and rising from the floor. They also fall down often and can't run properly, and their scapulae flare out (or "wing") when they raise their arms. They may use their arms when getting into a standing position (Gowers' sign). Calf muscles, especially, become enlarged and firm. Muscle deterioration progresses rapidly, and contractures develop. Usually, these children are confined to wheelchairs by age 12.

Late in the disease, progressive weakening of cardiac muscle causes tachycardia, electrocardiogram abnormalities, and pulmonary complications. Death commonly results from sudden heart failure, respiratory failure, or infection.

Becker's muscular dystrophy
Signs and symptoms of Becker's muscular dystrophy resemble those of Duchenne's muscular dystrophy, but they progress more slowly. Although symptoms start around age 5, the patient can still walk well beyond age 15 — sometimes into his 40s.

Facioscapulohumeral dystrophy
This is a slowly progressive and relatively benign form of muscular dystrophy that commonly begins before age 10 but may develop during early adolescence. It weakens the muscles of the face, shoulders, and upper arms at first but eventually spreads to all voluntary muscles, producing a pendulous lower lip and absence of the nasolabial fold.

Early symptoms include inability to pucker the mouth or whistle, abnormal facial movements, and absence of facial movements when laughing or crying. In infants there is inability to suckle. Other signs include inability to raise the arms above the head, diffuse facial flattening that leads to a masklike expression, winging of the scapulae, trunk weakness, difficulty rising from a chair, proximal weakness at the shoulder girdle, skeletal abnormalities, and fatigue.

Limb-girdle dystrophy
This form follows a similarly slow course and often causes only slight disability. Usually, it begins between ages 6 and 10; less often, in early adulthood. Muscle weakness first appears in the upper arm and pelvic muscles. Other symptoms include those of facioscapulohumeral dystrophy and may also include lordosis with abdominal protrusion, waddling gait, and poor balance.

Diagnostic tests

Typical clinical findings, family history, and test findings are used to diagnose the disease. If another family member has muscular dystrophy, its clinical characteristics can indicate the type of dystrophy the patient has and how he may be affected.

Electromyography typically demonstrates short, weak bursts of electrical activity in affected muscles. Muscle biopsy shows variations in the size of muscle fibers and, in later stages, fat and connective tissue deposits. In Duchenne's dystrophy, muscle biopsy reveals an absence of dystrophin.

Immunologic and molecular biological techniques now available in specialized medical centers facilitate accurate prenatal and postnatal diagnosis of Duchenne's and Becker's muscular dystrophies. These techniques also help to identify a person as a carrier. In addition, these newer techniques are replacing muscle biopsy and serum creatine kinase tests as diagnostic procedures.

Treatment

No treatment can stop the progressive muscle impairment of muscular dystrophy. However, orthopedic appliances as well as exercise, physical therapy, and surgery to correct contractures can help preserve the patient's mobility and independence.

Family members who are carriers of muscular dystrophy should receive genetic counseling regarding the risk of transmitting this disease.

Physical therapy considerations

• Comprehensive long-term care and follow-up, patient and family teaching, and psychological support can help the patient and family deal with this disorder.
• Provide a physical therapy program that includes strengthening exercises to maintain muscles as long as possible to encourage gait and promote independence.
• Encourage and assist with active and passive range-of-motion (ROM) exercises to preserve joint mobility and prevent muscle atrophy.
• Prevent contractures through passive and active ROM exercises and bracing. Surgery may also be appropriate.
• Encourage the use of splints, braces, trapeze bars, overhead slings, and a wheelchair to help preserve mobility.
• Use a footboard or high-topped sneakers and a foot cradle to increase comfort and prevent footdrop.
• When respiratory involvement occurs in Duchenne's muscular dystrophy, encourage coughing, deep-breathing exercises, and diaphragmatic breathing.
• For the patient requiring a wheelchair, ensure proper fit with appropriate accessories.

• Provide emotional support to help the patient cope with continual changes in body image.
• Encourage communication among family members to help them deal with the emotional strain caused by muscular dystrophy.

Teaching points
• Advise the patient to avoid long periods of bed rest and inactivity. If necessary, limit his television viewing and other sedentary activities.
• Train the patient in functionally independent wheelchair use.
• For the child with Duchenne's muscular dystrophy, teach parents how to recognize early signs of respiratory complications.
• Encourage parents to help the child with Duchenne's muscular dystrophy maintain peer relationships and realize his intellectual potential by remaining in a regular school as long as possible.
• For information on social services and financial assistance, refer patients and their families to the Muscular Dystrophy Association.
• Refer family members for genetic counseling.
• Be aware that cardiac or respiratory involvement of Duchenne's and Becker's muscular dystrophy types compromises endurance.

Neurogenic arthropathy

Most common in men over age 40, neurogenic arthropathy (Charcot's arthropathy) is a progressively degenerative disease of peripheral and axial joints, resulting from impaired sensory innervation. The loss of sensation in the joints causes progressive deterioration, resulting from unrecognized trauma (especially repeated minor episodes) or primary disease, which leads to laxity of supporting ligaments and eventual disintegration of the affected joints.

Causes

In adults, the most common cause of neurogenic arthropathy is diabetes mellitus. Other causes include tabes dorsalis (especially among patients ages 40 to 60), syringomyelia (which progresses to neurogenic arthropathy in about 25% of patients), myelopathy of pernicious anemia, spinal cord trauma, paraplegia, hereditary sensory neuropathy, and Charcot-Marie-Tooth disease. Rarely, amyloidosis, peripheral nerve injury, myelomeningocele (in children), leprosy, or alcoholism causes neurogenic arthropathy.

Frequent intra-articular injections of corticosteroids have also been linked to neurogenic arthropathy. The analgesic effect of the corticosteroids may mask symptoms and allow continuous damaging stress to accelerate joint destruction.

Signs and symptoms

Neurogenic arthropathy begins insidiously with swelling, warmth, increased mobility, and instability in a single joint or in many joints. It can progress to deformity. The first clue to vertebral neuroarthropathy, which progresses to gross spinal deformity, may be nothing more than a mild, persistent backache. Characteristically, pain is minimal despite obvious deformity.

The specific joint that's affected varies. Diabetes usually attacks the joints and bones of the feet; tabes dorsalis attacks the large weight-bearing joints, such as the knee, hip, ankle, or lumbar and dorsal vertebrae (Charcot spine); syringomyelia, the shoulder, elbow, or cervical intervertebral joint. Neurogenic arthropathy related to intra-articular injection

of corticosteroids usually develops in the hip or knee joint.

Diagnostic tests

A patient history of painless joint deformity and underlying primary disease suggests neurogenic arthropathy. The physical examination may reveal bone fragmentation in advanced disease. X-rays confirm the diagnosis and assess the severity of joint damage.

In the early stage of the disease, soft-tissue swelling or effusion may be the only overt effect; in the advanced stage, articular fracture, subluxation, erosion of articular cartilage, periosteal new bone formation, and excessive growth of marginal loose bodies (osteophytosis) or resorption may be evident.

Other diagnostic measures include:
• vertebral examination, which reveals narrowing of disk spaces, deterioration of vertebrae, and osteophyte formation, leading to ankylosis and deforming kyphoscoliosis
• synovial biopsy, which produces bony fragments and bits of calcified cartilage.

Treatment

Effective management relieves associated pain with analgesics and immobilization, using crutches, splints, braces, and restriction of weight bearing.

In severe disease, surgery may include arthrodesis or, in severe diabetic neuropathy, amputation. However, surgery risks further damage through nonunion and infection.

Physical therapy considerations

• Check sensory perception, ROM, alignment, joint swelling, and the status of underlying disease.

• Maintain ROM of affected joints.

Teaching points

• Advise the patient to report severe joint pain, swelling, or instability. Heat may be applied to relieve local pain and tenderness.

• Teach the patient the proper technique for using crutches or other orthopedic devices. Stress the importance of proper fit and regular professional readjustment of such devices. Warn that because of impaired sensation, the patient might sustain damage from these aids without discomfort.

• Explain the importance of daily foot inspection for the diabetic patient to prevent future ulceration.

• Emphasize the need to continue regular treatment of the underlying disease.

• Teach the patient joint protection techniques; to avoid physically stressful actions that may cause pathologic fractures; and to take safety precautions, such as removing throw rugs and clutter that might cause falls.

Osgood-Schlatter disease

Also known as osteochondrosis, Osgood-Schlatter disease is a painful, incomplete separation of the epiphysis of the tibial tubercle from the tibial shaft. It's most common in active adolescent boys, frequently affecting one or both knees. Severe disease may cause permanent tubercle enlargement.

Causes

Osgood-Schlatter disease probably results from trauma, before the complete fusion of the epiphysis to the main bone has occurred (between ages 10 and 15). Such trauma may be a single violent action or repeated knee flexion against a tight quadriceps muscle. Other causes include locally deficient blood supply and genetic factors.

Signs and symptoms

The patient complains of constant aching and pain and tenderness below the kneecap that worsens during any activity that causes forceful contraction of the patellar tendon on the tubercle, such as ascending or descending stairs. Such pain may be associated with some obvious soft-tissue swelling, localized heat, and local tenderness. (See *Epiphyseal degeneration.*)

Diagnostic tests

Physical examination supports the diagnosis. The examiner forces the tibia into internal rotation while slowly extending the patient's knee from 90 degrees of flexion; at about 30 degrees, such flexion produces pain that subsides immediately with external rotation of the tibia.

X-rays may be normal or show epiphyseal separation and soft-tissue swelling for up to 6 months after onset; eventually, they may show bone fragmentation.

Treatment

Treatment usually consists of immobilization of the leg for 6 to 8 weeks and supportive measures. Full extension immobilization of the leg using reinforced elastic knee support, plaster cast, or a splint allows revascularization and reossification of the tubercle and minimizes the pull of the quadriceps.

Supportive measures include activity restrictions, aspirin and, possibly, corticosteroid injections into the joint to relieve tenderness. In very mild cases, simple restriction of predisposing activities (bicycling, running) may suffice.

Rarely, conservative measures fail and surgery may be necessary. Such surgery includes removal or fixation of the epiphysis or drilling holes through the tubercle to the main bone to form channels for rapid revascularization.

Physical therapy considerations

• Coordinate therapy with administration of pain medication to ensure the patient's maximum effort with minimum discomfort.
• Give reassurance and emotional support because disruption of normal activities is difficult for an active teenager.

Teaching points

• Teach proper use of crutches, and provide gait training.
• Tell the patient to protect the injured knee with padding and to avoid trauma and repeated flexion, such as in running and contact sports.
• Maintain range of motion of knee joint through gentle stretching.
• Initiate strengthening exercises after any period of immobilization.
• Tell the patient that he may gradually return to activity with a supervised functional program. Emphasize, particularly to an active youth, that restrictions are temporary.

Osteoarthritis

The most common form of arthritis, osteoarthritis is chronic, causing deterioration of the joint cartilage and formation of reactive new bone at the margins and subchondral areas of the joints. This degeneration results from a breakdown of chondrocytes, most often in the hips and knees.

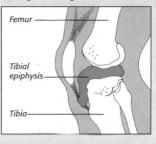

EPIPHYSEAL DEGENERATION

In Osgood-Schlatter disease, a piece of the tibial epiphysis degenerates, causing a swelling below the knee.

Femur

Tibial epiphysis

Tibia

Osteoarthritis is widespread, occurring equally in both sexes, and typically begins after age 40; symptoms generally begin in middle age and may progress with advancing age.

The degree of disability depends on the site and severity of involvement; it can range from minor limitation of the fingers to severe disability in persons with hip or knee involvement. The rate of progression varies, and joints may remain stable for years in an early stage of deterioration.

Causes

Primary osteoarthritis, a normal part of aging, results from many causes, including metabolic, genetic, chemical, and mechanical factors. Secondary osteoarthritis usually follows an identifiable predisposing event — most commonly trauma, congenital deformity, or obesity — and leads to degenerative changes. (See *What happens in osteoarthritis,* page 198.)

Signs and symptoms

The most common symptom of osteoarthritis is a deep, aching joint pain, particularly after exercise or

WHAT HAPPENS IN OSTEOARTHRITIS

The characteristic breakdown of articular cartilage is a gradual response to aging or to predisposing factors, such as joint abnormalities or traumatic injury.

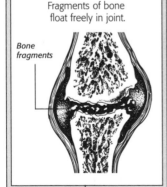

Chondrocytes break down.

↓

Cartilage degenerates.

Degeneration of cartilage

↓

Osteophytes (bony spurs) form.

↓

Fragments of bone float freely in joint.

Bone fragments

↓

Stiffness and decreased movement occur.

weight bearing, usually relieved by rest. Other symptoms include:
• stiffness in the morning and after exercise (relieved by rest)
• aching during changes in weather
• "grating" of the joint during motion
• altered gait contractures
• limited movement.

These symptoms increase with poor posture, obesity, and occupational stress.

Osteoarthritis of the interphalangeal joints produces irreversible changes in the distal joints (Heberden's nodes) and proximal joints (Bouchard's nodes). These nodes may be painless at first but eventually become red, swollen, and tender, causing numbness and loss of dexterity.

Diagnostic tests

A thorough physical examination confirms typical symptoms, and the absence of systemic symptoms rules out an inflammatory joint disorder. X-rays of the affected joint help confirm diagnosis of osteoarthritis but may be normal in the early stages. X-rays may require many views and typically show:
• narrowing of joint space or margin
• cystlike bony deposits in joint space and margins, sclerosis of the subchondral space
• joint deformity due to degeneration or articular damage
• bony growths at weight-bearing areas
• fusion of joints.

No laboratory test is specific for osteoarthritis.

Treatment

The goal of treatment is to relieve pain, maintain or improve mobility, and minimize disability. Medications include aspirin (or other nonnarcotic analgesics), phenylbutazone, indomethacin, fenoprofen, ibuprofen, propoxyphene and, in some cases, intra-articular injections of corticosteroids. Such injections, given every 4 to 6 months, may delay the development of nodes in the hands.

Effective treatment also reduces stress by supporting or stabilizing the joint with crutches, braces, cane, walker, cervical collar, or traction. Other supportive measures include massage, moist heat, paraffin dips for hands, protective techniques for preventing undue stress on the joints, adequate rest (particularly after activity) and, occasionally, exercise when the knees are affected.

Surgical treatment, reserved for patients who have severe disability or uncontrollable pain, may include the following:
• arthroplasty (partial or total) — replacement of deteriorated part of joint with prosthetic appliance
• arthrodesis — surgical fusion of bones; used primarily in the spine (laminectomy)
• osteoplasty — scraping and lavage of deteriorated bone from joint
• osteotomy — change in alignment of bone to relieve stress by removing a wedge of bone or cutting a bone.

Physical therapy considerations

• The goals of physical therapy are to relieve pain and muscle guarding, promote relaxation, maintain joint range of motion (ROM) and prevent deformity, prevent muscle weakness and atrophy, protect inflamed joints (assistive devices may be used), avoid excess fatigue, and improve endurance.
• Promote adequate rest, particularly after activity. Plan rest periods during the day, and provide for adequate sleep at night.
• Encourage the patient to perform gentle, isometric ROM exercises.

• Provide emotional support and reassurance to help the patient cope with limited mobility. Explain that osteoarthritis isn't a systemic disease.

Patient care specific to the affected joint
• *Hand:* Apply hot soaks and paraffin dips to relieve pain as necessary.
• *Spine (lumbar and sacral):* Provide McKenzie extension and Williams flexion exercises for range of motion and functional lumbar stabilization for strengthening.
• *Spine (cervical):* Initiate ROM exercises for cervical spine and upper extremities along with scapula strengthening exercises.
• *Hip:* Use moist heat pads to relieve pain. Assist with ROM and strengthening exercises, always making sure the patient gets the proper rest afterward. Check crutches, canes, braces, and walkers for proper fit, and teach the patient how to use his device correctly. For example, the patient with unilateral joint involvement should use an orthopedic appliance (such as a cane or walker) on the unaffected side. Advise the use of cushions when sitting as well as use of an elevated toilet seat.
• *Knee:* Twice daily, assist with prescribed ROM exercises, exercises to maintain muscle tone, and progressive resistance exercises to increase muscle strength. Provide elastic supports or braces if needed. After total knee arthroplasty, provide patellar mobilization and soft-tissue massage.

Teaching points
• Teach the patient to pace his daily activities; moderation is the key.
• To minimize the long-term effects of osteoarthritis, teach him to plan for adequate rest during the day, after exertion, and at night.
• Instruct him to take medication exactly as prescribed, and to report adverse reactions immediately.

• Teach the patient to avoid overexertion. He should take care to stand and walk correctly, to minimize weight-bearing activities, and to be especially careful when stooping or picking up objects.
• Advise the patient to always wear well-fitting supportive shoes; don't allow the heels to become too worn down.
• Tell him to avoid stretching during the acute inflammatory stage.

Osteoporosis

In osteoporosis, a metabolic bone disorder, the rate of bone resorption accelerates while the rate of bone formation slows down, causing a loss of bone mass. Bones affected by this disease lose calcium and phosphate salts and thus become porous, brittle, and abnormally vulnerable to fracture.

Osteoporosis may be primary or secondary to an underlying disease. Primary osteoporosis is often called senile or postmenopausal osteoporosis because it most commonly develops in elderly, postmenopausal women.

Causes

The cause of primary osteoporosis is unknown; however, a mild but prolonged negative calcium balance, resulting from an inadequate dietary intake of calcium, may be an important contributing factor — as may declining gonadal adrenal function, faulty protein metabolism due to estrogen deficiency, and a sedentary lifestyle.

Causes of secondary osteoporosis include prolonged therapy with steroids or heparin, total immobilization or disuse of a bone (as with hemiplegia, for example), alcoholism, malnutrition, malabsorption, scurvy, lactose intolerance, hyperthyroidism, osteogenesis imperfecta, and

Sudeck's atrophy (localized to hands and feet, with recurring attacks).

Signs and symptoms

Osteoporosis is usually discovered when an elderly person bends to lift something, hears a snapping sound, and then feels a sudden pain in the lower back. Vertebral collapse, producing a backache with pain that radiates around the trunk, is the most common presenting feature. Any movement or jarring aggravates the backache.

In another common pattern, osteoporosis can develop insidiously, with increasing deformity, kyphosis, loss of height, and a markedly aged appearance. As vertebral bodies weaken, spontaneous wedge fractures, pathologic fractures of the neck and femur, Colles' fractures after a minor fall, and hip fractures commonly occur.

Osteoporosis primarily affects the weight-bearing vertebrae. Only when the condition is advanced or severe, as in Cushing's syndrome or hyperthyroidism, do comparable changes occur in the skull, ribs, and long bones.

Diagnostic tests

Differential diagnosis must exclude other causes of rarefying bone disease, especially those affecting the spine, such as metastatic carcinoma and advanced multiple myeloma. Initial evaluation attempts to identify the specific cause of osteoporosis through the patient history. Diagnostic tests include the following:
• X-rays show typical degeneration in the lower thoracic and lumbar vertebrae. The vertebral bodies may appear flattened and may look denser than normal. Loss of bone mineral becomes apparent in later stages.
• Dual or single photon absorptiometry allows measurement of bone

mass, which helps to assess the extremities, hips, and spine.

• Serum calcium, phosphorus, and alkaline phosphatase levels are all within normal limits, but parathyroid hormone may be elevated.

• Bone biopsy shows thin, porous, but otherwise normal-looking bone.

Treatment

Effective treatment aims to prevent additional fractures and control pain. Physical therapy emphasizes gentle exercise and activity, an important part of the treatment. Estrogen may be started within 3 years after menopause to decrease the rate of bone resorption; antiosteoporotic drugs, to rebuild thinning bones; sodium fluoride, to stimulate bone formation; and calcium and vitamin D, to support normal bone metabolism.

Weakened vertebrae should be supported, usually with a back brace. Surgery can correct pathologic fractures of the femur by open reduction and internal fixation. Colles' fracture requires reduction with plaster immobilization for 4 to 10 weeks.

Prevention

The incidence of senile osteoporosis may be reduced through adequate intake of dietary calcium, antiosteoporotic drugs, and regular exercise. Hormonal and fluoride treatments may also offer some preventive benefit.

Secondary osteoporosis can be prevented through effective treatment of the underlying disease, as well as steroid therapy, early mobilization after surgery or trauma, decreased alcohol consumption, careful observation for signs of malabsorption, and prompt treatment of hyperthyroidism.

Physical therapy considerations

• Focus on the patient's fragility, stressing careful positioning, ambulation, and prescribed exercises.

• Check the patient's skin daily for redness, warmth, and new sites of pain, which may indicate new fractures. Encourage activity; help the patient walk several times daily.

• Perform passive range-of-motion exercises, or encourage the patient to perform active exercises. Make sure she regularly attends scheduled physical therapy sessions.

• Use weight-bearing exercises, such as closed kinetic chain activity for lower extremities and light weights for upper extremities.

• Institute safety precautions such as keeping side rails up.

• To prevent fractures, move the patient gently and carefully at all times.

• Ensure that the assistive device used is properly fitted so as not to increase secondary symptoms of kyphosis.

Teaching points

• Thoroughly explain osteoporosis to the patient and her family. If they don't understand the nature of this disease, they may feel that they could have prevented the fractures if they had been more careful.

• Explain to the patient's family and ancillary heath care personnel how easily an osteoporotic patient's bones can fracture.

• Instruct the patient in the proper use of the prescribed back brace.

• Teach the patient good body mechanics — to stoop before lifting anything and to avoid twisting movements and prolonged bending.

• Encourage ambulation.

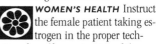 **WOMEN'S HEALTH** Instruct the female patient taking estrogen in the proper technique for self-examination of the breasts. Tell her to perform this ex-

amination at least once per month and to report any lumps immediately. Emphasize the need for regular gynecologic examinations. Tell her to report abnormal bleeding promptly because estrogen therapy is linked to increased risk of endometrial cancer.

Scoliosis

This lateral curvature of the spine may be found in the thoracic, lumbar, or thoracolumbar spinal segment. The curve may be convex to the right (more common in thoracic curves) or to the left (more common in lumbar curves). Rotation of the vertebral column around its axis occurs and may cause rib cage deformity. Scoliosis is often associated with kyphosis (humpback) and lordosis (swayback).

Causes

Scoliosis may be functional or structural. Functional (postural) scoliosis usually results from poor posture or a discrepancy in leg lengths, not fixed deformity of the spinal column. In structural scoliosis, curvature results from a deformity of the vertebral bodies.

Structural scoliosis may be:
• *congenital* — usually related to a congenital defect, such as wedge vertebrae, fused ribs or vertebrae, or hemivertebrae
• *paralytic or musculoskeletal* — develops several months after asymmetrical paralysis of the trunk muscles from polio, cerebral palsy, or muscular dystrophy
• *idiopathic (the most common form)* — may be transmitted as an autosomal dominant or multifactorial trait. This form appears in a previously straight spine during the growing years.

Idiopathic scoliosis can be classified as *infantile*, which affects mostly male infants between birth and age 3 and causes left thoracic and right lumbar curves; *juvenile*, which affects both sexes between ages 4 and 10 and causes varying types of curvature; or *adolescent*, which generally affects girls between age 10 and achievement of skeletal maturity and causes varying types of curvature.

Signs and symptoms

The most common curve in functional or structural scoliosis arises in the thoracic segment, with convexity to the right, and compensatory curves (S curves) in the cervical segment above and the lumbar segment below, both with convexity to the left. As the spine curves laterally, compensatory curves develop to maintain body balance and mark the deformity.

Scoliosis rarely produces subjective symptoms until it's well established; when symptoms do occur, they include backache, fatigue, and dyspnea. Because many teenagers are shy about their bodies, their parents may suspect that something is wrong only after they notice uneven hemlines, pant legs that appear unequal in length, or subtle physical signs like one hip appearing higher than the other.

Untreated scoliosis may result in pulmonary insufficiency (curvature may decrease lung capacity), back pain, degenerative arthritis of the spine, disk disease, and sciatica.

Diagnostic tests

Anterior, posterior, and lateral spinal X-rays, taken with the patient standing upright and bending over, confirm scoliosis and determine the degree of curvature (Cobb method) and flexibility of the spine (See *Measuring angle of curvature.*) A scoliometer can also be used to measure the angle of trunk rotation.

A physical examination reveals unequal shoulder heights, elbow levels, and heights of the iliac crests. Muscles on the convex side of the curve may be rounded; those on the concave side, flattened, producing asymmetry of paraspinal muscles.

Treatment

The severity of the deformity and potential spine growth determine appropriate treatment, which may include such noninvasive measures as close observation, exercise, or a brace. For more serious deformity, surgery or a combination of methods may be needed. To be most effective, treatment should begin early, when spinal deformity is still subtle.

Nonsurgical measures

A curve of less than 25 degrees is mild and can be monitored by X-rays and an examination every 3 months. An exercise program that includes situps, pelvic tilts, spine hyperextension, push-ups, and breathing exercises may strengthen torso muscles and prevent curve progression. A heel lift may help.

A curve of 30 to 50 degrees requires management with spinal exercises and a brace. (Transcutaneous electrical nerve stimulation may be used as an alternative.)

A brace halts progression in most patients but doesn't reverse the established curvature. Such devices passively strengthen the patient's spine by applying asymmetrical pressure to skin, muscles, and ribs. Braces can be adjusted as the patient grows and can be worn until bone growth is complete.

Surgery

A curve of 40 degrees or more requires surgery (spinal fusion with instrumentation), because a lateral

MEASURING ANGLE OF CURVATURE

The Cobb method measures the angle of curvature in scoliosis. The top vertebra in the curve (T6 in the illustration) is the uppermost vertebra whose upper face tilts toward the curve's concave side. The bottom vertebra in the curve (T12) is the lowest vertebra whose face tilts toward the curve's concave side. The angle at which perpendicular lines drawn from the upper face of the top vertebra and the lower face of the bottom vertebra intersect is the angle of the curve.

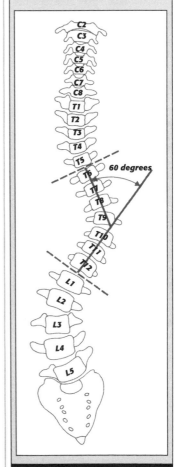

curve continues to progress at the rate of 1 degree a year even after skeletal maturity.

Some surgeons prescribe Cotrel dynamic traction for 7 to 10 days for preoperative preparation. This traction consists of a belt-pulley-weight system. While in traction, the patient should exercise for 10 minutes every hour, increasing muscle strength while keeping the vertebral column immobile.

Surgery corrects lateral curvature by posterior spinal fusion and internal stabilization with a Harrington rod. A distraction rod on the concave side of the curve "jacks" the spine into a straight position and provides an internal splint. A Cotrel-Dubousset rod system may also be used.

An alternative procedure, anterior spinal fusion with Dwyer or Zielke instrumentation, corrects curvature with vertebral staples and an anterior stabilizing cable. Some spinal fusions may require postoperative immobilization in a brace.

Postoperatively, periodic checkups are required for several months to monitor stability of the correction.

Physical therapy considerations

• Keep in mind that scoliosis often affects adolescent girls, who are likely to find activity limitations and the use of orthopedic appliances distressing. Therefore, provide emotional support, along with meticulous skin and cast care and patient teaching.
• If the patient needs traction or a cast before surgery, check the skin around the cast edge daily. Keep the cast clean and dry and edges of the cast "petaled."
After corrective surgery:
• Encourage deep-breathing exercises to avoid pulmonary complications.
• Give analgesics, as needed, especially before any activity.

• Promote active range-of-motion (ROM) arm exercises to help maintain muscle strength. Remember that any exercise, even brushing the hair or teeth, is helpful.
• Encourage the patient to perform quadriceps-setting, calf-pumping, and active ROM exercises of ankles and feet.
• Watch for skin breakdown and signs of cast syndrome.
• If you work in a school, screen children routinely for scoliosis during physical examinations.
• Aim physical therapy treatment at stretching shortened muscle tissue in the concave side of the curve, strengthening weak muscles in the convex side of curve, and postural reeducation. Include breathing exercises, posterior pelvic tilts, and spine elongation through weight shifting, exercises to strengthen trunk extensor muscles bilaterally through lifting trunk and lower extremities, and treating associated problems such as tight leg muscles.

Teaching points
• Explain to the patient that physical therapy alone can't stop the progression of scoliosis; its purpose is to strengthen back muscles and improve posture.
If the patient needs a brace:
• Explain what the brace does and how to care for it (checking screws for tightness and padding uprights to prevent excessive wear on clothing). Suggest wearing loose-fitting, oversized clothes for greater comfort.
• Tell the patient to wear the brace 23 hours a day and to remove it only for bathing and exercise.
• While the patient is still adjusting to the brace, tell her to lie down and rest several times a day. Suggest a soft mattress if a firm one is uncomfortable.
• Ensure the patient understands the importance of the brace and supply

the patient with the appropriate wearing schedule.

• To prevent skin breakdown, advise the patient not to use lotions, ointments, or powders on areas where the brace contacts the skin. Instead, suggest that she use rubbing alcohol or tincture of benzoin to toughen the skin. Tell her to keep the skin dry and clean and to wear a snug T-shirt under the brace.

• Advise her to increase activities gradually and to avoid strenuous sports. Emphasize the importance of performing prescribed exercises diligently. Recommend swimming during the 1 hour out of the brace but strongly warn against diving.

• Instruct the patient to turn her whole body, instead of just her head, when looking to the side. To make reading easier, tell her to hold the book so she can look straight ahead at it instead of down. If she finds this difficult, help her to obtain prism glasses.

If the patient needs traction or a cast before surgery:

• Explain preoperative procedures to the patient and family. Remember that application of a body cast can be traumatic because it's done on a special frame and the patient's head and face are covered throughout the procedure.

• Warn the patient not to insert anything under the cast or let anything get under it and to immediately report cracks in the cast, pain, burning, skin breakdown, numbness, or odor.

• Before surgery, assure the patient and family that she'll receive adequate pain control postoperatively.

• After surgery, teach the patient how to recognize signs of skin breakdown and cast syndrome.

Torticollis

Also called wryneck, torticollis is a neck deformity in which the sternocleidomastoid neck muscles are spastic or shortened, causing bending of the head to the affected side and rotation of the chin to the opposite side.

This disorder may be congenital or acquired. Incidence of congenital (muscular) torticollis is highest in infants after difficult delivery (breech presentation), in firstborn infants, and in girls. Acquired torticollis usually develops during the first 10 years of life or after age 40.

Causes

Possible causes of congenital torticollis include malposition of the head in utero, prenatal injury, fibroma, interruption of blood supply, or fibrotic rupture of the sternocleidomastoid muscle, with hematoma and scar formation.

The three types of acquired torticollis — acute, spasmodic, and hysterical — have differing causes.

• The *acute* form results from muscular damage caused by inflammatory diseases, such as myositis, lymphadenitis, and tuberculosis, and from cervical spinal injuries that produce scar tissue contracture.

• The *spasmodic* form results from rhythmic muscle spasms caused by an organic central nervous system disorder (probably due to irritation of the nerve root by arthritis or osteomyelitis).

• The *hysterical* form stems from a psychogenic inability to control neck muscles.

Signs and symptoms

The following features characterize congenital torticollis and acquired torticollis.

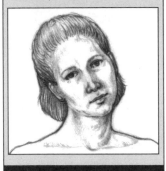

Congenital torticollis

The first sign of congenital torticollis is often a firm, nontender, palpable enlargement of the sternocleidomastoid muscle that is visible at birth and for several weeks afterward. It slowly regresses during a period of 6 months, although incomplete regression can cause permanent contracture.

If the deformity is severe, the infant's face and head flatten from sleeping on the affected side; this asymmetry gradually worsens. The infant's chin turns away from the side of the shortened muscle, and his head tilts to the shortened side. His shoulder may be elevated on the affected side, restricting neck movement.

Acquired torticollis

The first sign of acquired torticollis is usually recurring unilateral stiffness of neck muscles, followed by a drawing sensation and a momentary twitching or contraction that pulls the head to the affected side. This type of torticollis often produces severe neuralgic pain throughout the head and neck. *(See Recognizing torticollis.)*

Diagnostic tests

A history of painless neck deformity from birth suggests congenital torticollis; gradual onset of painful neck deformity suggests acquired torticollis. However, diagnosis must rule out tuberculosis of the cervical spine, pharyngeal or tonsillar inflammations, spinal accessory nerve damage, ruptured transverse ligaments, subdural hematoma, dislocations and fractures, scoliosis, congenital abnormalities of the cervical spine, rheumatoid arthritis, and osteomyelitis.

In acquired torticollis, cervical spine X-rays are negative for bone or joint disease but may reveal an associated disorder (such as tuberculosis, scar tissue formation, or arthritis).

Treatment

Congenital torticollis and acquired torticollis are treated in different ways.

Congenital torticollis

Therapy for congenital torticollis aims to stretch the shortened muscle. Nonsurgical treatment includes passive neck stretching and proper positioning during sleep for an infant and active stretching exercises for an older child—for example, touching the ear opposite the affected side to the shoulder and touching the chin to the same shoulder.

Surgical correction involves sectioning the sternocleidomastoid muscle; this should take place during preschool years and only if other therapies fail.

Acquired torticollis

Treatment of acquired torticollis aims to correct the underlying cause of the disease. In the acute form, application of heat, cervical traction, and gentle massage may help relieve pain. Stretching exercises and a neck brace may relieve symptoms of the spasmodic and hysterical forms.

Treatment of elderly patients with acquired torticollis may include administration of levodopa-carbidopa, carbamazepine, and haloperidol.

Physical therapy considerations

• To aid early diagnosis of congenital torticollis, observe the infant for limited neck movement, and thoroughly assess his degree of discomfort.
• Provide emotional support for the patient and family to relieve their anxiety due to fear, pain, limitations from the brace or traction, and an altered body image.
• Begin stretching exercises as soon as the patient can tolerate them.
• Provide physical therapy exercises that include inhibition and relaxation techniques to decrease the tone of the muscle in spasm.

Teaching point
• Instruct the patient and family in the application, wearing, and care of the cervical brace.

Neurologic disorders

Amyotrophic lateral sclerosis

Commonly called Lou Gehrig's disease, after the New York Yankees first baseman who died of this disorder, amyotrophic lateral sclerosis (ALS) is the most common motor neuron disease causing muscular atrophy. Other motor neuron diseases include progressive muscular atrophy and progressive bulbar palsy. Onset occurs between ages 40 and 70. A chronic,

progressively debilitating disease, ALS is rapidly fatal.

Causes

More than 30,000 Americans have ALS; about 5,000 new cases are diagnosed each year, with men affected three times more often than women. The exact cause of ALS is unknown, but about 5% to 10% of ALS cases have a genetic component. In these, it is an autosomal dominant trait and affects men and women equally.

ALS and other motor neuron diseases may result from:
• a slow-acting virus
• nutritional deficiency related to a disturbance in enzyme metabolism
• metabolic interference in nucleic acid production by the nerve fibers
• autoimmune disorders that affect immune complexes in the renal glomerulus and basement membrane.

Precipitating factors for acute deterioration include trauma, viral infections, and physical exhaustion.

Signs and symptoms

Patients with ALS develop fasciculations, accompanied by atrophy and weakness, especially in the muscles of the forearms and the hands. Other signs include impaired speech; difficulty chewing, swallowing, and breathing, particularly if the brain stem is affected; and, occasionally, choking and excessive drooling.

Mental deterioration doesn't usually occur, but patients may become depressed as a reaction to the disease. Progressive bulbar palsy may cause crying spells or inappropriate laughter.

Diagnostic tests

Characteristic clinical features indicate a combination of upper and lower motor neuron involvement without sensory impairment. Electromyography and a muscle biopsy help show nerve, rather than muscle, disease. The protein content of cerebrospinal fluid is increased in one-third of patients, but this finding alone doesn't confirm ALS.

Diagnosis must rule out multiple sclerosis, spinal cord neoplasm, polyarteritis, syringomyelia, myasthenia gravis, and progressive muscular dystrophy.

Treatment

Management aims to control symptoms and provide emotional, psychological, and physical support.

Physical therapy considerations

• Begin patient care with a complete neurologic assessment to serve as a baseline for future evaluations of progressing disease.
• Implement a rehabilitation program designed to maintain independence as long as possible.
• Help the patient obtain mobility equipment, such as a walker and a wheelchair.
• Provide emotional support. Prepare the patient and family for his eventual death, and encourage them to start the grieving process. Patients with ALS may benefit from hospice care.
• Be aware of early symptoms such as falling; loss of motor control in hands and arms; difficulty speaking, swallowing, and breathing; persistent fatigue; and twitching and cramping.
• Provide range-of-motion exercises to prevent contractures, transfer and gait assistance with appropriate assistive devices, orthotics, massage for spastic muscles, and energy conservation (no intense exercise).
• Suggest the use of adaptive equipment to increase functional independence.

Teaching points
• Teach the patient proper use of assistive devices.
• Teach the family or caregivers transfer techniques.
• Instruct the patient to pace his daily activities.

Cerebral palsy

The most common cause of crippling in children, cerebral palsy comprises a group of neuromuscular disorders resulting from prenatal, perinatal, or postnatal central nervous system (CNS) damage. Although nonprogressive, these disorders may become more obvious as an affected infant grows older.

There are three major types of cerebral palsy — spastic, athetoid, and ataxic — which sometimes occur in mixed forms. Motor impairment may be minimal (sometimes apparent only during physical activities such as running) or severely disabling. Associated defects, such as seizures, speech disorders, and mental retardation, are common.

The prognosis varies. In mild impairment, proper treatment may make a near-normal life possible.

Cerebral palsy occurs in an estimated 1.5 to 5:1,000 live births every year. Incidence is highest in premature infants (anoxia plays the greatest role in contributing to cerebral palsy) and in those who are small for their gestational age. Cerebral palsy is slightly more common in males than in females and occurs more often in whites.

Causes

Conditions that result in cerebral anoxia, hemorrhage, or other CNS damage are probably responsible for cerebral palsy.

Prenatal causes

Such causes include maternal infection (especially rubella), radiation, anoxia, toxemia, maternal diabetes, abnormal placental attachment, malnutrition, and isoimmunization.

Perinatal and birth difficulties

Examples of these causes include forceps delivery, breech presentation, placenta previa, abruptio placentae, depressed maternal vital signs from general or spinal anesthetic, and prolapsed cord with delay in the delivery of the head. Premature birth, prolonged or unusually rapid labor, and multiple birth (especially infants born last in a multiple birth) may also cause cerebral palsy.

Infection or trauma during infancy

Cerebral palsy may follow kernicterus resulting from erythroblastosis fetalis, brain infection, head trauma, prolonged anoxia, brain tumor, cerebral circulatory anomalies causing blood vessel rupture, and systemic disease resulting in cerebral thrombosis or embolus.

Signs and symptoms

Each type of cerebral palsy typically produces a distinctive set of clinical features, although some children display a mixed form of the disease.

Spastic cerebral palsy

This form of the disease affects about 70% of patients. Spastic cerebral palsy is characterized by hyperactive deep tendon reflexes, increased stretch reflexes, rapid alternating muscle contraction and relaxation, muscle weakness, underdevelopment of affected limbs, muscle contraction in response to manipulation, and a tendency toward contractures. Typically, a child with spastic cerebral palsy walks on his toes with a scissor gait, crossing one foot in front of the other.

Athetoid cerebral palsy

Affecting about 20% of patients, this form causes involuntary movements (grimacing, wormlike writhing, dystonia, and sharp jerks) that impair voluntary movement. Usually, these involuntary movements affect the arms more severely than the legs; involuntary facial movements may make speech difficult. These athetoid movements become more severe during stress, decrease with relaxation, and disappear entirely during sleep.

Ataxic cerebral palsy

Roughly 10% of patients have this form of the disease. Its characteristics include disturbed balance, incoordination (especially of the arms), hypoactive reflexes, nystagmus, muscle weakness, tremor, lack of leg movement during infancy, and a wide gait as the child begins to walk. Ataxia makes sudden or fine movements almost impossible.

Mixed form

Some children with cerebral palsy display a combination of these signs and symptoms. In most, impaired motor function makes eating, especially swallowing, difficult and retards growth and development. Up to 40% of these children are mentally retarded, about 25% have seizure disorders, and about 80% have impaired speech. Many also have dental abnormalities, vision and hearing defects, and reading disabilities.

Diagnostic tests

An early diagnosis is essential for effective treatment and requires careful clinical observation during infancy and precise neurologic assessment.

Suspect cerebral palsy whenever an infant:
• has difficulty sucking or keeping the nipple or food in his mouth
• seldom moves voluntarily, or has arm or leg tremors with voluntary movement
• crosses his legs when lifted from behind rather than pulling them up or "bicycling" like a normal infant
• has legs that are hard to separate, making diaper changing difficult
• persistently uses only one hand or, as he gets older, uses his hands well but not his legs.

Infants at particular risk include those with low birth weight, low Apgar scores at 5 minutes, seizures, and metabolic disturbances. However, all infants should have a screening test for cerebral palsy as a regular part of their 6-month checkup.

Treatment

Cerebral palsy can't be cured, but proper treatment can help affected children reach their full potential within the limits set by this disorder. Such treatment requires a comprehensive and cooperative effort involving doctors, nurses, teachers, psychologists, the child's family, and occupational, physical, and speech therapists. Home care is often possible.

Treatment usually includes:
• braces or splints and special appliances, such as adapted eating utensils and a low toilet seat with arms, to help these children perform activities independently
• an artificial urinary sphincter for the incontinent child who can use the hand controls
• range-of-motion (ROM) exercises to minimize contractures
• orthopedic surgery to correct contractures
• phenytoin, phenobarbital, or another anticonvulsant to control seizures

• sometimes muscle relaxants or neurosurgery to decrease spasticity.

Children with milder forms of cerebral palsy should attend regular school; children with severe forms need special education classes.

Physical therapy considerations

• Speak slowly and distinctly to the child hospitalized for orthopedic surgery or treatment of complications. Encourage him to ask for things he wants. Listen patiently and don't rush him.
• Give all care in an unhurried manner; otherwise, muscle spasticity may increase.
• Encourage the child and his family to participate in the patient's care so they can continue it at home.
• Use a team approach with appropriate referrals for occupational therapy, speech therapy, psychiatric treatment (behavioral therapy), and nutrition.
• Symptoms of cerebral palsy appear in the first few years of life and generally don't worsen over time; therefore, early intervention and maintenance programs are very important.
• Direct postsurgical physical therapy at maintaining ROM after tendon-lengthening procedures.
• Prevent musculoskeletal deformity of the spine with proper positioning, adequate exercise of trunk and limbs, and family education regarding posture.
• When working with patients with spastic cerebral palsy, look for speech deficits, poor extension in prone position, cocontractions at proximal joints, respiratory difficulty, increased energy expenditure with basic movements, poor head control, and inability to work in midline.
• When working with patients with athetoid cerebral palsy, look for lack of cocontraction for proximal stability, hypermobility of joints causing

possible subluxation, intermittent spasms, general low muscle tone, and delayed head control.

• With patients with ataxic cerebral palsy, look for symptoms in the lower extremities more than the upper extremities, deficits in gait later during development, balance deficits, and increased frequency of falls.

• When spasticity occurs, gently rotate the limb inward toward the spasticity and then rotate it outward. Repeating this motion will help relax the spastic extremity. Pressure on the tendons located in the joint socket while rotating will increase relaxation. Open a spastic hand by gently grabbing the lateral aspects and moving inward and out.

• When positioning the patient in bed, elongate the patient's down side, making sure the down shoulder is slightly pulled out for comfort and that all limbs are well supported.

• Consider hand and foot orthotics to help maintain mobility.

• Set realistic individual goals.

Teaching points

• Teach parents or caregivers how to perform appropriate exercises with the patient.

• Teach proper use of assistive devices.

• Refer parents to supportive community organizations. For more information, tell parents to contact the United Cerebral Palsy Association, Inc., or their local cerebral palsy agency.

Cerebrovascular accident

Commonly called a stroke, cerebrovascular accident (CVA) is a sudden impairment of cerebral circulation in one or more of the blood vessels supplying the brain. CVA interrupts or diminishes oxygen supply and often causes serious damage or necrosis in brain tissues.

The sooner circulation returns to normal after CVA, the better chances are for complete recovery. However, about half of those who survive a CVA remain permanently disabled and experience a recurrence within weeks, months, or years.

CVA is the third most common cause of death in the United States today and the most common cause of neurologic disability. It strikes 500,000 people each year; half of them die as a result.

Causes

Factors that increase the risk of CVA include history of transient ischemic attacks, atherosclerosis, hypertension, electrocardiogram changes, arrhythmias, rheumatic heart disease, diabetes mellitus, gout, postural hypotension, cardiac or myocardial enlargement, high serum triglyceride levels, lack of exercise, use of oral contraceptives, cigarette smoking, and family history of CVA.

The major causes of CVA are thrombosis, embolism, and hemorrhage.

Thrombosis

In middle-aged and elderly people, among whom there is a higher incidence of atherosclerosis, diabetes, and hypertension, thrombosis is the most common cause of CVA. Obstruction of a blood vessel causes the CVA. Typically, the main site of the obstruction is in extracerebral vessels, but sometimes it's intracerebral.

Thrombosis causes ischemia in brain tissue supplied by the affected vessel as well as congestion and edema. The latter may produce more clinical effects than thrombosis itself, but these symptoms subside as edema subsides.

Thrombosis may develop while the patient sleeps or soon after he awakens; it can also occur during surgery or after a myocardial infarction. The risk increases with obesity, smoking, or the use of oral contraceptives. Cocaine-induced ischemic stroke is now being seen in younger patients.

Embolism

The second most common cause of CVA, embolism is an occlusion of a blood vessel caused by a fragmented clot, a tumor, fat, bacteria, or air. It can occur at any age, especially among patients with a history of rheumatic heart disease, endocarditis, posttraumatic valvular disease, myocardial fibrillation and other cardiac arrhythmias, or following open-heart surgery.

The embolus usually develops rapidly — in 10 to 20 seconds — and without warning. When it reaches the cerebral vasculature, it cuts off circulation by lodging in a narrow portion of an artery, most often the middle cerebral artery, causing necrosis and edema.

If the embolus is septic and infection extends beyond the vessel wall, an abscess or encephalitis may develop. If the infection is within the vessel wall, an aneurysm may form, which could lead to cerebral hemorrhage.

Hemorrhage

The third most common cause of CVA is hemorrhage. Like embolism, it may occur suddenly, at any age. Such hemorrhage results from chronic hypertension or aneurysms, which cause sudden rupture of a cerebral artery. The rupture diminishes blood supply to the area served by this artery. In addition, blood accumulates deep within the brain, further compressing neural tissue and causing even greater damage.

CVA classification

CVAs are classified according to their course of progression. The least severe is the transient ischemic attack (TIA), or "little stroke," which results from a temporary interruption of blood flow, most often in the carotid and vertebrobasilar arteries. A progressive stroke (also known as a stroke-in-evolution or thrombus-in-evolution) begins with slight neurologic deficit and worsens in one or two days. In a completed stroke, neurologic deficits are maximal right at onset.

Signs and symptoms

Clinical features of CVA vary with the artery affected (and, consequently, the portion of the brain it supplies), the severity of damage, and the extent of collateral circulation that develops to help the brain compensate for decreased blood supply.

If the CVA occurs in the left hemisphere, it produces symptoms on the right side; if in the right hemisphere, symptoms are on the left side. However, a CVA that causes cranial nerve damage produces signs of cranial nerve dysfunction on the same side as the hemorrhage.

Symptoms are usually classified according to the artery affected:
• *middle cerebral artery:* aphasia, dysphasia, visual field cuts, and hemiparesis on the affected side (more severe in the face and arm than in the leg)
• *carotid artery:* weakness, paralysis, numbness, sensory changes, and visual disturbances on the affected side; altered level of consciousness (LOC), bruits, headaches, aphasia, and ptosis
• *vertebrobasilar artery:* weakness on the affected side, numbness around the lips and mouth, visual field cuts, diplopia, poor coordina-

tion, dysphagia, slurred speech, dizziness, amnesia, and ataxia
• *anterior cerebral artery:* confusion, weakness and numbness (especially in the leg) on the affected side, incontinence, loss of coordination, impaired motor and sensory functions, and personality changes
• *posterior cerebral arteries:* visual field cuts, sensory impairment, dyslexia, coma, and cortical blindness. Usually, paralysis is absent.

Symptoms can also be classified as premonitory, generalized, and focal. Premonitory symptoms, such as drowsiness, dizziness, headache, and mental confusion, are rare. Generalized symptoms, such as headache, vomiting, mental impairment, seizures, coma, nuchal rigidity, fever, and disorientation, are typical. Focal symptoms, such as sensory and reflex changes, reflect the site of hemorrhage or infarction and may worsen.

Diagnostic tests

Confirmation of CVA is based on observation of clinical features, a history of risk factors, and the results of diagnostic tests.
• Computed tomography scan shows evidence of hemorrhagic stroke immediately but may not show evidence of thrombotic infarction for 48 to 72 hours.
• Magnetic resonance imaging may help identify ischemic or infarcted areas and cerebral swelling.
• Brain scan shows ischemic areas but may not be positive for up to 2 weeks after the CVA.
• Lumbar puncture reveals bloody cerebrospinal fluid in hemorrhagic stroke.
• Ophthalmoscopy may show signs of hypertension and atherosclerotic changes in retinal arteries.
• Angiography outlines blood vessels and pinpoints occlusion or rupture site.

• EEG helps to localize the damaged area.
Other baseline laboratory studies include urinalysis, coagulation studies, complete blood count, serum osmolality, and electrolyte, glucose, triglyceride, creatinine, and blood urea nitrogen levels.

Treatment

Treatment options vary depending on the type of CVA and the patient's experiences. Early medical diagnosis of the type of CVA coupled with new drug treatments can greatly reduce the long-term disability secondary to ischemia.

Surgery performed to improve cerebral circulation in patients with thrombotic or embolic CVA includes an endarterectomy (removal of atherosclerotic plaque from the inner arterial wall) or a microvascular bypass (surgical anastomosis of an extracranial vessel to an intracranial vessel).

Medications useful in treating CVA include:
• alteplase (recombinant tissue plasminogen activator, tPA), effective in emergency treatment of embolic CVA. (Patients with emboli or thrombolytic CVA who aren't candidates for tPA [3 to 6 hours post-CVA] should receive aspirin or heparin.)
• long-term use of aspirin or ticlopidine, used as antiplatelet agents to prevent recurrent CVA
• anticoagulants (heparin and warfarin), which may be required to treat crescendo TIAs not responsive to antiplatelet agents
• antihypertensives, antiarrhythmics, and antidiabetic agents, which may be used to treat risk factors associated with recurrent CVA
• corticosteroids such as dexamethasone to minimize associated cerebral edema

• analgesics such as codeine to relieve the headache that typically follows hemorrhagic CVA.

Physical therapy considerations

• Watch for signs of pulmonary emboli, such as chest pains, shortness of breath, dusky color, tachycardia, fever, and changed sensorium.
• Watch for signs of other complications such as infection, cerebral edema, hydrocephalus, seizures, aspiration pneumonia, deep-vein thrombosis, pressure ulcers, urinary tract infections, contractures, and subluxation.
• To prevent aspiration pneumonia, place the patient in an upright and lateral position to allow secretions to drain. Turn him frequently.
• When positioning the patient, align his extremities correctly. Use rolls to prevent external rotation. Use high-topped sneakers to prevent footdrop when the patient is sitting up and his feet are on the floor.
• Provide range-of-motion (ROM) exercises throughout the day.
• Assist in minimizing long-term disability. Deficits can include motor weakness, coordination and balance problems, diminished corneal reflex, visual field deficits, dysarthria, dysphasia, impaired memory and concentration, and pain.
• Establish and maintain communication with the patient. If he is aphasic, set up a simple method of communicating basic needs. Remember to phrase your questions so he'll be able to answer using this system. Repeat yourself quietly and calmly (remember, he isn't deaf) and use gestures if necessary to help him understand. Even the unresponsive patient can hear, so don't say anything in his presence you wouldn't want him to hear and remember.

• Provide psychological support. Set realistic short-term goals. Involve the patient's family in his care when possible, and explain his deficits and strengths.
• For the patient with hemiparesis, arrange the room with objects of interest located on the affected side. This will encourage him to look in that direction.
• Position the patient in bed in a side-lying position on the affected side. This can help him decrease hypertonicity and increase awareness on the hemiparetic side.
• Be aware of orthopedic problems that can occur, such as:
– *subluxation of the shoulder:* occurs when any biomechanical factors contributing to glenohumeral joint stability are interrupted
– *pain:* due to muscle imbalance, loss of joint ROM, improper movement patterns, and improper weight-bearing patterns. (It may lead to reflex sympathetic dystrophy. Taking extra care with ROM can prevent it.)
• Establish rapport with the patient. Spend time with him, and provide a means of communication. Simplify your language, asking yes-or-no questions whenever possible. Don't correct his speech or treat him like a child. Remember that building rapport may be difficult because of the mood changes that may result from brain damage or as a reaction to being dependent.

Evaluating the patient
Some physical therapy considerations to remember during the evaluation of the patient include:
• Thoroughly review the chart to understand the patient's condition, treatment, and progress.
• Interview the family to better understand the prior functional level of the patient.
• Assess cognitive and mental status by determining level of consciousness

(alert to comatose); orientation to person, place, and time; presence of confusion (decreased understanding of the environment); higher cortical functions (serial subtraction); short-term memory; ability to follow simple or multiple-step commands; and presence of confabulation.
• Assess ROM and document passive and active motion of extremities and trunk.
• Assess strength. Because muscle groups can't be isolated, you can't perform true manual muscle testing. Don't use resistance in the acute stage of CVA because of the risk of another CVA with exertion or Valsalva's maneuver. Document against-gravity strength.
• Assess sensation. Test for light touch, kinesthesia, deep pressure, 2-point discrimination, hot and cold sensation, and proprioception. Keep in mind proprioception is important for normal movement. Sensation may appear to change with changes in cognition.
• Assess coordination of fine and gross motor development through finger-to-nose, opposition, and rapid alternating movement tests. Determine presence of ataxia.
• Assess tone through resistance of passive stretch. Typically, the CVA patient begins with hypotonicity, which then turns to hypertonicity, and eventually reduces to more normal tone with increased voluntary control of muscles. Positional changes may induce spasticity.
• Assess static and dynamic balance in all positions (supported and unsupported).
• Assess endurance by observing for fatigue, shortness of breath (due to paralysis of thorax), and decrease in lung capacity.
• Assess skin for evidence of pressure and pitting edema. Position the patient properly to maintain skin integrity.

• Assess abnormal righting and extensor reflexes. Tendon reflexes may be slow, brisk, or normal.
• Assess wheelchair mobility. The patient needs to be able to independently move and manage his wheelchair on all surfaces.
• Assess transfers and instruct in all types, but focus on the most functional.
• Assess gait and evaluate deviations on all surfaces and stairs. Instruct in the proper use of assistive devices and orthoses or braces as appropriate.
• Refer to speech and occupational therapy for evaluation and appropriate treatment.

Teaching points
• If necessary, teach the patient to comb his hair, dress, and wash.
• Instruct in the use of assistive devices, such as walking frames, hand bars by the toilet, and ramps, as needed.
• To reinforce teaching, involve the patient's family in all aspects of rehabilitation. With their cooperation and support, devise realistic discharge goals, and let them help decide when the patient can return home.

Multiple sclerosis

This progressive disease is caused by demyelination of the white matter of the brain and spinal cord. In multiple sclerosis (MS), sporadic patches of demyelination throughout the central nervous system induce widely disseminated and varied neurologic dysfunction. Characterized by exacerbations and remissions, MS is a major cause of chronic disability in young adults.

The prognosis varies. MS may progress rapidly, disabling the patient by early adulthood or causing death within months of onset. However,

70% of patients lead active, productive lives with prolonged remissions.

Causes

The exact cause of MS is unknown, but current theories suggest a slow-acting or latent viral infection and an autoimmune response. Other theories have linked MS to environmental and genetic factors.

Emotional stress, overwork, fatigue, pregnancy, and acute respiratory infections may precede the onset of this illness.

MS usually begins between ages 20 and 40 (the average age of onset is 27). It affects three women for every two men and five whites for every black. Incidence is low in Japan; it's generally higher among urban populations and upper socioeconomic groups. A family history of MS and living in a cold, damp climate increase the risk.

Signs and symptoms

Clinical findings in MS depend on the extent and site of myelin destruction, the extent of remyelination, and the adequacy of subsequent restored synaptic transmission.

Signs and symptoms in MS may be transient, or they may last for hours or weeks. They may wax and wane with no predictable pattern, vary from day to day, and be bizarre and difficult for the patient to describe.

In most patients, visual problems and sensory impairment, such as paresthesia, are the first signs that something may be wrong.

Other characteristic changes include the following:

• *ocular disturbances* — optic neuritis, diplopia, ophthalmoplegia, blurred vision, and nystagmus
• *muscle dysfunction* — weakness, paralysis ranging from monoplegia to quadriplegia, spasticity, hyper-reflexia, intention tremor, and gait ataxia
• *urinary disturbances* — incontinence, frequency, urgency, and frequent infections
• *emotional lability* — characteristic mood swings, irritability, euphoria, or depression.

Associated signs and symptoms include poorly articulated or scanning speech and dysphagia. Clinical effects may be so mild that the patient is unaware of them or so bizarre that he appears hysterical.

Diagnostic tests

Because early symptoms may be mild, years may elapse between onset of the first signs and the diagnosis. Diagnosis of this disorder requires evidence of multiple neurologic attacks and characteristic remissions and exacerbations. Periodic testing and close observation of the patient are necessary, perhaps for years, depending on the course of the disease.

The following tests may be performed:

• Magnetic resonance imaging may detect MS lesions.
• EEG is abnormal in one-third of patients.
• Lumbar puncture shows an elevated gamma globulin fraction of immunoglobulin G but normal total cerebrospinal fluid (CSF) protein levels. An elevated CSF gamma globulin level is significant only when serum gamma globulin levels are normal; it reflects hyperactivity of the immune system due to chronic demyelination. In addition, the white blood cell level in CSF may be elevated.
• Electrophoresis can detect oligoclonal bands of immunoglobulin in CSF. Present in most patients, they can be found even when the percentage of gamma globulin in CSF is normal.

A differential diagnosis must rule out spinal cord compression, foramen magnum tumor (which may mimic the exacerbations and remissions of MS), multiple small strokes, syphilis or another infection, and psychological disturbances.

Treatment

The aim of treatment is to shorten exacerbations and relieve neurologic deficits so that the patient can resume a normal lifestyle.

Drug therapy

Corticotropin, prednisone, or dexamethasone is used to reduce the associated edema of the myelin sheath during exacerbations. Corticotropin and corticosteroids may relieve symptoms and hasten remission, but they don't prevent future exacerbations.

Other drugs used include chlordiazepoxide to mitigate mood swings, baclofen or dantrolene to relieve spasticity, and bethanechol or oxybutynin to relieve urine retention and minimize frequency and urgency.

Interferon beta-lb may be used for ambulatory patients with relapsing-remitting MS to reduce the frequency of exacerbations. Immunosuppressants, such as azathioprine or cyclophosphamide, may suppress the immune response.

Supportive measures

During acute exacerbations, supportive measures include bed rest, comfort measures such as massages, prevention of fatigue, prevention of pressure ulcers, bowel and bladder training (if necessary), administration of antibiotics for bladder infections, physical therapy, and counseling.

Physical therapy considerations

• Active, resistive, and stretching exercises maintain muscle tone and joint mobility, decrease spasticity, improve coordination, and boost morale.
• Regulate the patient's activity level. Encourage daily physical exercise with regular rest periods to prevent fatigue.
• Remember that exacerbating factors include heat, stress, and trauma.

Physical therapy management of common MS symptoms include:
• *Sensory disturbances:* Desensitize limb with vigorous rubbing or tapping, biofeedback for loss of proprioception, and pressure relief education.
• *Pain due to malalignment:* Manage with stretching, postural training, orthotics, adaptive seating equipment, and modalities.
• *Fatigue:* Manage by increasing strength or endurance, isokinetic exercises, tone reduction, and energy conservation techniques. Exercising to fatigue level is contraindicated. Morning exercise is most beneficial.
• *Spasticity:* Manage with cryotherapy, therapeutic exercise (passive elongation of spastic muscle), relaxation techniques, mat activities for trunk rotation, and peripheral neuromuscular facilitation (PNF) and neurodevelopmental technique (NDT) to encourage trunk flexion.
• *Cerebellar disturbances:* Encourage postural stability with weight-bearing activities and weight shifting. Ataxic limb movement can be decreased by using cuff weights to increase proprioceptive feedback.
• *Range-of-motion (ROM) deficits:* Manage with passive ROM several times daily and joint mobilization
• *Gait problems:* Manage with proximal stability exercises, weight transfer, trunk rotation, assistive devices,

orthotics, rocker shoes, and wheel-chair training if appropriate.

Teaching points

• Inform the patient that exacerbations are unpredictable, necessitating physical and emotional adjustments in his lifestyle.

• For more information, refer the patient to the National Multiple Sclerosis Society.

Myelitis and acute transverse myelitis

Myelitis, or inflammation of the spinal cord, can result from several diseases. Poliomyelitis affects the cord's gray matter and produces motor dysfunction; leukomyelitis affects only the white matter and produces sensory dysfunction. These types of myelitis can attack any level of the spinal cord, causing partial destruction or scattered lesions.

Acute transverse myelitis, which affects the entire thickness of the spinal cord, produces both motor and sensory dysfunctions. This form of myelitis, which has a rapid onset, is the most devastating.

The prognosis depends on the severity of cord damage and prevention of complications. If spinal cord necrosis occurs, the prognosis for complete recovery is poor. Even without necrosis, residual neurologic deficits usually persist after recovery. Patients who develop spastic reflexes early in the illness are more likely to recover than those who don't.

Causes

Acute transverse myelitis has a variety of causes. It often follows acute infectious diseases, such as measles or pneumonia (the inflammation occurs after the infection has subsided), and primary infections of the spinal cord itself, such as syphilis or acute disseminated encephalomyelitis.

Acute transverse myelitis can accompany demyelinating diseases such as acute multiple sclerosis and inflammatory and necrotizing disorders of the spinal cord such as hematomyelia.

Certain toxic agents (such as carbon monoxide, lead, and arsenic) can cause a type of myelitis in which acute inflammation (followed by hemorrhage and possible necrosis) destroys the entire circumference (myelin, axis cylinders, and neurons) of the spinal cord.

Other forms of myelitis may result from poliovirus, herpes zoster, herpesvirus B, or rabies virus; disorders that cause meningeal inflammation, such as syphilis, abscesses and other suppurative conditions, and tuberculosis; smallpox or polio vaccination; parasitic and fungal infections; and chronic adhesive arachnoiditis.

Signs and symptoms

In acute transverse myelitis, onset is rapid, with motor and sensory dysfunctions below the level of spinal cord damage appearing in 1 to 2 days.

Patients with acute transverse myelitis develop flaccid paralysis of the legs (sometimes beginning in just one leg) with loss of sensory and sphincter function. Such sensory loss may follow pain in the legs or trunk. Reflexes disappear in the early stages but may reappear later. The extent of damage depends on which level of the spinal cord is affected; transverse myelitis rarely involves the arms. If spinal cord damage is severe, it may cause shock (hypotension and hypothermia).

Diagnostic tests

Paraplegia of rapid onset usually points to acute transverse myelitis. In such patients, neurologic examination confirms paraplegia or neurologic deficit below the level of the spinal cord lesion and absent or, later, hyperactive reflexes. Cerebrospinal fluid may be normal or show increased lymphocyte or protein levels.

Diagnostic evaluation must rule out a spinal cord tumor and identify the cause of any underlying infection.

Treatment

No effective treatment exists for acute transverse myelitis. However, this condition requires appropriate treatment of any underlying infection. Some patients with postinfectious or multiple sclerosis-induced myelitis have received steroid therapy, but its benefits aren't clear.

Physical therapy considerations

• Frequently assess vital signs. Watch carefully for signs of spinal shock (hypotension and excessive sweating).
• Prevent contractures with range-of-motion exercises and proper alignment.
• Prevent skin infections and pressure ulcers with meticulous skin care. Check pressure points often and keep skin clean and dry; use a waterbed or another pressure-relieving device.
• Initiate rehabilitation immediately. Assist the patient with bowel and bladder training, and any lifestyle changes that his condition requires.
• For additional physical therapy considerations, see the "Spinal injuries" entry in Chapter 7.

Teaching point
• Instruct the patient and family in proper positioning to prevent pressure ulcers.

Parkinson's disease

Named for James Parkinson, the English doctor who first accurately described the disease in 1817, Parkinson's disease (also known as parkinsonism, paralysis agitans, and shaking palsy) is a slowly progressive movement disorder that characteristically produces progressive muscle rigidity, akinesia, and involuntary tremor. The disorder isn't fatal but death may result from aspiration pneumonia or some other infection.

Parkinson's disease, one of the most common crippling diseases in the United States, affects men more often than women. According to current statistics, it strikes 1 in every 100 people over age 60. Because of increased longevity, this amounts to roughly 60,000 new cases diagnosed annually in the United States alone.

Causes

Although the cause of Parkinson's disease is unknown, study of the extrapyramidal brain nuclei (corpus striatum, globus pallidus, substantia nigra) has established that a dopamine deficiency prevents affected brain cells from performing their normal inhibitory function within the central nervous system.

Signs and symptoms

The cardinal symptoms of Parkinson's disease are muscle rigidity and akinesia, and an insidious tremor that begins in the fingers (unilateral pill-roll tremor), increases during stress or anxiety, and decreases with purposeful movement and sleep.

Muscle rigidity results in resistance to passive muscle stretching, which may be uniform (lead-pipe rigidity) or jerky (cogwheel rigidity). Akinesia causes the patient to walk with difficulty (gait lacks normal parallel motion and may be retropulsive or propulsive).

Parkinson's disease also produces a high-pitched, monotone voice; drooling; a masklike facial expression; loss of posture control (the patient walks with body bent forward); and dysarthria, dysphagia, or both. Occasionally, akinesia may also cause oculogyric crises (eyes are fixed upward, with involuntary tonic movements) or blepharospasm (eyelids are completely closed). Parkinson's disease itself doesn't impair the intellect, but a coexisting disorder, such as arteriosclerosis, may.

Diagnostic tests

Generally, laboratory data are of little value in identifying Parkinson's disease; diagnosis is based on the patient's age and history and on the characteristic clinical picture. However, urinalysis may support the diagnosis by revealing decreased dopamine levels.

A conclusive diagnosis is possible only after ruling out other causes of tremor, involutional depression, cerebral arteriosclerosis, and, in patients under age 30, intracranial tumors, Wilson's disease, or phenothiazine or other drug toxicity.

Treatment

Because there is no cure for Parkinson's disease, the primary aim of treatment is to relieve symptoms and keep the patient functional as long as possible. Treatment consists of drugs, physical therapy and, in severe disease states unresponsive to drugs, stereotactic neurosurgery.

Drug therapy

Drug therapy usually includes levodopa, a dopamine replacement that is most effective during early stages. It's given in increasing doses until symptoms are relieved or adverse effects appear. Because adverse effects can be serious, levodopa is frequently given in combination with carbidopa to halt peripheral dopamine synthesis.

When levodopa proves ineffective or too toxic, alternative drug therapy includes anticholinergics such as trihexyphenidyl; antihistamines such as diphenhydramine; and amantadine, an antiviral agent. Selegiline, an enzyme inhibiting agent, allows conservation of dopamine and enhances the therapeutic effect of levodopa.

Stereotactic neurosurgery

When drug therapy fails, stereotactic neurosurgery may be an alternative. In this procedure, electrical coagulation, freezing, radioactivity, or ultrasound destroys the ventrolateral nucleus of the thalamus to prevent involuntary movement. This is most effective in young, otherwise healthy persons with unilateral tremor or muscle rigidity. Neurosurgery can only relieve symptoms.

Physical therapy considerations

• Individually planned physical therapy complements drug treatment and neurosurgery to maintain normal muscle tone and function. Appropriate physical therapy includes both active and passive range-of-motion (ROM) exercises and routine daily activities, walking, and baths and massage to help relax muscles.
• To help manage rigidity, instruct the patient in diaphragmatic breathing to increase thoracic mobility and in relaxation techniques, and perform slow rhythmic rocking, passive ROM exercises, and active ROM exercises with rotational component.
• Gait disturbances commonly present with stooped posture, retropulsion, festering gait, bradykinesia, poor balance, and decreased initia-

tion of movement. To treat these, provide postural reeducation, balance activities to incorporate trunk rotation, coordination exercises to emphasize changes in direction, and training with assistive device.
• Use a wheeled walker to promote fluidity of gait.
• Give the patient and family emotional support.
• Help them express their feelings and frustrations about the progressively debilitating effects of the disease.
• Establish long- and short-term treatment goals, and be aware of the patient's need for intellectual stimulation and diversion.

Teaching points
• Teach the patient and family about the disease, its progressive stages, and the adverse effects of drug therapy.
• Show them how to prevent pressure ulcers and contractures by proper positioning. Inform them of the dietary restrictions necessary for levodopa treatment, and explain household safety measures to prevent accidents.
• To obtain more information, refer the patient and family to the National Parkinson Foundation or the United Parkinson Foundation.

Peripheral neuritis

Also known as multiple neuritis, peripheral neuropathy, and polyneuritis, peripheral neuritis is the degeneration of peripheral nerves supplying mainly the distal muscles of the extremities. It results in muscle weakness with sensory loss and atrophy, and decreased or absent deep tendon reflexes. This syndrome is associated with a noninflammatory degeneration of the axon and myelin sheaths, chiefly affecting the distal muscles of the extremities.

Although peripheral neuritis can occur at any age, its incidence is highest in men between ages 30 and 50. Because onset is usually insidious, patients may compensate by overusing unaffected muscles; however, onset is rapid with severe infection and chronic alcohol intoxication. If the cause can be identified and eliminated, the prognosis is good.

Causes

Causes of peripheral neuritis include:
• chronic intoxication (ethyl alcohol, arsenic, lead, carbon disulfide, benzene, phosphorus, and sulfonamides)
• infectious diseases (meningitis, diphtheria, syphilis, tuberculosis, pneumonia, mumps, and Guillain-Barré syndrome)
• metabolic and inflammatory disorders (gout, diabetes mellitus, rheumatoid arthritis, polyarteritis nodosa, systemic lupus erythematosus)
• nutritive diseases (beriberi and other vitamin deficiencies, and cachectic states).

Signs and symptoms

The clinical effects of peripheral neuritis develop slowly, and the disease usually affects the motor and sensory nerve fibers. Neuritis typically produces flaccid paralysis, wasting, loss of reflexes, pain of varying intensity, loss of ability to perceive vibratory sensations, and paresthesia, hyperesthesia, or anesthesia in the hands and feet.

Deep tendon reflexes are diminished or absent, and atrophied muscles are tender or hypersensitive to pressure or palpation. Footdrop may also be present. Cutaneous manifestations include glossy, red skin and decreased sweating. Patients often have a history of clumsiness and may complain of frequent vague sensations.

Diagnostic tests

The patient history and physical examination delineate characteristic distribution of motor and sensory deficits. Electromyography may show a delayed action potential if this condition impairs motor nerve function.

Treatment

Effective treatment of peripheral neuritis consists of supportive measures to relieve pain, adequate bed rest, and physical therapy as needed. Most important, the underlying cause must be identified and corrected. For instance, it's essential to identify and remove the toxic agent, correct nutritional and vitamin deficiencies (the patient needs a high-calorie diet rich in vitamins, especially B complex), or counsel the patient to avoid alcohol.

Physical therapy considerations

• Relieve pain with correct positioning, analgesics, or possibly phenytoin, which has been used experimentally for neuritic pain, especially if associated with diabetic neuropathy.
• To prevent pressure ulcers, apply a foot cradle. To prevent contractures, arrange for the patient to obtain splints, boards, braces, or other orthopedic appliances. Provide orthotic, protective, or supportive devices, as needed.
• After the pain subsides, provide passive range-of-motion exercises, massage to promote soft tissue mobilization, and possibly electrotherapy for nerve and muscle stimulation.
• Provide neuromuscular reeducation, such as biofeedback or electrical stimulation.
• Initiate an exercise program, including balance or coordination exercises, stretching, aerobic endurance activities, active strengthening exer-

cises, and exercise with resistive equipment
• Encourage functional activities to improve independence and safety of daily tasks.

Teaching points
• Instruct the patient to rest and refrain from using the affected extremity.
• Teach him how to use an assistive device as appropriate.

Cardiovascular disorders

Arterial occlusive disease

In this disorder, the obstruction or narrowing of the lumen of the aorta and its major branches causes an interruption of blood flow, usually to the legs and feet. Arterial occlusive disease may affect the carotid, vertebral, innominate, subclavian, mesenteric, and celiac arteries. Occlusions may be acute or chronic, and often cause severe ischemia, skin ulceration, and gangrene.

Arterial occlusive disease is more common in males than in females. The prognosis depends on the location of the occlusion, the development of collateral circulation to counteract reduced blood flow, and, in acute disease, the time elapsed between occlusion and its removal.

Causes

Arterial occlusive disease is a frequent complication of atherosclerosis. The occlusive mechanism may be endogenous, due to emboli formation or thrombosis, or exogenous, due to trauma or fracture. Predisposing factors include smoking; aging; conditions such as hypertension, hyperlipidemia, and diabetes; and a family history of vascular disorders, myocardial infarction, or cerebrovascular accident.

Signs and symptoms

Evidence of this disease varies widely, according to the occlusion site. (See *Clinical features of arterial occlusive disease,* page 224.)

Diagnostic tests

In arterial occlusive disease, the diagnosis is usually based on the patient history and physical examination.

Pertinent supportive diagnostic tests include the following:
• Arteriography demonstrates the type of occlusion (thrombus or embolus), location, and degree of obstruction, and collateral circulation. Arteriography is particularly useful in chronic disease or for evaluating candidates for reconstructive surgery.
• Doppler ultrasonography and plethysmography are noninvasive tests that, in acute disease, show decreased blood flow distal to the occlusion.
• Ophthalmodynamometry helps determine the degree of obstruction in the internal carotid artery by comparing ophthalmic artery pressure to brachial artery pressure on the affected side. More than a 20% difference between pressures suggests insufficiency.
• EEG and a computed tomography scan may be necessary to rule out brain lesions.

Treatment

Effective treatment depends on the cause, location, and size of the obstruction. For mild chronic disease, supportive measures include elimination of smoking, hypertension control, and walking exercise. For carotid artery occlusion, antiplatelet therapy may begin with aspirin. For intermittent claudication of chronic occlusive disease, pentoxifylline may improve blood flow through the capillaries, particularly for patients who are poor candidates for surgery.

Acute arterial occlusive disease usually requires surgery to restore circulation to the affected area. Possible procedures include the following:
• embolectomy — removal of thrombotic material from the artery using a balloon-tipped catheter; mainly used for mesenteric, femoral, or popliteal artery occlusion
• thromboendarterectomy — opening of the occluded artery and direct removal of the obstructing thrombus and the medial layer of the arterial wall; usually performed after angiography and often used with autogenous vein or Dacron bypass surgery (femoral popliteal or aortofemoral)
• patch grafting — removal of the thrombosed arterial segment and replacement with an autogenous vein or Dacron graft
• bypass graft — diverting blood flow through an anastomosed autogenous or Dacron graft past the thrombosed segment
• thrombolytic therapy — lysis of any clot around or in the plaque by urokinase, streptokinase, or alteplase
• atherectomy — excision of plaque using a drill or slicing mechanism
• balloon angioplasty — compression of the obstruction using balloon inflation
• laser angioplasty — use of excision and hot-tipped lasers to vaporize the obstruction
• stents — insertion of a mesh of wires that stretch and mold to the arterial wall to prevent reocclusion
• combined therapy — concomitant use of any of the above treatments
• lumbar sympathectomy — an adjunct to surgery, depending on the condition of the sympathetic nervous system.

Amputation becomes necessary with failure of arterial reconstructive surgery or with the development of

CLINICAL FEATURES OF ARTERIAL OCCLUSIVE DISEASE

Site of occlusion	Signs and symptoms
Carotid arterial system • Internal carotid arteries • External carotid arteries	Neurologic dysfunction: transient ischemic attacks (TIAs) due to reduced cerebral circulation produce unilateral sensory or motor dysfunction (transient monocular blindness, hemiparesis), possible aphasia or dysarthria, confusion, decreased mentation, and headache; these recurrent clinical features usually last 5 to 10 minutes but may persist up to 24 hours and may herald a stroke) absent or decreased pulsation with an auscultatory bruit over the affected vessels.
Vertebrobasilar system • Vertebral arteries • Basilar arteries	Neurologic dysfunction: TIAs of brain stem and cerebellum produce binocular visual disturbances, vertigo, dysarthria, and "drop attacks" (falling down without loss of consciousness). Less common than carotid TIA.
Innominate artery • Brachiocephalic artery	Neurologic dysfunction: signs and symptoms of vertebrobasilar occlusion. Indications of ischemia (claudication) of right arm; possible bruit over right side of neck.
Subclavian artery	Subclavian steal syndrome (characterized by the backflow of blood from the brain through the vertebral artery on the same side as the occlusion, into the subclavian artery distal to the occlusion); clinical effects of vertebrobasilar occlusion and exercise-induced arm claudication; possible gangrene, usually limited to the digits.
Mesenteric artery • Superior (most commonly affected) • Celiac axis • Inferior	Bowel ischemia, infarct necrosis, and gangrene; sudden, acute abdominal pain; nausea and vomiting; diarrhea; leukocytosis; and shock due to massive intraluminal fluid and plasma loss.
Aortic bifurcation (saddle block occlusion, an emergency associated with cardiac embolization)	Sensory and motor deficits (muscle weakness, numbness, paresthesia, paralysis) and signs of ischemia in both legs (sudden pain; cold, pale legs with decreased or absent peripheral pulses).
Iliac artery (Leriche's syndrome)	Intermittent claudication of lower back, buttocks, and thighs, relieved by rest; absent or reduced femoral or distal pulses; possible bruit over femoral arteries; impotence in males.
Femoral and popliteal artery (associated with aneurysm formation)	Intermittent claudication of the calves on exertion; ischemic pain in feet; pretrophic pain (heralds necrosis and ulceration); leg pallor and coolness; blanching of feet on elevation; gangrene; no palpable pulses in ankles and feet.

gangrene, persistent infection, or intractable pain.

Other treatments include heparin to prevent emboli (for embolic occlusion) and bowel resection after restoration of blood flow (for mesenteric artery occlusion).

Physical therapy considerations

• Remember that the patient is unable to produce normal increases in peripheral blood flow essential for increasing the oxygen supply to exercising muscles. If oxygen supply is inadequate to meet demand, ischemia and pain develop along with shortness of breath when central circulation is affected.

• Monitor the heart rate and blood pressure of patients with peripheral vascular disease, who are assumed to have atherosclerotic disease.

• Provide closer monitoring for patients who have undergone amputation because disease progression is assumed.

• Start daily exercise training to increase pain-free walking tolerance and decrease extremity pain at rest.

• Gradually increase exercise time and intensity while providing frequent rest periods.

• Be aware that blood pressure may rise during exercise secondary to a diminished vascular bed.

• Use a subjective pain response to express claudication discomfort.

• *Preoperatively (during an acute episode):* Assess the patient's circulatory status by checking for the most distal pulses and by inspecting his skin color and temperature.

• *Postoperatively:* Monitor the patient's vital signs. Continuously assess his circulatory function by inspecting skin color and temperature and by checking for distal pulses. In charting, compare earlier assessments and observations. Watch closely for signs of hemorrhage (tachycardia and hypotension), and check dressings for excessive bleeding.

• In both femoral and popliteal artery occlusions, assist with early ambulation, and discourage prolonged sitting.

Teaching points

• Tell the patient not to exercise past moderate discomfort levels; any higher exacerbates symptoms.

• Provide comprehensive patient teaching such as proper foot care.

• Explain all diagnostic tests and procedures.

• Advise the patient to stop smoking and to follow the prescribed medical regimen.

Buerger's disease

Also known as thromboangiitis obliterans, this inflammatory, nonatheromatous occlusive condition causes segmental lesions and subsequent thrombus formation in the small and medium arteries (and sometimes the veins), resulting in decreased blood flow to the feet and legs. Buerger's disease may produce ulceration and, eventually, gangrene.

Causes

Although the cause of Buerger's disease is unknown, a definite link exists to smoking, suggesting a hypersensitivity reaction to nicotine. Incidence is highest among men of Jewish ancestry, ages 20 to 40, who smoke heavily.

Signs and symptoms

Buerger's disease typically produces intermittent claudication of the instep, which is aggravated by exercise and relieved by rest. During exposure to low temperature, the feet initially become cold, cyanotic, and numb; later, they redden, become hot, and tingle. Occasionally, Buerger's disease also affects the hands, possibly resulting in painful fingertip ulcerations.

Associated signs and symptoms may include impaired peripheral pulses, migratory superficial thrombophlebitis and, in later stages, ulceration, muscle atrophy, and gangrene.

Diagnostic tests

Patient history and physical examination strongly suggest Buerger's

disease. Supportive diagnostic tests include:
• Doppler ultrasonography to show diminished circulation in the peripheral vessels
• plethysmography to help detect decreased circulation in the peripheral vessels
• arteriography to locate lesions and rule out atherosclerosis.

Treatment

Therapy may include an exercise program that uses gravity to fill and drain the blood vessels or, in severe disease, a lumbar sympathectomy to increase blood supply to the skin. Amputation may be necessary for nonhealing ulcers, intractable pain, or gangrene.

Physical therapy considerations

• Provide emotional support. If necessary, refer the patient for psychological counseling to help him cope with imposed restrictions.
• If the patient has undergone amputation, assess rehabilitative needs, especially regarding changes in body image. Refer him to occupational therapists and social service agencies as needed.
• See the entry "Arterial occlusive disease" in this chapter for further considerations.

Teaching points

• Strongly urge the patient to discontinue smoking permanently to enhance the effectiveness of treatment. If necessary, refer him to a self-help group to stop smoking.
• Warn the patient to avoid precipitating factors, such as emotional stress, exposure to extreme temperatures, and trauma.
• Teach proper foot care, especially the importance of wearing well-fitting shoes and cotton or wool socks. Show the patient how to inspect his feet daily for cuts, abrasions, and signs of skin breakdown, such as redness and soreness. Remind him to seek medical attention right after any trauma.

Coronary artery disease

The dominant effect of coronary artery disease (CAD) is the loss of oxygen and nutrients to myocardial tissue because of diminished coronary blood flow. This disease is near epidemic in the Western world.

CAD occurs more often in men than in women, in whites, and in middle-aged and elderly people. In the past, this disorder rarely affected women who were premenopausal; however, that is no longer the case, perhaps because many women now take oral contraceptives, smoke cigarettes, and are employed in stressful jobs that used to be held exclusively by men.

Causes

Atherosclerosis is the usual cause of CAD. In this form of arteriosclerosis, fatty, fibrous plaques narrow the lumen of the coronary arteries, reduce the volume of blood that can flow through them, and lead to myocardial ischemia. Plaque formation also predisposes to thrombosis, which can provoke myocardial infarction (MI).

Atherosclerosis usually develops in high-flow, high-pressure arteries, such as those in the heart, brain, kidneys, and aorta, especially at bifurcation points. It has been linked to many risk factors: family history, hypertension, obesity, smoking, diabetes mellitus, stress, a sedentary lifestyle, and high serum cholesterol and triglyceride levels.

Uncommon causes of reduced coronary artery blood flow include dissecting aneurysms, infectious vasculitis, syphilis, and congenital defects in the coronary vascular system. Coronary artery spasms may also impede blood flow.

Signs and symptoms

The classic symptom of CAD is angina, the direct result of inadequate flow of oxygen to the myocardium. It's usually described as a burning, squeezing, or tight feeling in the substernal or precordial chest that may radiate to the left arm, neck, jaw, or shoulder blade.

Typically, the patient clenches his fist over his chest or rubs his left arm when describing the pain, which may be accompanied by nausea, vomiting, fainting, sweating, and cool extremities. Anginal episodes most often follow physical exertion but may also follow emotional excitement, exposure to cold, or a large meal.

Angina has three major forms:
• *Stable* angina causes pain that is predictable in frequency and duration and can be relieved with nitrates and rest.
• *Unstable* angina causes pain that increases in frequency and duration. It's more easily induced.
• *Prinzmetal's* angina causes unpredictable coronary artery spasm.

Severe and prolonged anginal pain generally suggests MI, with potentially fatal arrhythmias and mechanical failure.

Diagnostic tests

The patient history — including the frequency and duration of angina and the presence of associated risk factors — is crucial in evaluating CAD. Additional diagnostic measures include the following:

• Electrocardiography (ECG) during angina may show ischemia or may be normal; it may also show arrhythmias such as premature ventricular contractions. The ECG is apt to be normal when the patient is pain-free.
• Treadmill or bicycle exercise test may provoke chest pain and ECG signs of myocardial ischemia (ST-segment depression).
• Coronary angiography reveals narrowing or occlusion of the coronary artery, with possible collateral circulation.
• Myocardial perfusion imaging with thallium-201 or cardiolite during treadmill exercise detects ischemic areas of the myocardium, visualized as "cold spots."

Treatment

The goal of treatment in patients with angina is to either reduce myocardial oxygen demand or increase oxygen supply. Therapy consists primarily of nitrates, such as nitroglycerin (given sublingually, orally, transdermally, or topically in ointment form), isosorbide dinitrate (given sublingually or orally), beta-adrenergic blockers (given orally), or calcium channel blockers (given orally). Obstructive lesions may necessitate coronary artery bypass surgery and the use of vein grafts.

Angioplasty may be performed during cardiac catheterization to compress fatty deposits and relieve occlusion in patients with no calcification and partial occlusion. A certain risk is associated with this procedure, but its morbidity is lower than that for surgery. Percutaneous transluminal coronary angioplasty may be done in combination with coronary stenting. Stents provide a framework to hold an artery open by securing flaps of tunica media and intima against the artery wall.

Prevention

Because CAD is so widespread, prevention is of incalculable importance. Dietary restrictions aimed at reducing intake of calories (in obesity) and of dietary fats and cholesterol serve to minimize the risk, especially when supplemented with regular exercise. Abstention from smoking and reduction of stress are also beneficial.

Other preventive actions include control of hypertension (with sympathetic blocking agents, such as methyldopa and propranolol, or diuretics such as hydrochlorothiazide), control of elevated serum cholesterol or triglyceride levels (with antilipemics such as atorvastatin calcium [Lipitor], pravastatin sodium [Pravachol], or simvastatin [Zocor]), and measures to minimize platelet aggregation and the danger of blood clots (with aspirin).

Physical therapy considerations

• Upper extremity exercises elicit different responses than lower extremity exercises. Myocardial efficiency is lower, oxygen uptake is higher, myocardial oxygen consumption (heart rate × systolic blood pressure) is higher, and 35% less exercise can be done before symptoms are produced.
• Encourage participation in a cardiac rehabilitation program.
— *Phase I activities*: Aerobic, submaximal exercises performed using less than 2 metabolic equivalents (METS) of energy. Exercise can determine risk for repeat cardiovascular events if monitored in early stage.
— *Phase II activities*: Aerobic and anaerobic exercises, performed at less than 3 to 4 METS and gradually increased to 5 to 7 METS, and interval training to decrease oxygen debt, with a stress test administered at the end of phase II.

— *Phase III activities*: Jogging, hiking, cycling, skiing, swimming, and other sports.

Teaching points
• Tell the patient not to exercise past moderate discomfort levels; any higher level exacerbates symptoms.
• Teach the patient to pace his daily activities.

Heart failure

A syndrome characterized by myocardial dysfunction, heart failure leads to impaired pump performance (reduced cardiac output) or to frank heart failure and abnormal circulatory congestion. Congestion of systemic venous circulation may result in peripheral edema or hepatomegaly; congestion of pulmonary circulation may cause pulmonary edema, an acute, life-threatening emergency.

Pump failure usually occurs in a damaged left ventricle (left-sided heart failure) but may occur in the right ventricle (right-sided heart failure) either as a primary disorder or secondary to left-sided heart failure. Sometimes, left- and right-sided heart failure develop simultaneously.

Although heart failure may be acute (as a direct result of myocardial infarction), it's generally a chronic disorder associated with retention of sodium and water by the kidneys. Advances in diagnostic and therapeutic techniques have greatly improved the outlook for patients with heart failure, but the prognosis still depends on the underlying cause and its response to treatment.

Causes

Heart failure may result from a primary abnormality of the heart muscle, such as an infarction, inadequate myocardial perfusion due to coronary artery disease, or cardiomyopathy. Other causes include:

• mechanical disturbances in ventricular filling during diastole when there is too little blood for the ventricle to pump, as in mitral stenosis secondary to rheumatic heart disease or constrictive pericarditis and atrial fibrillation

• systolic hemodynamic disturbances, such as excessive cardiac workload due to volume overloading or pressure overload, that limit the heart's pumping ability.

These disturbances can result from mitral or aortic insufficiency, which causes volume overloading, and aortic stenosis or systemic hypertension, which results in increased resistance to ventricular emptying.

Reduced cardiac output triggers three compensatory mechanisms: ventricular dilation, hypertrophy, and increased sympathetic activity. These mechanisms improve cardiac output at the expense of increased ventricular work.

Ventricular dilation

In ventricular dilation, an increase in end-diastolic ventricular volume (preload) causes increased stroke work and stroke volume during contraction, stretching cardiac muscle fibers beyond optimum limits and producing pulmonary congestion and pulmonary hypertension, which in turn lead to right-sided heart failure.

Ventricular hypertrophy

In ventricular hypertrophy, an increase in muscle mass or diameter of the left ventricle allows the heart to pump against increased resistance (impedance) to the outflow of blood.

An increase in ventricular diastolic pressure necessary to fill the enlarged ventricle may compromise diastolic coronary blood flow, limiting the oxygen supply to the ventricle and causing ischemia and impaired myocardial contractility.

Increased sympathetic activity

As a response to decreased cardiac output and blood pressure, increased sympathetic activity occurs by enhancing peripheral vascular resistance, contractility, heart rate, and venous return.

Signs of increased sympathetic activity, such as cool extremities and clamminess, may indicate impending heart failure. Increased sympathetic activity also restricts blood flow to the kidneys, which respond by reducing the glomerular filtration rate and increasing tubular reabsorption of sodium and water, in turn expanding the circulating blood volume. This renal mechanism, if unchecked, can aggravate congestion and produce overt edema.

Chronic heart failure may worsen as a result of respiratory tract infections, pulmonary embolism, stress, increased sodium or water intake, or failure to comply with the prescribed treatment regimen.

Signs and symptoms

Left-sided heart failure primarily produces pulmonary signs and symptoms; right-sided heart failure, primarily systemic signs and symptoms. However, heart failure often affects both sides of the heart.

Left-sided heart failure

Clinical signs of left-sided heart failure include dyspnea, orthopnea, crackles, possibly wheezing, hypoxia, respiratory acidosis, cough, cyanosis or pallor, palpitations, arrhythmias, elevated blood pressure, and pulsus alternans.

Right-sided heart failure

Clinical signs of right-sided heart failure include dependent peripheral edema, hepatomegaly, splenomegaly, jugular vein distention, ascites, slow weight gain, arrhythmias, hepato-jugular reflex, abdominal distention, nausea, vomiting, anorexia, weakness, fatigue, dizziness, and syncope.

Complications

These typically include pulmonary edema, venostasis with a predisposition to thromboembolism (associated primarily with prolonged bed rest), cerebral insufficiency, and renal insufficiency with severe electrolyte imbalance.

Diagnostic tests

The following tests are used to diagnose heart failure:

• Electrocardiography reflects heart strain, enlargement, or ischemia. It may also reveal atrial enlargement, tachycardia, and extrasystole.
• Chest X-ray shows increased pulmonary vascular markings, interstitial edema, or pleural effusion and cardiomegaly.
• Pulmonary artery monitoring typically demonstrates elevated pulmonary artery and pulmonary artery wedge pressures, left ventricular end-diastolic pressure in left-sided heart failure, and elevated right atrial pressure or central venous pressure in right-sided heart failure.

Treatment

The aim of therapy is to improve pump function by reversing the compensatory mechanisms producing the symptoms. Heart failure can be controlled quickly by treatment consisting of:

• diuresis to reduce total blood volume and circulatory congestion
• prolonged bed rest
• digoxin to strengthen myocardial contractility

• vasodilators to increase cardiac output by reducing the impedance to ventricular outflow (afterload)
• antiembolism stockings to prevent venostasis and thromboembolism formation.

Physical therapy considerations

• The status of patients with heart failure can change daily; therefore, exercise prescriptions must also change to meet the needs of the patient.
• Exercise is contraindicated in cases of acute heart failure.
• With chronic heart failure, gradual progressive exercise training is appropriate, with intensity determined by tolerance.
• Even low-intensity walking for short periods of time will elicit a training effect in heart failure patients because their activity level has previously been limited to bed rest or short walks to the bathroom.
• Closely monitor vital signs; which include heart rate, blood pressure, oxygen saturation levels, and respiration rate. Include electrocardiogram (ECG) readings if the patient is on a telemetry monitor.
• Be aware of vital sign responses to exercise:
– *Heart rate:* Make sure the patient is working at 60% to 65% of maximal heart rate. Determine this value by subtracting the patient's age from 220.
– *Blood pressure:* Systolic pressures should increase as exertion increases. Diastolic pressures shouldn't vary more than 8 to 10 mm Hg with exercise. An abnormally high value is approximately 140/90 mm Hg and a low value is 70/40 mm Hg.
– *Respirations:* Perform the "talk test," in which the patient should be able to converse normally during exercise without a sense of shortness of

breath. Oxygen saturation shouldn't fall below 90% with exercise.

— *ECG:* The exercise should be stopped if signs of the following appear: ventricular tachycardia, ST-segment depression or elevation greater than 4 mm, onset of second-degree heart block, multifocal premature ventricular contractions, or left bundle-branch block (not seen at baseline).

• Other indications for stopping exercise include progressive angina; signs of light-headedness, confusion, pallor, ataxia, cyanosis, nausea, or severe circulatory impairment; patient requests; and failure of any part of the monitoring systems.

When monitoring vital signs, consider the following:

• Heart failure patients may have renal dysfunction, which will reduce maximal heart rate by 20 to 40 beats/minute.

• Systolic blood pressures may be lowered due to autonomic dysfunction.

• Cardiac medications such as beta blockers may reduce heart rate and blood pressure readings, giving a false response to exercise.

Teaching points

• Teach the patient to pace his daily activities.

• Instruct the patient to take medication exactly as prescribed and to report any adverse reactions immediately.

• Teach the patient and family about the disease and energy reducing activities.

Myocardial infarction

In myocardial infarction (MI), also known as heart attack, reduced blood flow through one of the coronary arteries results in myocardial ischemia and necrosis. In cardiovascular disease, the leading cause of death in the United States and Western Europe, death usually results from the cardiac damage or complications of MI.

Mortality is high when treatment is delayed; almost half of all sudden deaths due to an MI occur before hospitalization, within 1 hour of the onset of symptoms. The prognosis improves if vigorous treatment begins immediately.

Causes

Predisposing factors include:
• positive family history
• hypertension
• smoking
• elevated serum triglyceride, total cholesterol, and low-density lipoprotein levels
• diabetes mellitus
• obesity or excessive intake of saturated fats, carbohydrates, or salt
• sedentary lifestyle
• aging
• stress or a type A personality (aggressive, ambitious, competitive, addicted to work, chronically impatient)
• drug use, especially cocaine.

Men and postmenopausal women are more susceptible to MI than premenopausal women, although incidence is rising among females, especially those who smoke and take oral contraceptives.

The site of the MI depends on the vessels involved. Occlusion of the circumflex branch of the left coronary artery causes a lateral wall infarction; occlusion of the anterior descending branch of the left coronary artery, an anterior wall infarction.

True posterior or inferior wall infarctions generally result from occlusion of the right coronary artery or one of its branches. Right ventricular infarctions can also result from right coronary artery occlusion, can accompany inferior infarctions, and may cause right-sided heart failure. In transmural MI, tissue damage extends through all myocardial layers;

in subendocardial MI, only in the innermost and possibly the middle layers.

Signs and symptoms

The cardinal symptoms of MI is persistent, crushing substernal pain that may radiate to the left arm, jaw, neck, or shoulder blades. Such pain is often described as heavy, squeezing, or crushing, and may persist for 12 hours or more. However, in some MI patients — particularly older adults or diabetics — pain may not occur at all; in others, it may be mild and confused with indigestion.

In patients with coronary artery disease, angina of increasing frequency, severity, or duration (especially if not provoked by exertion, a heavy meal, or cold and wind) may signal impending infarction.

Other features

Other clinical effects include a feeling of impending doom, fatigue, nausea, vomiting, and shortness of breath. Some patients may have no symptoms. The patient may experience catecholamine responses, such as coolness in extremities, perspiration, anxiety, and restlessness. Fever is unusual at the onset of a MI, but a low-grade fever may develop during the next few days. Blood pressure varies; hypotension or hypertension may be present.

Complications

The most common post-MI complications include recurrent or persistent chest pain, arrhythmias, left-sided heart failure, and cardiogenic shock. Unusual but potentially lethal complications that may develop soon after infarction include thromboembolism, papillary muscle insufficiency, rupture of the ventricular septal defect, rupture of the myocardium, and ventricular aneurysm.

Up to several months after infarction, Dressler's syndrome may develop (pericarditis, pericardial friction rub, chest pain, fever, leukocytosis and, possibly, pleurisy or pneumonitis).

Diagnostic tests

Persistent chest pain, ST-segment changes on the electrocardiogram (ECG), and elevated levels of total creatine kinase (CK) and the CK-MB isoenzyme over a 72-hour period usually confirm MI. Auscultation may reveal diminished heart sounds, gallops and, in papillary dysfunction, the apical systolic murmur of mitral insufficiency over the mitral valve area.

When clinical features are equivocal, assume that the patient has had an MI until tests rule it out. Diagnostic test results include the following:
• Serial 12-lead ECG abnormalities may be absent or inconclusive during the first few hours after an MI. When present, characteristic abnormalities include serial ST-segment depression in subendocardial MI and ST-segment elevation in transmural MI.
• Serial serum enzyme levels show elevated CK levels, specifically, CK-MB.
• Echocardiography may show ventricular wall motion abnormalities in patients with a transmural MI.

Scans using I.V. technetium 99 can identify acutely damaged muscle by picking up radioactive nucleotide, which appears as a "hot spot" on the film. They are useful in localizing a recent MI.

Treatment

The goals of treatment are to relieve chest pain, to stabilize heart rhythm, to reduce cardiac workload, to revascularize the coronary artery, and to preserve myocardial tissue. Arrhythmias, the predominant problem during the first 48 hours after the infarction, may require antiarrhythmics, possibly a pacemaker and, rarely, cardioversion.

To preserve myocardial tissue, thrombolytic therapy should be started I.V. within 6 hours after the onset of symptoms (unless contraindications exist). Thrombolytic therapy includes either streptokinase, alteplase, or urokinase.

Percutaneous transluminal coronary angioplasty (PTCA) may be another option. If PTCA is performed soon after the onset of symptoms, the thrombolytic agent may be administered directly into the coronary artery.

Other treatments consist of:
• lidocaine or other drugs, such as procainamide, quinidine, bretylium, or disopyramide, for ventricular arrhythmias
• atropine I.V. or a temporary pacemaker for heart block or bradycardia
• nitroglycerin (sublingual, topical, transdermal, or I.V.); calcium channel blockers, such as nifedipine, verapamil, or diltiazem (sublingual, oral, or I.V.); or isosorbide dinitrate (sublingual, oral, or I.V.) to relieve pain by redistributing blood to ischemic areas of the myocardium, increasing cardiac output, and reducing myocardial workload
• heparin I.V. (usually follows thrombolytic therapy); morphine I.V. for pain and sedation; bed rest with bedside commode to decrease cardiac workload
• oxygen administration at a modest flow rate for 24 to 48 hours (a lower concentration is necessary if the patient has chronic obstructive pulmonary disease)
• drugs to increase myocardial contractility or blood pressure
• beta-adrenergic blockers, such as propranolol or timolol, after acute MI to help prevent reinfarction

• aspirin to inhibit platelet aggregation (should be initiated within 24 hours after the onset of symptoms)
• pulmonary artery catheterization to detect left- or right-sided heart failure and to monitor the patient's response to treatment.

Physical therapy considerations

• Care for patients who have suffered an MI is directed toward detecting complications, preventing further myocardial damage, and promoting comfort, rest, and emotional well-being. Most MI patients receive treatment in the coronary care unit, where they're under constant observation for complications.
• Exercise is an absolute contraindication for a recent MI (less than 2 days since the episode).
• When the patient is cleared for exercise by the doctor, begin low-level activities. These may include relaxation techniques such as deep breathing, coughing, and diaphragmatic breathing. Also begin antiembolic exercises, and include ankle pumps and gentle range of motion.
• Increase the patient's activity, as tolerated, to improve endurance. Monitor ambulation. (Refer to the previous entry, "Heart failure," for considerations for monitoring vital signs and when to stop exercise.)
• Watch for signs and symptoms of fluid retention (crackles, cough, tachypnea, edema) which may indicate impending heart failure.
• Auscultate for adventitious breath sounds periodically (patients on bed rest frequently have atelectatic crackles, which may disappear after coughing) and for S_3 or S_4 gallops.
• Be aware that post-MI syndrome may develop, producing chest pain that must be differentiated from recurrent MI, pulmonary infarct, or heart failure.

Teaching points
- Inform the patient about adverse reactions to drugs, and advise him to watch for and report signs of toxicity (anorexia, nausea, vomiting, and yellow vision, if the patient is receiving digoxin).
- Review dietary restrictions with the patient. If he must follow a low-sodium or low-fat and low-cholesterol diet, provide a list of foods that he should avoid. Ask the dietitian to speak to the patient and his family.
- Counsel the patient to resume sexual activity progressively. Advise him to report typical or atypical chest pain.
- Stress the need to stop smoking.
- Encourage participation in a cardiac rehabilitation program.

CHAPTER

7

Traumatic injury
Restoring function
without complications

Common traumatic injuries

Acceleration-deceleration cervical injuries

Acceleration-deceleration cervical injuries (commonly known as whiplash) result from sharp hyperextension and flexion of the neck that damages muscles, ligaments, disks, and nerve tissue. The prognosis for this type of injury is excellent; symptoms usually subside with treatment.

Causes

Whiplash commonly results from rear-end automobile accidents. Fortunately, the padded headrests, air bags, and seat belts with shoulder harnesses now common in cars have reduced the incidence of this type of traumatic injury.

Signs and symptoms

Although symptoms may develop immediately, they're often delayed 12 to 24 hours if the injury is mild. Whiplash produces moderate to severe anterior and posterior neck pain. Within several days, the anterior pain diminishes, but the posterior pain persists or even intensifies, causing patients to seek medical attention if they didn't do so before. Whiplash may also cause dizziness, gait disturbances, vomiting, headache, nuchal rigidity, neck muscle asymmetry, and rigidity or numbness in the arms.

Diagnostic tests

Full cervical spine X-rays are required to rule out cervical fractures. If the X-rays are negative, the physical examination focuses on motor ability and sensation below the cervical spine to detect signs of nerve root compression.

Treatment

In all suspected spinal injuries, assume that the spine is injured until proven otherwise. Any patient with suspected whiplash or other injuries requires careful transportation from the accident scene. Until an X-ray rules out a cervical fracture, move the patient as little as possible.

Physical therapy considerations

• Before evaluating the cervical region, test the alar and transverse ligaments for possible laxity. Don't proceed with range-of-motion exercises if laxity is found.
• Use cervical collars for a short period of time to ensure the affected area doesn't heal in a faulty position.
• Use massage and muscle-setting techniques to maintain circulation and promote relaxation.
• If you find muscle guarding, don't do any stretching.

Teaching points

• Before discharge, teach the patient to watch for possible drug adverse effects; to avoid alcohol if he's receiving diazepam, narcotics, or muscle relaxants; and to rest for a few days and avoid lifting heavy objects.
• Instruct him to return to the hospital immediately if he experiences persistent pain or develops numbness, tingling, or weakness on one side.

Arm and leg fractures

Fractures of the arms and legs usually result from trauma and often cause substantial muscle, nerve, and other soft-tissue damage. The prognosis varies with the extent of disablement or deformity, the amount of tissue and vascular damage, the adequacy of reduction and immobilization, and the patient's age, health, and nutritional status.

Children's bones usually heal rapidly and without deformity. Bones of adults in poor health and with impaired circulation may never heal properly. Severe open fractures, especially of the femoral shaft, may cause substantial blood loss and life-threatening hypovolemic shock.

Causes

Most arm and leg fractures result from major trauma; for example, a fall on an outstretched arm, a skiing accident, or child abuse (shown by multiple or repeated episodes of fractures). However, in a person with a pathologic bone-weakening condition, such as osteoporosis, bone tumors, or metabolic disease, a mere cough or sneeze can also produce a fracture. Prolonged standing, walking, or running can cause stress fractures of the foot and ankle — usually in nurses, postal workers, soldiers, and joggers.

Signs and symptoms

Arm and leg fractures may produce any or all of the "5 Ps": pain and point tenderness, pallor, pulse loss, paresthesia, and paralysis. (The last three are distal to the fracture site.) Other signs include deformity, swelling, discoloration, crepitus, and loss of limb function. Numbness and tingling, mottled cyanosis, cool skin at the end of the extremity, and loss of pulses distal to the injury indicate possible arterial compromise or nerve damage. Open fractures also produce an obvious skin wound.

Complications of arm and leg fractures include:
• permanent deformity and dysfunction if bones fail to heal (nonunion) or heal improperly (malunion)
• aseptic necrosis of bone segments from impaired circulation
• hypovolemic shock as a result of blood vessel damage (especially likely in patients with a fractured femur)
• muscle contractures
• renal calculi from decalcification (produced by prolonged immobility)
• fat embolism
• myositis ossificans — calcification of soft tissue surrounding the fracture (due to trauma to the muscle).

Diagnostic tests

A history of trauma and a physical examination, including gentle palpation and a cautious attempt by the patient to move parts distal to the injury, suggest an arm or leg fracture.

When performing the physical examination, also check for other injuries. Anteroposterior and lateral X-rays of the suspected fracture, as well as X-rays of the joints above and below it, confirm the diagnosis.

Treatment

The following treatments are performed in arm and leg fractures.

Emergency treatment

In an emergency, the limb is splinted above and below the suspected fracture, a cold pack is applied, and the limb is elevated to reduce edema and pain.

In severe fractures that cause blood loss, direct pressure is applied to control bleeding, and replacement fluids are administered as soon as possible to prevent or treat hypovolemic shock.

Reduction

After a fracture has been confirmed, treatment begins with reduction (which involves restoring displaced bone segments to their normal position).

• After reduction, the fractured arm or leg must be immobilized by a splint or a cast or with traction.

• X-rays confirm that reduction has been successful and that proper bone alignment has been achieved.

• When closed reduction is impossible, open reduction during surgery reduces and immobilizes the fracture by means of rods, plates, or screws. Afterward, a plaster cast is usually applied.

• When a splint or cast fails to maintain the reduction, immobilization requires skin or skeletal traction, using a series of weights and pulleys.

Physical therapy considerations

• Coordinate pain medication with therapy to ensure the best effort by the patient.

During the acute phase, follow these guidelines:

• Keep muscles proximal to the injury strong with active exercises.

• Discuss functional obstacles with the patient and family, such as stair management.

During the posthealing-clinical union phase (bone appears united, but fracture is still visible on the X-ray), follow these guidelines:

• Use active and active-assistive exercise. Avoid passive stretching and resistive exercises at this time.

• Mobilization of grades 1 and 2 is recommended.

• Allow only partial weight bearing for this period.

During the posthealing-complete union phase (fracture line not visible on X-ray and callus is ossified), follow these guidelines:

• Use resistive exercise and stretching.

• Mobilization of grades 3 and 4 is recommended.

• Allow full weight bearing during this phase.

The factors that affect union are:

• increasing age or diabetes (slows healing)

• use of steroids (impedes healing)

• weight bearing (facilitates healing if fragments are aligned and immobilized adequately).

Teaching points

• Teach the patient how to use the assistive device. Because he'll use it for 8 to 12 weeks, make sure that it's the least restrictive device appropriate for his weight-bearing status.

Burns

A major burn is a horrifying injury, necessitating painful treatment and a long period of rehabilitation. It's often fatal or permanently disfiguring and incapacitating (both emotionally and physically). In the United States, about 2 million persons annually suffer burns. Of these, 100,000 are burned seriously and over 6,000 are fatalities, making burns this nation's third-leading cause of accidental death.

Causes

Thermal burns, the most common type, are frequently the result of residential fires, automobile accidents, playing with matches, improperly stored gasoline, space heater or electrical malfunctions, or arson. Other causes include improper handling of firecrackers, scalding accidents, and kitchen accidents (such as a child climbing on top of a stove or grabbing a hot iron). Burns in children are sometimes traced to parental abuse.

GAUGING BURN DEPTH

One method of assessing burns is by determining the burn's depth. A partial-thickness burn damages the epidemis and part of the dermis, whereas a full-thickness burn damages the epidermis, dermis, subcutaneous tissue, and muscle, as shown.

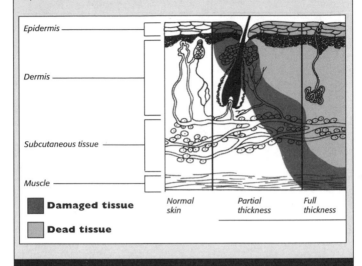

Epidermis

Dermis

Subcutaneous tissue

Muscle

■ **Damaged tissue**

■ **Dead tissue**

Normal skin | Partial thickness | Full thickness

Chemical burns result from the contact, ingestion, inhalation, or injection of acids, alkalis, or vesicants. Electrical burns usually occur after contact with faulty electrical wiring or with high voltage power lines, or when electric cords are chewed (by young children). Friction or abrasion burns happen when the skin is rubbed harshly against a coarse surface. Sunburn, of course, follows excessive exposure to sunlight.

Signs and symptoms

The depth of damage to the skin and tissue and the size of the burn are important factors in burn assessment.

Depth of skin and tissue damage

A traditional method gauges burn depth by degrees, although most burns are a combination of different degrees and thicknesses.

• *First-degree* — Damage is limited to the epidermis, causing erythema and pain.
• *Second-degree* — The epidermis and part of the dermis are damaged, producing blisters and mild to moderate edema and pain.
• *Third-degree* — The epidermis and the dermis are damaged; no blisters appear, but white, brown, or black leathery tissue and thrombosed vessels are visible.
• *Fourth-degree* — Damage extends through deeply charred subcutaneous tissue to muscle and bone. (See *Gauging burn depth*.)

Diagnostic tests

Assessing burn size

The size of a burn is usually expressed as the percentage of body surface area (BSA) covered by the burn. The Rule of Nines chart most commonly provides this estimate, but the

Lund and Browder chart is more accurate, because it allows for BSA changes with age.

A correlation of the burn's depth and size permits an estimate of its severity, as follows:

• *major* — third-degree burns on more than 10% of BSA; second-degree burns on more than 25% of adult BSA (more than 20% in children); burns of hands, face, feet, or genitalia; burns complicated by fractures or respiratory damage; electrical burns; all burns in poor risk patients
• *moderate* — third-degree burns on 2% to 10% of BSA; second-degree burns on 15% to 25% of adult BSA (10% to 20% in children)
• *minor* — third-degree burns on less than 2% of BSA; second-degree burns on less than 15% of adult BSA (10% in children).

Other considerations

When evaluating burns, these factors must also be considered:

• Location — Burns on the face, hands, feet, and genitalia are most serious, because of possible loss of function.
• Configuration — Circumferential burns can cause total occlusion of circulation in extremity as a result of edema. Burns on the neck can produce airway obstruction, whereas burns on the chest can lead to restricted respiratory expansion.
• History of complicating medical problems — Note disorders that impair peripheral circulation, especially diabetes, peripheral vascular disease, and chronic alcohol abuse.
• Patient age — Victims under age 4 or over age 60 have a higher incidence of complications and, consequently, a higher mortality.
• Pulmonary injury — Smoke inhalation can cause pulmonary injury.
• Other injuries sustained at the time of the burn can affect the burn.

Treatment

Immediate, aggressive burn treatment increases the patient's chance for survival. Later, supportive measures and strict aseptic technique can minimize infection. Meticulous, comprehensive burn care can make the difference between life and death.

If the patient's burns are minor, immerse the burned area in cool saline solution (55° F [12.8° C]) or apply cool compresses. Administer pain medication as needed. Debride the devitalized tissue, taking care not to break any blisters. Cover the wound with an antimicrobial agent and a nonstick bulky dressing, and administer tetanus prophylaxis as needed.

In moderate and major burns, immediately assess the patient's airway, breathing, and circulation. Be especially alert for signs of smoke inhalation and pulmonary damage: singed nasal hairs, mucosal burns, voice changes, coughing, wheezing, soot in the mouth or nose, and darkened sputum. Assist with endotracheal intubation and administer 100% oxygen.

Electrical and chemical burns demand special attention. Tissue damage from electrical burns is difficult to assess because internal destruction along the conduction pathway is usually greater than the surface burn would indicate. Electrical burns that ignite the patient's clothes may cause thermal burns as well. Irrigate a chemical burn with copious amounts of water or normal saline solution.

Physical therapy considerations

• The goals of physical therapy in managing a patient with burns are to prevent deformity, maintain range of motion (ROM) and strength, and achieve maximum functional status.
• Ensure proper alignment of limbs.

• General positioning of the shoulders is abducted to 90 degrees, horizontal adducted to 20 to 30 degrees, and elbows extended.

• General positioning of the legs is knees in extension, hip in neutral rotation, abduction to 15 degrees, and ankles neutral.

• Splinting prevents flexion contractures and maintains range of motion. Splints are applied over dressings at night and removed for exercise.

• Initiate exercise as soon as possible to maintain length of healing skin. Exercise also decreases edema, maintains ROM and strength, increases endurance, and avoids complications of bed rest.

• After grafting and as prescribed, begin passive and active-assisted motion as soon as 1 day postoperative. Active motion can begin 4 to 5 days postoperatively.

• Parameters for ambulation depend on the location of the graft. Ambulation may begin 2 to 3 days after an upper extremity graft, 5 to 6 days after a buttocks graft, or 8 to 10 days after a lower extremity graft.

• Apply pressure garments — in the form of Jobst garments, Ace wraps, or splints — as soon as healing allows and keep them on the patient 24 hours a day. Healing occurs in the form of hypertrophic scarring (undesirable excess collagen production), and pressure makes the collagen fibers more organized.

• Use deep breathing exercises, transcutaneous electrical nerve stimulation on nonburned areas, and ROM to help relieve pain.

• Increase strength and endurance through conditioning programs, continued through outpatient and home stages.

Teaching points
• Provide thorough teaching and complete aftercare instructions for the patient.
• Stress the importance of keeping the dressing dry and clean, elevating the burned extremity for the first 24 hours, taking prescribed analgesics, and returning for a wound check in 1 to 2 days.

Dislocations and subluxations

Dislocations displace joint bones so that their articulating surfaces totally lose contact; subluxations partially displace the articulating surfaces. Dislocations and subluxations occur at the joints of the shoulders, elbows, wrists, digits, hips, knees, ankles, and feet; these injuries may accompany joint fractures or result in deposition of fracture fragments between joint surfaces. Prompt reduction can limit the resulting damage to soft tissue, nerves, and blood vessels.

Causes

A dislocation or subluxation may be congenital (as in congenital dislocation of the hip), or it may follow trauma or disease of surrounding joint tissues (for example, Paget's disease).

Signs and symptoms

Dislocations and subluxations produce deformity around the joint, change the length of the involved extremity, impair joint mobility, and cause point tenderness.

When the injury results from trauma, it's extremely painful and often accompanies joint surface fractures. Even in the absence of concomitant fractures, the displaced bone may damage surrounding muscles, liga-

COMMON DISLOCATION

Normal elbow joint

Elbow joint with lateral dislocation

ments, nerves, and blood vessels and may cause bone necrosis, especially if reduction is delayed. (See *Common dislocation*.)

Diagnostic tests

Patient history, X-rays, and a physical examination rule out or confirm a fracture.

Treatment

Immediate reduction (before tissue edema and muscle spasm make reduction difficult) can prevent additional tissue damage and vascular impairment.

Closed reduction consists of manual traction under general anesthesia (or local anesthesia and sedatives). During such reduction, morphine I.V. controls pain; midazolam I.V. controls muscle spasm and facilitates muscle stretching during traction.

Some injuries require open reduction under regional block or general anesthesia. Such surgery may include wire fixation of the joint, skeletal traction, and ligament repair.

After reduction, a splint, cast, or traction immobilizes the joint. Generally, immobilizing the digits for 2 weeks, hips for 6 to 8 weeks, and oth-

er dislocated joints for 3 to 6 weeks allows surrounding ligaments to heal.

Physical therapy considerations

• Dislocations and subluxations are typically followed by a period of immobilization. Once the patient is cleared by the doctor for therapy, focus on restoring normal joint range of motion.
• Strength training plays a large role in rehabilitation to prevent future reinjury. The more diverse the exercises, the more stability the joint will have. Recommended techniques include closed kinetic chain exercises, open-chain exercises, peripheral neuromuscular facilitation (PNF), functional reintegration, sport-specific activities, weight training, and other treatments as needed.

Electric shock

When an electric current passes through the body, the damage it does depends on the intensity of the current (amperes, milliamperes, or microamperes), the resistance of the tissues it passes through, the kind of current (AC, DC, or mixed), and the frequency and duration of current flow.

Electric shock may cause ventricular fibrillation, respiratory paralysis, burns, and death. The prognosis depends on the site and extent of damage, the patient's state of health, and the speed and adequacy of treatment. In the United States, about 1,000 people die of electric shock each year.

Causes

Electric shock usually follows accidental contact with exposed parts of electrical appliances or wiring, but it may also result from lightning or the flash of electric arcs from high-voltage power lines or machines.

Electric current can cause injury in three ways: true electrical injury as the current passes through the body, arc or flash burns from current that doesn't pass through the body, and thermal surface burns caused by associated heat and flames.

Signs and symptoms

Severe electric shock usually causes muscle contraction, followed by unconsciousness and loss of reflex control, sometimes with respiratory paralysis (by way of prolonged contraction of respiratory muscles, or a direct effect on the respiratory nerve center).

After momentary shock, hyperventilation may follow initial muscle contraction. Passage of even the smallest electric current — if it passes through the heart — may induce ventricular fibrillation or another arrhythmia that progresses to fibrillation or myocardial infarction.

Electric shock from a high-frequency current (which generates more heat in tissues than a low-frequency current) usually causes burns and local tissue coagulation and necrosis. Low-frequency currents can also cause serious burns if the contact with the current is concentrated in a small area (for example, when a toddler bites into an electrical cord).

Contusions, fractures, and other injuries can result from violent muscle contractions or falls during the shock; later, the patient may develop renal shutdown. Residual hearing impairment, cataracts, and vision loss may persist after severe electric shock.

Diagnostic tests

Usually, the cause of electrical injuries is either obvious or suspected. However, an accurate history can define the voltage and the length of contact.

Treatment

Immediate emergency treatment includes carefully separating the victim from the current source, quickly assessing vital functions, and emergency measures, such as cardiopulmonary resuscitation (CPR) and defibrillation.

To separate the victim from the current source, immediately turn it off or unplug it. If this isn't possible, pull the victim free with a nonconductive device, such as a loop of dry cloth or rubber, a dry rope, or a leather belt.

Physical therapy considerations

• Assess the patient's neurologic status frequently because central nervous system damage may result from ischemia or demyelination. If neurologic compromise is present, see "Spinal injuries" in this chapter or "Peripheral neuritis" in Chapter 6 for physical therapy considerations.
• Check for neurovascular damage in the extremities by assessing peripheral pulses and capillary refill and by asking about numbness, tingling, or pain. Elevate any injured extremities.
• Refer to the entry "Burns" in this chapter for specific physical therapy considerations when caring for wounds and skin damage.
• Protect patients from electric shock in the hospital.

Teaching points
• Before an accident occurs, tell patients, family members, and friends how to avoid electrical hazards at home and at work. Advise parents of small children to put safety guards on all electrical outlets and keep children away from electrical devices. Warn all patients not to use electrical appliances while showering or wet.
• Also warn patients never to touch electrical appliances while touching faucets or cold water pipes in the kitchen because these pipes often provide the ground for all electrical circuits in the house.

Spinal injuries

Spinal injuries (without cord damage) include fractures, contusions, and compressions of the vertebral column, usually as a result of trauma to the head or neck. The real danger lies in possible spinal cord damage. Spinal fractures most commonly occur in the fifth, sixth, and seventh cervical, twelfth thoracic, and first lumbar vertebrae.

Causes

Most serious spinal injuries result from motor vehicle accidents, falls, diving into shallow water, and gunshot wounds; less serious injuries, from lifting heavy objects and minor falls. Spinal dysfunction may also result from hyperparathyroidism and neoplastic lesions.

Signs and symptoms

The most obvious symptom of spinal injury is muscle spasm and back pain that worsen with movement. In cervical fractures, pain may produce point tenderness; in dorsal and lumbar fractures, it may radiate to other body areas such as the legs.

If the injury damages the spinal cord, clinical effects range from mild paresthesia to quadriplegia and shock. After milder injuries, such symptoms may be delayed for several days or weeks.

Effects of cord injury include:
• spastic paralysis
• loss of sensation
• autonomic dysfunctions, such as neurogenic bladder, loss of rectal sphincter control, impaired perspiration (danger of heat stress), and altered sexual function
• respiratory dysfunctions: C2 to C4 sites of injury affect control of the phrenic nerve; T2 to T12 areas control intercostal muscles; and T6 to T12 areas control abdominal muscles
• orthostatic hypotension
• impaired body temperature regulation
• metabolic change, such as bone demineralization, hypercalcemia, or autonomic dysreflexia (above T6).

Potential complications include:
• urinary tract infections
• pressure ulcers
• heterotrophic bone formation
• spasticity
• dysesthetic pain.

Diagnostic tests

• Typically, diagnosis is based on patient history, physical examination, X-rays and, possibly, lumbar puncture, computed tomography (CT) scan, and magnetic resonance imaging (MRI).
• Patient history may reveal trauma, a metastatic lesion, an infection that could produce a spinal abscess, or an endocrine disorder.
• Physical examination (including a neurologic evaluation) locates the level of injury and detects cord damage.
• Spinal X-rays, the most important diagnostic measure, locate the fracture.

- Lumbar puncture may show increased cerebrospinal fluid pressure from a lesion or trauma in spinal compression.
- CT scan or MRI can locate the spinal mass.

Treatment

The primary treatment after spinal injury is immediate immobilization to stabilize the spine and prevent cord damage; other treatment is supportive. Cervical injuries require immobilization, using sandbags on both sides of the patient's head, a hard cervical collar, or skeletal traction with skull tongs or a halo device.

Supportive measures
Treatment of stable lumbar and dorsal fractures consists of bed rest on firm support (such as a bed board), analgesics, and muscle relaxants until the fracture stabilizes (usually 10 to 12 weeks). Later treatment includes exercises to strengthen the back muscles and a back brace or corset to provide support for walking.

An unstable dorsal or lumbar fracture requires a plaster cast, a turning frame and, in severe fracture, laminectomy and spinal fusion.

Other measures
When spinal injury results in compression of the spinal column, neurosurgery may relieve the pressure. If a metastatic lesion causes compression, chemotherapy and radiation may relieve it. Surface wounds accompanying the spinal injury require tetanus prophylaxis unless the patient has had recent immunization.

Physical therapy considerations

- Management of spinal cord injuries primarily addresses complications that can arise.

- Respiratory compromise can result in decreased inspiration, expiration, and cough due to paralysis. For effective management, position the patient to increase breathing capacity. Maintain bronchiole hygiene through chest physiotherapy, postural drainage, breathing exercises with assisted cough, and continued chest mobility.
- Preserve skin integrity and prevent pressure ulcers by using pressure-relieving beds, changing the patient's position every 2 hours, padding pressure points in the bed and wheelchair, and teaching weight shifting techniques. Be aware that common points of skin pressure include the heels, malleoli, knees, trochanters, ischial tuberosities, sacrum, coccyx, scapula, and acromion processes. Poor sensation adds to the risk of pressure ulcers.
- Address pain syndromes with transcutaneous electrical nerve stimulation (TENS) or relaxation techniques.
- Address postural hypotension by having the patient use the tilt table as tolerated while pulse and blood pressure are monitored to determine effects of the treatment. Elastic garments can also be applied to the lower extremities.
- Include range of motion (ROM) as an important part of rehabilitation. A few degrees of limitation can greatly impact function. However, know that heterotrophic bone formation commonly interferes with ROM at the knee, shoulder, and elbow. It may also interfere with sitting posture and therefore interfere with pressure relief. Passive ROM may create pseudoarthrosis.
- Once the patient has achieved normal passive ROM, daily activities may preserve the needed range.
- Strengthen muscles that remain innervated. These muscles must compensate for those that have been paralyzed. Focus on muscles used to ex-

tend elbows, to flex or horizontally adduct the shoulders, and to protract or depress the scapula.

Teaching points
• For pain relief, teach the patient about TENS or relaxation techniques.
• Initiate functional training early. The patient must learn muscle substitution and acrobatic maneuvers used to move the body. As activity increases, so will strength and flexibility.
• Teach the patient about transfers. Address transfers from even and uneven surfaces and from all locations the patient encounters (such as wheelchair to floor, toilet, bed, or car), including the reverse (such as floor to wheelchair).
• Show the patient how to do bed mobility exercises that include rolling, coming to a sitting position, and leg management.
• When teaching maneuvering of the wheelchair, include propulsion on level and unleveled surfaces and management of curbs, ramps, stairs, and narrow doorways. Also address managing wheelchair accessories as well as returning safely to the chair after a fall.
• In the ambulation program, include standing properly from a wheelchair, falling safely to the floor, and returning to a standing position.
• Be sure to teach the patient how to use appropriate assistive devices on all surfaces.

Sprains and strains

A *sprain* is a complete or incomplete tear in the supporting ligaments surrounding a joint that usually follows a sharp twist. A *strain* is an injury to a muscle or tendinous attachment. Both usually heal without surgical repair.

Signs and symptoms
Sprains

A sprain causes local pain (especially during joint movement), swelling, loss of mobility (which may not occur until several hours after the injury), and a black-and-blue discoloration from blood extravasating into surrounding tissues. A sprained ankle is the most common joint injury.

Strains

A strain may be acute (an immediate result of vigorous muscle overuse or overstress) or chronic (a result of repeated overuse).

An acute strain causes a sharp, transient pain (the patient may say he heard a snapping noise) and rapid swelling. When severe pain subsides, the muscle is tender; after several days, ecchymoses appear.

A chronic strain causes stiffness, soreness, and generalized tenderness. These conditions appear several hours after the injury.

Diagnostic tests

A history of recent injury or chronic overuse, clinical findings, and an X-ray to rule out fractures establish the diagnosis.

Treatment
Sprains

Sprains call for control of pain and swelling and immobilization of the injured joint to promote healing. Immediately after the injury, elevating the joint above the level of the heart and intermittently applying ice for 12 to 48 hours controls swelling. A towel between the ice pack and the skin prevents cold injuries.

An immobilized sprain usually heals in 2 to 3 weeks, and the patient can then gradually resume normal activities. Occasionally, however, torn ligaments don't heal properly and cause recurrent dislocation, necessitating surgical repair.

Some athletes may request immediate surgical repair to hasten healing. To prevent sprains, they may tape their wrists and ankles before sports activities.

Strains
Acute strains require analgesics and application of ice for up to 48 hours, then heat. Complete muscle rupture may require surgery.

Chronic strains usually don't need treatment, but heat application, nonsteroidal anti-inflammatory drugs, or an analgesic muscle relaxant can relieve discomfort.

Physical therapy considerations
• For sprains, immobilize the joint, using an elastic bandage or cast or, for severe sprains, a soft cast or splint.
• Strength training plays a large role in rehabilitation to prevent future reinjury. The more diverse the exercises, the more stability the joint will have. Recommended techniques include closed kinetic chain exercises, open kinetic chain exercises, peripheral neuromuscular facilitation (PNF), functional reintegration, sport-specific activities, weight training, and other modalities as needed.

Teaching points
• If the patient has a sprained ankle, make sure he receives crutch gait training. Because patients with sprains seldom require hospitalization, provide patient teaching.
• Tell the patient with a sprain to elevate the joint for 48 to 72 hours after the injury (pillows can be used while sleeping) and to apply ice intermittently for 12 to 48 hours.
• If the patient has an elastic bandage in place, teach him how to reapply it by wrapping from below to above the injury, forming a figure eight. For a sprained ankle, demonstrate applying the bandage from toes to midcalf. Tell the patient to remove the bandage before going to sleep and to loosen it if it causes the leg to become pale, numb, or painful.
• Instruct the patient to call if pain worsens or persists. He may need an additional X-ray to detect a fracture originally overlooked.
• Inform the patient about bracing options for return to sports or other activities.
• Instruct the patient how to perform exercises at home.

Traumatic amputation

This type of injury involves accidental loss of a body part, usually a finger, toe, arm, or leg. In complete amputation, the member is totally severed; in partial amputation, some soft-tissue connection remains.

Acute care physical therapy includes positioning, transfer skills, an exercise program, and early ambulation. The prognosis has improved as a result of early improved emergency and critical care management, new surgical techniques, early rehabilitation, prosthesis fitting, and new prosthesis design. New limb reimplantation techniques have been moderately successful, but incomplete nerve regeneration remains a major limiting factor.

Causes
Traumatic amputations usually result from factory, farm, power tool, or motor vehicle accidents.

Assessment
Every traumatic amputee requires careful monitoring of vital signs. If

amputation involves more than just a finger or toe, assessment of airway, breathing, and circulation is also required. Because profuse bleeding is likely, watch for signs of hypovolemic shock, and draw blood for hemoglobin, hematocrit, and typing and crossmatching. In partial amputation, check for pulses distal to the amputation. After any traumatic amputation, assess for other traumatic injuries as well.

Treatment

Because the greatest immediate threat after traumatic amputation is blood loss and hypovolemic shock, emergency treatment consists of local measures to control bleeding, fluid replacement with normal saline solution and colloids, and blood replacement as needed.

Reimplantation remains controversial, but it's becoming more common and successful because of advances in microsurgery. If reconstruction or reimplantation is possible, surgical intervention attempts to preserve usable joints. When arm or leg amputations are done, the surgeon creates a stump to be fitted with prosthesis. A rigid dressing permits early prosthesis fitting and rehabilitation.

Physical therapy considerations

• Preoperative care aims to prevent complications by:
– providing sound limb care
– preventing further trauma
– inspecting and cleaning the skin daily
– limiting skin exposure to moisture
– avoiding friction and shearing forces that could injure the skin.
• Postoperative care aims to facilitate healing without complications by:
– reducing edema to promote cylindrical residual limbs

– preventing skin infection and ensuring skin graft viability by using sterile technique in dressing changes
– preventing loss of motion
– increasing upper and lower extremity strength
– promoting mobility and self-care
– helping the amputee cope with his altered body image.
– promoting sound limb care.

Rehabilitation goals
• Focus rehabilitation on working toward a prosthetic device.
• Use ambulation for balance control, weight bearing, increasing endurance, and improving coordination.
• Increase strength of the residual limb, the sound limb, and the arms.
• Maintain full range of motion and promote normal gait pattern.

Prosthetic training (outpatient basis)
• Ensure good prosthetic fit by working closely with prosthesis.

Teaching points
• Teach the patient how to use crutches to increase balance and upper extremity strength early.
• Provide daily training to improve tolerance, and closely observe skin changes or pressure areas with the prosthesis. Be sure to cover:
– putting on and taking off the prosthesis independently,
– walking without assistive device on stairs, ramps, curbs, and unleveled surfaces
– transfers from floor, chair, and car
– backward walking, picking up objects from the floor, kneeling, and driving.
• Continue training until the patient can perform all functional activities with skill and can wear the prosthesis 8 hours a day without skin compromise.

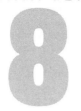

Cardiac rehabilitation

Increasing endurance

Overview of cardiac rehabilitation

The cardiac rehabilitation team

Cardiac rehabilitation is a comprehensive program of exercise, counseling, risk factor reduction, and education designed to help patients with cardiac disease achieve optimal physical, psychological, and functional status within the confines of their disease. It follows the acute recovery phase after myocardial infarction and consists of successive phases that move from the inpatient setting of subacute recovery (Phase I) to the outpatient setting (Phases II, III, and IV). Each phase has specific goals related to education, lifestyle modification, amount of supervision, and performance of activities and exercises. The Agency for Health Care Policy and Research lists as the leading benefits of cardiac rehabilitation:

• improved exercise tolerance
• reduced symptoms
• improved blood lipid levels
• reduced cigarette smoking
• improved psychosocial well-being and reduced stress
• reduced mortality.

A cardiac rehabilitation team is multidisciplinary. In addition to the patient and the family, it includes the patient's primary care provider; the cardiac rehabilitation medical director; and other health care specialists, such as physical and behavioral therapists, an exercise physiologist, a nurse, and a dietitian.

Each member of the team has specific responsibilities. The patient — the most important member of the team — is responsible for his own recovery and lifestyle modifications. His primary care provider retains responsibility for the patient's medical care during the program. The cardiac rehabilitation medical director is responsible for medical consultation and program development. Roles and responsibilities of other team members vary depending on the patient's needs. (See *Roles of team members.*)

Overall, the cardiac rehabilitation team should be knowledgeable about cardiac emergency procedures, medical management of cardiovascular disease, exercise training, dietary modifications, pharmacology, stress management, behavior modification, and risk factor management.

Cardiac rehabilitation services

Inpatient programs

Cardiac rehabilitation services are provided in a variety of inpatient and outpatient settings. Inpatient cardiac rehabilitation (Phase I) is provided in the acute care setting. Physical activity and education can be done at the patient's bedside, while progressive ambulation can be performed in the hallway. Hospitals serving large populations of cardiac rehabilitation patients may provide these services in an inpatient exercise room.

At discharge from the acute care setting, patients may be referred to transitional programs or to an outpatient cardiac rehabilitation program. Because the length of hospital stay has generally been decreasing under managed care pressures, some patients with comorbidities and age-related frailty may be referred outside the acute care hospital to a skilled nursing facility, a rehabilitation hospital, or home care.

ROLES OF TEAM MEMBERS

The cardiac rehabilitation team is multidisciplinary and usually includes members that function in these roles.

Role	Function
Cardiac educator (Registered nurse, physical therapist, exercise physiologist, other allied health staff)	Responsible for teaching about diagnostic procedures, preventive strategies, recovery from medical-surgical procedures, and home exercise
Rehabilitation specialist (Physical therapist, exercise physiologist, registered nurse, other allied health staff)	Responsible for evaluation, exercise training, and exercise progression
Dietitian	Responsible for nutritional assessment and dietary counseling
Vocational rehabilitation, health psychologist, social worker, behavioral specialist	Responsible for behavioral evaluation and counseling (This requires knowledge in community services.)

Outpatient programs

Outpatient cardiac rehabilitation programs take place in a variety of settings depending upon the needs of the patient. In addition to hospitals, locations include community colleges, Young Men's Christian Associations, Jewish community centers, private facilities, and patients' homes

Historically, outpatient cardiac rehabilitation has been divided into three phases: Phase II (with 12 weeks of continuous electrocardiogram [ECG] monitoring), Phase III (variable length of programming with intermittent or no ECG monitoring), and Phase IV (no monitoring with limited supervision). Because these designations are inconsistently applied from one program to the next, they have been confusing for patients, health care providers, and third-party payers. Changes in health care delivery, new evidence of the safety of exercise, and new theories of risk stratification have led to individualization of the degree of ECG monitoring and the length of programming. Patients requiring close clinical supervision and ECG monitoring

generally participate in a setting where appropriate medical support, such as advanced cardiac life support, may be provided. All such programs, regardless of location, must have personnel able to deliver emergency services, such as basic life support, as well as some emergency equipment. Third-party-reimbursement issues usually dictate where the patient may be assigned.

Indications for cardiac rehabilitation

In the last several years the variety of patients eligible for cardiac rehabilitation services has expanded. Many patients once thought to be poor candidates for cardiac rehabilitation can now benefit from it if services are tailored to the patient's individual needs.

Clinical indications for a cardiac rehabilitation program currently include:
• medically stable condition after myocardial infarction (MI)
• stable angina
• coronary artery bypass graft surgery

• percutaneous transluminal coronary angioplasty
• compensated heart failure
• cardiomyopathy
• heart or other organ transplantation
• other cardiac surgery, such as prosthetic valve, pacemaker, and implantable cardioverter-defibrillator insertion
• peripheral vascular disease
• high-risk cardiovascular disease that is ineligible for surgical intervention
• sudden cardiac death syndrome
• end-stage renal disease
• patients at risk for coronary artery disease who are diagnosed with diabetes mellitus, hyperlipidemia, or hypertension
• other patients who may benefit from structured exercise, patient education, or both (based on physician referral and consensus of the rehabilitation team).

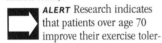 **ALERT** Research indicates that patients over age 70 improve their exercise tolerance as well as younger patients without increasing their risk of complications or adverse outcomes related to the exercise training.

Inpatients can be stratified by onset and severity of complicating factors following MI. These factors are useful to identify a high-risk cardiac inpatient.
• Low-risk patients:
  No complicating factors by day 4
• Moderate-risk patients:
  Poor ventricular function (ejection fraction less than 30%) or significant ischemia with low-level (2 to 3 metabolic equivalents) activity beyond day 4
• High-risk patients:
  Continued ischemia, left-sided heart failure, episode of shock, or serious arrhythmias

Contraindications

These conditions have been identified as contraindications for participation in cardiac rehabilitation.
• Unstable angina
• Resting systolic blood pressure greater than 200 mm Hg or resting diastolic blood pressure greater than 110 mm Hg (evaluate on an individual basis)
• Orthostatic blood pressure drop of greater than 20 mm Hg with symptoms
• Critical aortic stenosis
• Acute systemic illness or fever
• Uncontrolled atrial or ventricular arrhythmias
• Uncontrolled sinus tachycardia (greater than 120 beats/minute)
• Uncompensated heart failure
• Third-degree atrioventricular block (without pacemaker)
• Active pericarditis or myocarditis
• Recent embolism
• Thrombophlebitis
• Resting ST-segment displacement (greater than 2 mm)
• Uncontrolled diabetes (resting blood glucose greater than 400 mg/dl)
• Severe orthopedic problems that prohibit exercise
• Other metabolic problems, such as acute thyroiditis, hypokalemia, hyperkalemia, and hypovolemia.

Implementing a therapeutic plan

Inpatient cardiac rehabilitation program

Referral to a cardiac rehabilitation program is made by the patient's doctor and can be done either individually or via standing orders. After the order is received, the cardiac rehabilitation team begins collecting data about the patient. These data include the following:

- a chart review
- a patient assessment
- an activity evaluation
- an assessment of cardiac disease risk factors
- the patient's and family's goals.

The primary goals of inpatient cardiac rehabilitation are to educate the patient about the cardiac disease process and how to manage cardiac risk factors, and to initiate functional activities and assess the patient's response to these activities.

A general appraisal of activities includes assessment of the response to activities of daily living, such as showering, toileting, dressing, and brushing teeth. Activity assessment also includes arm and leg range-of-motion exercises and progresses from supine to sitting to standing. Finally, the patient's ability to ambulate is assessed.

Any adverse responses to activity are noted; responses that may require termination of the activity include the following:

- heart rate greater then 130 beats/ minute or greater than 30 beats/ minute above preexercise level
- diastolic blood pressure greater than 110 mm Hg
- decrease in systolic blood pressure greater than 10 mm Hg
- significant ventricular or atrial arrhythmias
- second- or third-degree heart block
- signs and symptoms of exercise intolerance, including angina pectoris and marked dyspnea.

Cardiac rehabilitation involves a progression of activity to strengthen the patient's endurance. This progression depends on clinical signs and symptoms, the patient's medical history, and the initial assessment. Patients who are at low risk (as in uncomplicated myocardial infarction) may progress in activity levels more

---

CRITERIA FOR EXERCISE PROGRESSION

The following general exercise criteria may be used to guide activity progression for inpatients.

Intensity
- Rating of perceived exertion less than 13 (on 6 to 20 scale)
- After myocardial infarction: heart rate less than 120 beats/minute or 20 beats above resting heart rate
- After surgery: 30 beats above resting heart rate
- To tolerance if asymptomatic

Duration
- Intermittent bouts lasting 3 to 5 minutes
- Rest periods
- At patient's discretion
- Lasting 1 to 2 minutes
- Shorter than exercise bout duration
- Total duration of up to 20 minutes

Frequency
- Early mobilization: 3 to 4 times per day (days 1 to 3)
- Later mobilization: 2 times per day (beginning on day 3)

Progression
- Initially increasing duration up to 10 to 15 minutes of continuous exercise; then increasing intensity

---

Adapted with permission from American College of Sports Medicine. *ACSM's Guidelines for Exercise Testing and Prescription,* 5th ed. Philadelphia: Lippincott Williams & Wilkins, 1995.

---

rapidly than a higher-risk patient. (See *Criteria for exercise progression.*)

In the past, inpatient cardiac rehabilitation programs consisted of rigid 7- to 14-day programs with multiple steps for progression of activity. Because of the decreasing length of hospital stays, these programs are no longer feasible. The result is a simpli-

5-DAY PROGRESSIVE ACTIVITY PLAN

The chart shows a sample program of progressive activity for shortened hospital stays.

Day and level of acuity	Metabolic equivalents (METS)	Activity
Day 1 0 to 16 hours High level	1.2	• Bedrest until stable • Active or passive range of motion (ROM) in the upper extremity (UE) and lower extremity (LE) (supine) • Plantar flexion and dorsiflexion
16 to 24 hours High level or step down level, depending on patient stability	1.2 to 1.5	• Dangle at side of the bed as tolerated • Plantar flexion and dorsiflexion • Active ROM in UE and LE (sitting) as tolerated • Transfer sit to stand as tolerated • Turning self in bed • Stand to void • Bedside commode with assistance and continual observation • Deep breathe and cough 10 times per hour
Days 2 to 3 Step down level, depending on patient stability	1.5 to 2.5	• Out of bed in chair for meals for 20 to 30 minutes • Active ROM in UE and LE (sitting or standing) as tolerated • Ambulate in room twice per day with assistance • Bedside commode with assistance and continual observation
Days 3 to 4 Med-surg level, depending on patient stability	2.5 to 3.5	• Out of bed in chair sitting • Active ROM in UE and LE (standing) as tolerated • Ambulate in hall for 3 to 5 minutes • Ambulate in room ad lib
Days 4 to 5 Med-surg level, depending on patient stability	3.5 to 4.0	• Active ROM in UE and LE • Ambulate in hall for 7 to 10 minutes • Up and down one flight of stairs

Adapted from *Myocardial Infarction Activity Protocol,* courtesy of Lehigh Valley Hospital, Allentown, Pa.

fied approach to cardiac rehabilitation for the inpatient. (See *5-day progressive activity plan.*)

In addition to exercise, patients begin receiving information and education regarding management of cardiac risk factors, such as hyperlipidemia, hypertension, smoking, stress, and diabetes.

Determination of cardiac risk factors is accomplished at the initial assessment of the patient and appropriate interventions are identified to assist the patient with risk factor reduction.

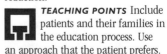 **TEACHING POINTS** Include patients and their families in the education process. Use an approach that the patient prefers.

GAUGING EXERCISE RISK

This model, developed by the American Association of Cardiovascular and Pulmonary Rehabilitation (AACVPR), helps identify cardiac patients who are at risk for both safety and disease progression during exercise.

Low risk
• No significant left ventricular (LV) dysfunction (ejection fraction [EF] of 50% or more)
• No resting or exercise-induced complex arrhythmias
• Uncomplicated myocardial infarction (MI), coronary artery bypass graft, angioplasty, atherectomy, or stent (absence of heart failure signs and symptoms indicating postevent ischemia)
• Normal hemodynamics with exercise or recovery
• Asymptomatic, including the absence of angina with exertion or recovery
• Functional capacity of 7 metabolic equivalents (METS) or more
• Absence of clinical depression

Intermediate (moderate risk)
• Mild to moderately depressed LV function (EF equals 40% to 49%)

• Signs and symptoms, including angina at moderate levels of exercise (5 to 6.9 METS) or in recovery

High risk
• Decreased LV function (EF less than 40%)
• Survivor of cardiac arrest or sudden death
• Complex ventricular arrhythmias at rest or with exercise
• MI complicated by HF, cardiogenic shock, or complex signs and symptoms of postprocedure ischemia
• Abnormal hemodynamics with exercise (especially flat or decreasing systolic blood pressure or chronotropic incompetence with increasing workload)
• Signs and symptoms, including angina pectoris at low levels of exercise (less than 5 METS) or in recovery
• Functional capacity less than 5 METS
• Clinically significant depression

Adapted with permission from AACVPR. *Guidelines for Cardiac Rehabilitation and Secondary Prevention Programs.* Champaign, Ill.: Human Kinetics Publishers, Inc., 1999.

This may include one-on-one instruction, handouts, videos, or pamphlets.

At discharge, the patient should be provided information about:
• understanding the cardiac disease process
• functional activity levels
• self-monitoring skills, such as using nitroglycerin and recognizing signs and symptoms of angina
• medication schedules, dosages, and indications for medications
• home exercise equipment options for outpatient exercise programs.

Outpatient cardiac rehabilitation program

After an evaluation for readiness, patients can begin outpatient cardiac rehabilitation as early as 24 hours after their hospital discharge. (See *Gauging exercise risk.*) The goals of outpatient cardiac rehabilitation are to:
• enhance cardiovascular function and physical work capacity
• teach proper exercise techniques
• provide long-term exercise guidelines
• establish healthy lifestyles in the patient and family

E.C.G. MONITORING DURING EXERCISE

This chart helps determine the optimum length of ECG monitoring for patients based on their level of risk for complications during exercise.

Monitoring	Low risk	Moderate risk	High risk
Initial continuous ECG monitoring and close supervision	6 to 18 sessions	12 to 24 sessions	18 to 24 sessions
Decreased intensity of ECG monitoring to intermittent monitoring	During sessions 8 to 12	During later sessions	During later sessions
Minimal close clinical supervision	30 days after the event	60 to 90 days after the event	90 days or more after the event
Expected response to exercise	Normal hemodynamic response: appropriately increasing systolic blood pressure level or falling diastolic blood pressure, appropriately increasing heart rate, and no symptoms indicating exercise intolerance Regular periodic progression of the exercise prescription: increasing functional capacity and well-tolerated exercise without undue fatigue		

Adapted with permission from American Association of Cardiovascular and Pulmonary Rehabilitation. *Guidelines for Cardiac Rehabilitation and Secondary Prevention Programs.* Champaign, Ill.: Human Kinetics Publishers, Inc., 1999.

• enhance the patient's psychological function
• prepare the patient for resumption of normal roles (work, family, and social).

Before beginning the program, patients should be assessed for risk of complications. This risk stratification identifies patients who may be at risk for an adverse event during exercise as well as patients at risk for progression of cardiac disease.

Traditionally, in early outpatient cardiac rehabilitation (Phase II), patients exercise with continuous ECG monitoring for 36 sessions. However, the duration of ECG monitoring may now depend on the patient's risk stratification. Although there is evidence that continuous ECG monitoring may be inversely linked with risk, no firm predictors accurately identify patients for whom ECG monitoring is useful. The use of continuous ECG monitoring may also be dictated by insurance and Medicare guidelines. The decision to terminate continuous ECG monitoring should be made after consultation between the patient's doctor and cardiac rehabilitation staff. (See *ECG monitoring during exercise.*)

Upon admittance to the outpatient program, an exercise prescription should be devised for the patient. This is usually determined by the exercise specialist, based upon the results of exercise testing. An exercise prescription consists of:
• an exercise intensity goal or target heart rate
• a mode of exercise
• the frequency and duration of exercise

• any special instructions related to the patient's condition.

Determining exercise intensity

The results of an exercise stress test are used to determine the exercise intensity. If the patient hasn't had a stress test before entering the outpatient program, the guidelines for exercise intensity for inpatients may be used until the test is performed. (See *Criteria for exercise progression,* page 253.)

Several methods can be used to determine the exercise intensity of the patient. They include using a percentage of heart rate $(HR)_{max}$, the HR reserve method (Karvonen's formula), the rating of perceived exertion (RPE) method, or using METS (metabolic equivalents).

Percentage of HR$_{max}$

A target heart rate (HR) is prescribed as a percentage of the maximal heart rate (HR_{max}) obtained during the exercise stress test. A patient with a very low fitness level may be prescribed an exercise intensity of between 40% to 50% of HR_{max}, but a person with a higher fitness level may be prescribed an exercise intensity of 60% to 80% of HR_{max}. Possible influences on HR, such as the use of beta-adrenergic blockers, need to be considered. For example, a patient taking a nonselective beta-adrenergic blocker such as propranolol would be expected to have a blunted HR response to exercise and a limited exercise capacity.

HR reserve method (Karvonen's formula)

Heart rate (HR) reserve is the difference between the maximum heart rate (HR_{max}) and the resting heart rate (HR_{rest}). The HR_{max} is obtained from the exercise stress test and the HR_{rest} is obtained while the subject is seated and at rest. This method assumes that 60% to 90% of HR_{max} is equal to 50% to 85% of maximal oxygen consumption, or HR reserve. For example:

   HR_{rest} = 80 beats/minute and
   HR_{max} = 170 beats/minute.
To calculate an exercise prescription of 60% to 80% of HR reserve:
   $HR_{max} - HR_{rest}$ = HR reserve.
   170 beats/minute − 80 beats/minute = 90 beats/minute.
Take 60% and 80% of HR reserve:
   0.60 X 90 beats/minute = 54 beats/minute; 0.80 × 90 beats/minute = 72 beats/minute.
Then add HR_{rest} to both of these values to determine the HR range:
   80 beats/minute + 54 beats/minute = 134 beats/minute
   80 beats/minute + 72 beats/minute = 152 beats/minute.
The exercise target heart rate is 134 to 152 beats/minute.

Borg rating of perceived exertion scale

The Borg rating of perceived exertion (RPE) scale is an objective measure of fatigue. This scale can also be used to monitor exercise intensity. The patient is asked to rate his fatigue with a number on the scale based on his perception of the difficulty of the activity. Based on this determination of exertion, he monitors exercise intensity to reach a target intensity.

There are two RPE scales currently in use. The older scale rates exercise intensity on a scale of 6 to 20; the newer scale rates exercise intensity on a scale of 0 to 10. The latter was developed to simplify terms and make the scale easier to understand. (See *Rating perceived exertion,* page 258.)

RATING PERCEIVED EXERTION

The Borg rating of perceived exertion (RPE) scale, an objective method of rating fatigue, can be used to monitor exercise intensity. Two RPE scales are currently used.

Original 15-grade scale	Revised 10-grade scale
6 No exertion at all	0 Nothing at all
7 Extremely light	0.5 Very, very light (just noticeable)
8	1 Very weak
9 Very light	2 Weak (light)
10	3 Moderate
11 Light	4 Somewhat strong
12	5 Strong (heavy)
13 Somewhat hard	6
14	7 Very strong
15 Hard (heavy)	8
16	9
17 Very hard	10 Extremely strong (maximal)
18	
19 Extremely hard	
20 Maximal exertion	

Adapted with permission from Borg, G. *An Introduction to Borg's RPE Scale*. Ithaca, N.Y.: Movement Publications, 1985.

It has been determined that a training effect can be achieved by exercising at a level of "somewhat hard" (13 to 16 on the older scale) or "somewhat strong" (4 to 5 on the newer scale). The RPE method of monitoring exercise intensity is useful for patients who have difficulty palpating their pulse and those for whom monitoring HR isn't a reliable indicator of exercise intensity, such as patients taking medications that affect HR and those with cardiac transplants, silent ischemia, or severe left ventricular dysfunction. An obese patient who is unable to monitor his own pulse could be taught to correlate his perceived level of exertion on the scale with his HR as determined by cardiac monitoring. After practicing several times, this patient may be able to reliably determine his target HR as a level on the RPE scale.

Metabolic equivalents

Metabolic equivalents (METS) can also be used to prescribe exercise intensity. This method is best when used in a controlled environment. One MET is the amount of oxygen a person consumes while at rest and is equal to approximately 3.5 ml of oxygen per kg of body weight per minute. These values can be used to compare the energy cost of various activities versus the energy cost at rest. For example, if an activity is estimated to be 4 METS, the energy cost of this activity is approximately 4 times that of the energy cost at rest. If a person's maximal MET level from an exercise stress test is known, then an exercise prescription can be determined.

For example, assume a person has a maximal MET level of 4 METS and a prescribed exercise intensity of 50% to 70%. To obtain the lower end of the exercise prescription, add the

MET LEVELS FOR SELECTED ACTIVITIES

Knowledge of a person's maximal metabolic equivalent (MET) levels and of the metabolic cost of a variety of activities is useful in helping patients choose activities in which it is safe for them to participate.

Activity	METS	Activity	METS
Backpacking	5 to 11	Music playing	2 to 3
Basketball (game)	7 to 12+	Racquetball	7 to 10
Bathing	2 to 3	Running	
Billiards	2.5	(12-minute mile)	8.7
Bowling	3 to 4	(11-minute mile)	9.4
Canoeing, rowing,		(10-minute mile)	10.2
kayaking	3 to 8	(9-minute mile)	11.2
Carpentry (light)	4 to 5	Sailing	2 to 5
Cleaning windows	3	Sexual intercourse	5 to 5.5+
Climbing hills	5 to 10	Showering	3.5 to 4.2
Cycling (pleasure)	3 to 8+	Skiing, snow	
Dancing (aerobic)	6 to 9	(downhill)	5 to 8
Desk work	1.5 to 2	(cross-country)	6 to 12+
Dressing	2 to 2.3	Snow shoveling	
Fishing		(wet snow)	8 to 15
(from bank)	2 to 4	(powder snow)	6 to 9
(wading in stream)	5 to 6	Stair climbing	4 to 8
Gardening (weeding)	3 to 5	Swimming	4 to 8+
Golf		Tennis	4 to 9+
(powercart)	2 to 3	Toileting	1 to 2
(carrying bag or		Vacuuming carpets	3 to 4
pulling cart)	4 to 7	Walking, flat surface	
Hiking (cross-country)	3 to 7	(2 mph)	2 to 2.5
Housework		(2.5 mph)	2.5 to 2.9
(heavy: scrubbing,		(3 mph)	3 to 3.3
making beds)	3 to 6	(4 mph)	4.6
(light: sweeping,		Washing car	6 to 7
polishing)	2 to 4	Washing and hanging	
Ironing (standing)	3.5	clothes	2.5 to 3.5
Leg calisthenics	2.5 to 4.5	Watching TV	1 to 2
Mopping	3.5		
Mowing lawn (power			
mower)	4 to 5		

maximal MET level to 50 and divide this quantity by 100:

$$(50 + 4)/100 = 0.54$$

Repeat for the high end of exercise intensity:

$$(70 + 4)/100 = 0.74$$

Then multiply each of these results by the maximal MET level:

$$0.54 \times 4 = 2.16 \text{ METS}$$

and

$$0.74 \times 4 = 2.96 \text{ METS}.$$

The exercise intensity is between 2.16 METS and 2.96 METS.

Considerable variation in the actual MET cost of activities can occur depending upon how intensely a person performs the activity. Close observation of the intensity of the activity must be done when using the METS method of exercise prescription. In general, prescribing with MET levels is less applicable to persons with cardiac disease or those with low functional capacities. However, knowledge of a person's maximal MET level and of the metabolic cost of a variety of activities is useful in helping patients choose activities that are safe for them. (See *MET levels for selected activities.*)

Exercise types

Aerobic exercise training, involving both upper and lower limb muscles, is most beneficial for patients with heart disease. Walking is the most practical and easiest form of aerobic training, but other activities, such as swimming, biking, and aerobic dancing, may be equally effective, depending on the needs and preferences of the patient. The physical therapy treatment may consist of active range-of-motion exercises, periods of walking or stair climbing, or riding a stationary bike. Including warm-up and cool-down periods, each exercise session generally lasts 1 hour and is performed three times per week.

Strength training has only been used to a limited extent in outpatient cardiac rehabilitation because it causes acute increases in diastolic blood pressure. Unlike aerobic exercise, strength training hasn't been shown to lower total cholesterol, increase high-density lipoproteins, or lower blood pressure.

 WOMEN'S HEALTH Strength training may be useful for women, who commonly have less muscle mass and strength compared to men. Reduced strength often limits the performance of physical activity and activities of daily living in women. Strength training should be emphasized when muscle mass and strength are low.

Exercise progression

Exercise progression should be based on the patient's medical condition and response to exercise. Heart rate (HR) is the most reliable method of measuring the patient's response to exercise. Normally, the HR increases moderately after a submaximal bout of exercise. A dramatic increase in HR and little or no increase in HR signal cardiovascular intolerance to the stress. Patients with a higher exercise capacity may progress at a faster rate than patients with a lower exercise capacity. In general, increase exercise every 1 to 3 weeks, with the goal of achieving 20 to 30 minutes of continuous exercise, before prescribing an increase in exercise intensity.

Among cardiac rehabilitation patients, several diagnoses warrant clinical supervision and special consideration. (See *Considerations for early rehabilitation.*)

During the outpatient cardiac rehabilitation phase, patients should be taught the basics of self-monitoring. These include the use of HR, the rating of perceived exertion (RPE), and cardiac signs and symptoms, such as anginal pain, breathlessness, diaphoresis, syncope, and leg pain indicative of claudication. Further instruction includes the components of an exercise session — warm-up, aerobic phase, and cool-down.

The patient should also be instructed in the following:
• interventions for improving cardiac risk factors
• understanding the cardiac disease process
• knowledge and techniques for maintaining good mental health
• understanding cardiac medications
• restrictions in activity secondary to cardiac disease.

 ALERT Because older patients compose the majority of cardiac patients, consider using teaching aids, such as large print for impaired vision and printed instructions for those who are hearing-impaired.

For a variety of reasons, not all patients can participate in a supervised exercise program. Low-risk patients may be candidates for a home exercise program. Patients who exercise at home should be provided detailed instruction regarding exercise guide-

CONSIDERATIONS FOR EARLY REHABILITATION

Cardiac rehabilitation patients with certain diagnoses warrant special consideration regarding the type of exercise and amount of clinical supervision advised. The table below shows these diagnoses with their key factors and recommendations.

Diagnosis	Key factors	Recommendations
Coronary artery bypass graft or valvular surgery	• Incisional discomfort • Infectious process	• Rating of perceived exertion (RPE) of 11 to 14 (on 6 to 20 scale) • Resting heart rate (HR) + 30 beats/minute (if HR is a desired limitation for intensity) • Range of motion for trunk and upper extremities • Muscular strength and endurance for upper extremities
Percutaneous transluminal coronary angioplasty (or similar procedure), myocardial infarction, or angina	• Signs or symptoms of continued ischemia • Anxiety • Symptom denial • New ischemia • Resting angina	• HR criteria if below ECG signs of ischemia • Limited by symptoms • RPE
Silent ischemia	• Associated signs (shortness of breath [SOB], nausea, general malaise) • Sudden decrease in exercise capacity • Sudden changes in overall condition or sense of well-being	• RPE preferred monitoring
Severe left ventricular dysfunction and heart failure	• Significant weight gain (greater than 4 lb) over short duration (1 to 2 days) • Decrease (or lack of increase) in systolic blood pressure (SBP) during exercise • Resting or abnormal exercise SOB	• RPE • SBP response to exertion • Symptoms
Pacemaker or implantable cardioverter-defibrillator (ICD)	• ICD or pacemaker type and method of function • Symptoms similar to those at insertion • Ectopy	• RPE • HR and intensity threshold for exercise-induced ventricular tachycardia • Ventricular ectopy patterns

Adapted with permission from American College of Sports Medicine. *ACSM's Guidelines for Exercise Testing and Prescription,* 5th ed. Philadelphia: Lippincott Williams & Wilkins, 1995.

COMMON COMPLICATIONS DURING EXERCISE

You and other members of the cardiac rehabilitation staff need to recognize possibly life-threatening problems that may arise during the patient's program. The most common medical problems during cardiac rehabilitation include:

- new or changing angina patterns
- changing arrhythmia patterns
- hypertension or hypotension
- hyperglycemia or hypoglycemia
- signs or symptoms of heart failure
- syncopal or near-syncopal episodes.

lines, self-monitoring techniques, medications, and emergency responses. A member of the cardiac rehabilitation team should telephone the patient weekly to discuss progress and potential problems. Some cardiac facilities are able to monitor the patient's ECG over the telephone line. With all home exercise programs, family members should be taught CPR and how to activate the 911 emergency response system.

Medical emergencies

Proper screening and risk stratification minimize the potential risk of myocardial infarction and other complications during exercise training in cardiac rehabilitation programs. Research shows that these incidents are rare. Nevertheless, all patients should have advance directives on file with the entity in charge of their cardiac rehabilitation program. Prior to each session, patients should be monitored for blood pressure; ECG, if appropriate; changes in medications; and patient-reported signs and symptoms since the last visit. (See *Common complications during exercise.*)

Staff should be trained to recognize potential problems. An emergency plan with appropriate equipment should always be available. All team members should be trained in basic life support and at least one person should be trained in advanced cardiac life support and have medical and legal authority to implement these measures if needed.

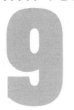

CHAPTER 9

Therapeutic exercise

Restoring strength and flexibility

Understanding therapeutic exercise

Designing a therapeutic exercise program

The use of therapeutic exercise is one of the primary interventions that sets the physical therapist apart from other health care providers. The term *therapeutic* implies treatment for an injury, a pathology, or a disease; *exercise* is the repeated, purposeful movement or action of the body or a body part. Therapeutic exercises are designed primarily to restore function to a body part affected by an injury, a pathology, or a disease. However, they can also be beneficial for nonpatients, such as recreational and serious athletes, and members of specific age groups, such as the young and the elderly.

This chapter provides a brief overview of exercise physiology and exercise principles as well as therapeutic exercise guidelines to facilitate clinical decision-making. These guidelines include the design and proper implementation of selected exercises along with their advantages and disadvantages.

In therapeutic exercise, the patient uses a program of specific muscle contractions or body movements designed to correct or improve impaired musculoskeletal and neurologic function and to maintain a state of well-being. Based on the patient's needs, specific exercises can be used to achieve different goals.

The therapeutic exercise treatment plan is developed and implemented by the physical therapist after a comprehensive evaluation of the patient. This assessment helps to identify spe-

cific problem areas that will need to be addressed. The therapist must thoroughly understand the condition or pathology for which the exercise program is devised and must ascertain whether the patient's condition is acute, subacute, or chronic. In addition, the therapist must understand the effects of various types of exercise on the particular condition and be aware of any contraindications that may apply. A thorough understanding of kinesiology, biomechanics, anatomy, and physiology is mandatory prior to the implementation of any type of exercise regime.

As they participate in an exercise program, patients will learn to understand the signs and symptoms of their pathology as well as the limits and restrictions imposed by their condition and the extent at which they can progress in their program. Patients who learn to actively "listen to their bodies" will eventually reap the rewards of knowing how far to push themselves and when to rest. This knowledge aids the progression of the therapeutic exercise program and helps avoid further damage or reinjury of the involved area.

Program objectives and goals

The objectives of long- and short-term therapeutic exercises are to:
• increase range of motion (ROM) and flexibility
• increase strength, muscle control, and muscle endurance
• improve cardiovascular fitness and endurance
• improve coordination, proprioception, agility, and balance
• increase performance of functional skills and activities
• improve joint stability
• promote relaxation.

Types of therapeutic exercises discussed in this chapter include mobility, strengthening, conditioning, relaxation, and plyometric exercises.

The physical therapist should instruct the patient about certain aspects of the exercise, including:
- frequency, duration, and repetitions
- types and amounts of resistance
- sequence of progression
- exercise equipment needed, if any
- warm-up and cool-down periods.

Other factors to be considered in the program include pain, medical conditions, any general contraindications, and patient compliance.

Long-term goals are the expected responses to the therapeutic exercise program over an extended period. Long-term goals usually have a functional basis and often refer to an activity of daily living or a return to play or work criteria. The *functional outcome* refers to the full restoration or limitations of function based on the disability at the conclusion of the physical therapy program. Such an outcome might be written as: "The patient will achieve full restoration of shoulder ROM following the completion of 12 weeks of physical therapy."

Short-term goals are identified as measurable, objective treatment outcomes. They often reflect portions of the long-term goals or functional outcome. A short-term goal might be written as: "The patient will increase shoulder flexion ROM by 25% over a 4-week period."

Physiologic response to exercise

Any kind of physical exertion makes demands on the body's physiologic systems. Therapeutic exercises, with their emphasis on repetitive, rhythmic activity, have immediate systemic effects on the body, including:

- increased blood flow to muscles
- increased heart rate
- increased arterial pressure with heavy exercise
- increased oxygen demand and consumption
- increased rate and depth of respirations
- decreased insulin secretion and increased glucagon secretion
- increased secretion of catecholamines.

A period of consistent, sustained exercise results in a steady state in heart rate, blood pressure, and cardiac output. When this exercise is stopped, there is an initial rapid decrease in heart rate followed by a slower return to normal. The body should be allowed to adjust gradually to changes in exertion. Typically, a preexercise warm-up period is recommended to avoid the risk of ECG abnormalities or syncopal episodes, and a postexercise cool-down period is recommended to avoid a sudden drop in blood pressure.

If active, rhythmic exercise continues beyond the body's ability to maintain it, fatigue and muscle soreness ensue. In muscle fatigue, the muscle contracts repeatedly; eventually, the force the muscle is able to exert diminishes as a result of the depletion of oxygen and other energy sources, lactic acid and chemical waste product accumulation, or decreased synaptic impulses. Recovery time from local muscle fatigue usually occurs within minutes depending on the body's ability to restore the oxygen and synaptic responses to the muscles. The amount of muscle or tissue breakdown that takes place and the ability to remove accumulated lactic acid will also determine the recovery time of a muscle.

Acute muscle soreness is caused by local muscle fatigue, in which the muscle tires and can no longer contract. Delayed-onset muscle soreness (DOMS) results from microscopic tearing of the muscle fibers. In DOMS, the pain generally worsens within 48 hours after completing an exercise program but subsides over the next few days. Swelling in and around the muscle may also contribute to delayed soreness, causing more stiffness and pain.

DOMS can be minimized by performing low-level aerobic exercises followed by gentle stretching of the muscles during the warm-up prior to an activity. Gradually increasing the demands applied to the joints and muscles helps to acclimate the body to the stresses of the designated activity, thereby reducing the risk of delayed soreness.

Basic exercise principles

This section briefly reviews basic terms used to describe muscle training and exercise regimens.

Muscle strength is the force that results from the tension created by muscular contractions. Depending on the type of exercise desired, a muscular contraction produces an internal force that shortens the muscle (*concentric isotonic contraction*), lengthens the muscle (*eccentric isotonic contraction*), or is static in length (*isometric contraction*). Strength testing to analyze these properties of muscle can be done by the physical therapist using manual muscle testing (See chapter 1, Assessment: Reviewing the techniques).

Two types of muscle strength are recognized — *dynamic* and *static*. Dynamic strength is applied in muscle contractions that are used to lift, load, or move a weight or object. Concentric and eccentric isotonic ex-

ercises are considered dynamic strength exercises.

Static strength is applied when the muscle creates a force within itself or an internal force against an immovable object but without any joint movement. Isometric or "setting" exercises are types of static strength exercises.

Power is used in conjunction with strength. It's defined mechanically as the rate of performing work. *Muscle power* is the speed at which the muscle contracts and creates tension and force. Any musculoskeletal activity that requires moving an object in a brief amount of time requires power. Increasing the speed of muscle contractions during a therapeutic exercise program aids in approximating the activity or function that the patient is attempting to improve.

Load describes the weight or other source of resistance that is applied to the body or body part during exercises. The load may be the weight of the limb or the body itself, gravity, or another source, such as a dumbbell, cuff weight, and a machine. Typically, when working against a load, the patient performs a series of muscle contractions. Each is called a *repetition;* a group of repetitions is called a *set.* In a therapeutic exercise program, the patient performs one or more sets of repetitions of a specific motion or action. An example for a patient performing elbow curls would be three sets of 10 repetitions at a particular load or weight.

Overload describes the progressive increase of the load used to stress and challenge the muscles being exercised. Muscle strength increases when the demands placed on the muscle are more than those normally encountered in activities of daily living. Overloading can be achieved in many different ways — increasing weight or resistance, increasing the number of sets and repetitions, increasing the rate of the exercise, decreasing rest periods, or increasing the duration of the exercise period. All methods of overload should be gradual and incremental to allow the patient to adapt to the exercise changes.

Flexibility describes the ability of a muscle to lengthen, thereby allowing a joint (or more than one joint in a series) to move through a range of motion. Exercises that enhance flexibility can reduce the risk of injury, enhance activity performance, and assist in rehabilitation of many orthopedic and musculoskeletal injuries.

Endurance describes how many times a muscle can contract at its maximum level before fatigue occurs. There are two types of endurance: muscular endurance and total body endurance. *Muscular endurance* is the ability of a muscle to contract and exert tension over a prolonged, specific interval of time. *Total body endurance* results from cardiovascular conditioning that allows the body to deliver enough oxygen and nutrients to the muscles to allow them to perform repetitively for a prolonged period.

Coordination is the patient's ability to effortlessly perform smooth and controlled movements (optimal interaction of muscle function). The physical therapist can increase the complexity of such movements to challenge the neuromuscular system and to approximate the activity that the patient is attempting to master.

Agility describes the combination of coordination and speed that allows the patient to perform activities that require a rapid change in movement or direction.

Balance and *proprioception* are, respectively, the ability to maintain one's center of gravity over the base of support and the ability of the body to know its position in space. The ability to perform complex movements, such as walking, running, twisting, and turning, requires enhanced balance and proprioception. Patients can be trained to perform such complex tasks through therapeutic exercise techniques using, among other things, balance and wobble boards.

Specificity of training and *functional exercise training* are terms used to describe a therapeutic exercise program designed to improve a specific task or function. Although a patient will develop strength, power, and endurance during a training program, this may not necessarily improve his performance at the task or sport he desires. Therefore, the physical therapist should design a specific training program that includes repeated use of partial or complete movements specific to the patient's desired activity. The physical therapist must thoroughly understand the movements required by the patient's activity so that the patient can be properly trained. Improper training could lead to reinjury or further injury.

Types of exercise
Mobility exercises

Mobility exercises are used to maintain or restore the mobility of soft tissue and joints so the patient can perform normal functional movements. They can be active, active assisted, or passive. Mobility exercises include range-of-motion, or flexibility, exercises and static and dynamic stretching exercises.

Range of motion

Range-of-motion (ROM) exercises increase joint and soft tissue mobility.

PASSIVE AND ACTIVE RANGE OF MOTION

In the illustration on the right, the physical therapist manually flexes the patient's leg at the hip to increase the length of the hamstring using a passive range-of-motion exercise.

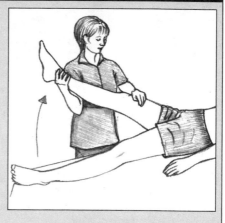

In the illustration below, the patient is performing an active range-of-motion exercise of her elbow.

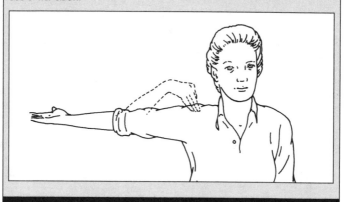

These exercises are designed to move a patient's muscles, joints, and soft tissues through their full, usual amount of movement. There are three types of ROM exercises — passive ROM (PROM), active ROM (AROM), and active assisted ROM (AAROM). In PROM, the patient uses another person or a machine to move the muscles and joints through the exercises. The patient doesn't activate muscle contractions or volitional movements but relies on an external agent in an effort to increase the amount of joint motion and soft tissue extensibility. PROM is indicated for many reasons, including maintaining muscle and soft tissue integrity, minimizing soft tissue contractures, decreasing pain, improving circulation and vascularity, and enhancing the healing process. (See *Passive and active range of motion.*)

In AROM, the patient uses his own muscle power to initiate movements of a body part throughout the available ROM. The benefits are the same as those of PROM, but AROM also brings additional muscle contraction, sensory feedback from the muscle and joint movement, and increased circulation from the muscle pumping action. The patient is also more aware of bone and joint movements. AROM allows the patient to develop coordination of motor skills and, in those patients who have been immobilized, enhances muscle reeducation for functional activities.

In AAROM, AROM is performed by the patient with help from another person or device. AAROM can be used when the muscle is too weak to perform the task or motion completely; the patient will attempt to move the body part as far into the ROM as possible but may be limited by weakness or loss of ROM. The outside force can then be applied by the physical therapist or by the patient, using the opposite limb for assistance. (See *Active assisted range of motion*.)

Stretching

Stretching exercises aim to increase joint ROM and flexibility. In *static stretching,* the patient's joint is moved through the available ROM and held momentarily as gentle but firm force is applied at the point of maximal stretch. Static stretching exercises typically use a slow, prolonged stretch of 30 to 60 seconds.

In *dynamic stretching,* the patient acts unassisted to use the force of the antagonist muscle, such as the triceps, to increase the length of the agonist, such as the biceps. Dynamic stretching exercises attempt to facilitate the speed of the motor response system as the muscle responds at higher velocities, which will simulate functional activities. The patient progresses from a slow-velocity stretch to a high-velocity stretch that approximates the functional activity. To en-

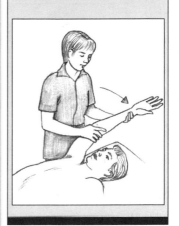

ACTIVE ASSISTED RANGE OF MOTION

In this illustration, the patient actively elevates and flexes his shoulder. Then the therapist assists him in completing the range of motion.

hance dynamic flexibility, the physical therapist must incorporate a ballistic type of stretching (using quick, rapid movement) while gradually increasing the velocity of the stretch. Increased stretching velocity enhances the ability of the muscle and soft tissue to adapt to the demands of the patient's activity.

Strengthening exercises

Strengthening exercises are primarily used to increase muscle strength and may increase endurance. They are based on the overload principle. Isometric, isotonic, and isokinetic are types of strengthening exercises.

 ALERT Strength training has been shown to improve the physical function of older adults by 50% and should be a part of every exercise program, unless con-

ISOMETRIC EXERCISE

In this example of isometric exercise, the patient uses his hand to apply self-resistance to shoulder flexion and shoulder abduction on the opposite arm.

Flexion

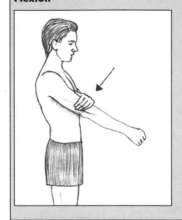

Abduction

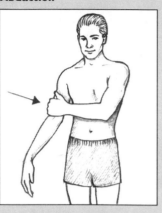

traindicated. Exercises, such as lifting weights, performed even once or twice per week, can keep the older adult from losing muscle tissue, strengthen the bones, and protect the knees and other joints.

Isometrics

In isometric exercises the muscle fibers shorten slightly during contraction, but there is no joint motion. A muscle may be contracted at any point during ROM to stabilize a joint. This can be done with or without applying external resistance. (See *Isometric exercise*.)

Isometric contractions are beneficial in early rehabilitation when regaining muscle control and reeducation of the muscle is crucial. Isometric exercises increase static muscle strength, which is critical for the functional stability of involved joints.

The advantages of isometric exercises in a therapeutic exercise program include:
• minimal joint irritation
• stimulation of joint mechanoreceptors
• muscular "pumping" action, which decreases swelling and edema
• minimal neural dissociation and atrophy
• slightly increased static muscle strength
• improved functional stability of involved joints.

The disadvantages of isometric exercises include:
• lack of eccentric work
• difficulty increasing endurance
• increased strength only at the joint angle at which the patient is training
• minimal joint feedback with only slight compression
• difficulty motivating the patient.

ISOTONIC EXERCISE

In this illustration of isotonic exercise, the patient grasps a hand weight to improve dynamic strength of the shoulder girdle retractors. To lift the weight, he uses a *concentric* contraction; to lower it, he uses an *eccentric* contraction.

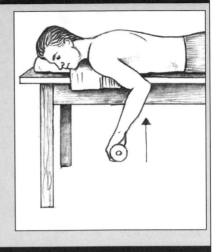

Isometric exercise regimen

An example of a multiple-angle isometric exercise regimen uses Davies's "Rule of 10s": the patient performs 10 sets of 10 contractions, holding each contraction for 10 seconds at every 10 degrees of the ROM. By performing a contraction at every 10 degrees of the ROM, the patient gains strength at different angles in the ROM. This type of regimen can only be performed if the joint to be trained has a permissible ROM.

Isotonics

In contrast to isometric muscle contractions, *isotonic* contractions include joint motion; in addition, some exercises utilize *concentric* (shortening) muscle contractions and some utilize *eccentric* (lengthening) muscle contractions.

Concentric isotonic exercise

Concentric isotonic exercises are muscle-shortening exercises that utilize a fixed resistance and a variable speed. The insertion of the muscle will move toward its origin. The concentric isotonic exercises are often referred to as progressive resistance exercises. The fixed resistance may be the weight of the limb, the effect of gravity on the body part, or the type of load applied, such as dumbbells, cuff weights, and free weights. (See *Isotonic exercise*.)

The advantages of concentric isotonic exercises include:
• ease of access
• ability to perform work through full or partial ROM
• use of small or large overload increments
• objective documentation of increases in strength or overload
• significant strength augmentation
• improvement of muscle reeducation to minimize atrophy.

The disadvantages of concentric isotonic exercises include:
• load always at weakest point in ROM
• difficulty reproducing speed, power, and work

• possibility of using momentum to initiate movement
• muscle soreness caused by muscle fiber breakdown and tissue ischemia
• speed of exercise much slower than the speed of functional activities.

Eccentric isotonic exercises

In contrast to concentric isotonic exercises, eccentric isotonic exercises utilize a lengthening contraction where the insertion of the muscle moves away from the origin. The speed of the work is variable, but the resistance remains fixed.

The advantages of eccentric isotonic exercises include:
• usefulness in early and late stages of rehabilitation
• effectiveness of concentric exercise combined with eccentric exercise
• ROM sometimes increased because of muscle lengthening.

The disadvantage of this type of exercise is that it causes residual muscular soreness.

Isotonic exercise regimens

The type of isotonic exercise to be used depends on the patient's diagnosis and physical condition as well as muscle grade, endurance, and joint mobility. This section reviews several regimens now in use.

Progressive resistive exercise (DeLorme technique).

In the DeLorme technique, the physical therapist determines a 10-repetition maximum (10 RM) for each muscle group to be trained. The *repetition maximum* is the maximum amount of weight that a patient can lift 10 times through the available ROM.

The process of determining a 10 RM can be arduous and time-consuming and may lead to erroneous results unless it has been carefully monitored. The patient performs an exercise at a selected load and attempts as many repetitions as possible. If the patient lifts more than 12 repetitions or less than 8, the weight is either too light or too heavy. The weight is adjusted after this set and, after a brief rest, the patient tries again to establish the 10 RM (between 8 and 12 repetitions). The patient must determine his 10 RM for each muscle group to be trained. After this is done, the patient then performs three sets of 10 repetitions as follows:

Set 1: 10 repetitions at one-half the weight of the 10 RM
Set 2: 10 repetitions at three-quarters of the weight of the 10 RM
Set 3: 10 repetitions at the weight of the full 10 RM

After the patient trains at this first 10 RM for 3 to 5 days, a new 10 RM is determined.

Oxford technique

Like the DeLorme technique, the Oxford technique utilizes a 10 RM; however, the sets are performed in reverse order — fatigue is minimized by *decreasing* the weight with each successive set as the patient becomes tired.

Both the DeLorme and Oxford techniques are effective in increasing the patient's muscle strength, but program adjustments must be made to meet the individual's needs. Either way, the goal is to apply the overload principle by increasing the weight and the load on the muscles to be strengthened. The DeLorme and Oxford techniques should be used together with closed kinetic chain exercises (see "Closed kinetic chain exercises," page 275) and functional training activities, such as stair climbing and walking.

Knight technique

The Knight technique, also known as daily adjustable progressive resistance exercise (DAPRE), helps the therapist and the patient to determine when and by how much a weight or resistance should be increased. The suggested initial working weight recommended by Knight is a 6 RM. After the weight of the 6 RM is determined, the patient then performs the following regimen:

Set 1: 10 repetitions at one-half the working weight

Set 2: 6 repetitions at three-quarters of the working weight

Set 3: As many repetitions as possible of the full working weight

Set 4: As many repetitions as possible of the adjusted working weight.

The adjusted working weight is set by the number of repetitions performed in Set 3, as shown here.

Repetitions in Set 3	Set 4	Next Day
0 to 2	Decrease 5 to 10 lb. Repeat set.	Decrease 5 to 10 lb.
3 to 4	Decrease 0 to 5 lb.	Keep the same weight.
5 to 6	Keep the same weight.	Increase 5 to 10 lb.
7 to 10	Increase 5 to 10 lb.	Increase 5 to 15 lb.
11	Increase 10 to 15 lb.	Increase 10 to 20 lb.

The patient is asked to perform as many repetitions as possible; ideally the number of repetitions before the onset of fatigue should be between 5 and 7.

The Knight technique helps to eliminate guesswork and tries to objectively determine the increases and decreases of load for the next day's training. This program can be used with free weights or weight machines and requires accurate record keeping.

Circuit training

Circuit training is a program designed for increasing muscle strength and total body conditioning. The resistance exercises are usually isotonic, concentric, and eccentric in nature. Circuit training is designed for the patient to follow a specific sequence on various machines and allows the training of as many large muscle groups as possible. The circuit can include a diminished rest period to induce cardiovascular conditioning as well. The circuit is most often utilized in gyms and workout rooms that have a large variety of isotonic machines. Any of the techniques (Delorme, Oxford, or Knight) can be used.

One example of a circuit training program is a 6 RM of these exercises, resting 30 to 60 seconds between each one.

- Leg press
- Bench press
- Leg curls
- Latissimus pull down
- Abdominal crunches
- Squats
- Military press
- Heel raises
- Biceps curls

Isokinetic exercises

Isokinetic exercise is a form of exercise that requires a rate-limiting device that limits the speed of the body part being tested or trained. The term *isokinetic* refers to movement that occurs at a constant speed. In these exercises, the speed of movement remains constant, but the resistance to the movement varies according to the force applied to the resistance lever of the device. Therefore, the muscle is

OPEN KINETIC CHAIN EXERCISE

In this illustration of an open kinetic chain exercise, the patient performs a straight leg raise with resistance (such as a shoe, cuff weight, or Wright boot) added at the ankle while the foot remains free to move.

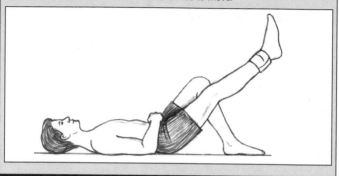

loaded maximally throughout the entire ROM. Isokinetic devices are typically used in conjunction with isotonic techniques, such as the De-Lorme and Oxford techniques. Isokinetic exercises are used in conjunction with all types of exercises — isotonic and eccentric as well as isometric.

There are many benefits to using an isokinetic device.
• The muscle is maximally loaded throughout the entire ROM.
• The joint ROM can be limited, if desired.
• Resistance is never more than the patient can tolerate.
• The isokinetic device allows a patient to reduce muscle tension to avoid causing pain. Because the reduced muscle tension will be less than the device's preset speed, there is little or no resistance against which the patient may injure himself.
• Isokinetic devices are usually computerized and can record and store data for comparison following treatment sessions. Objective, reproducible data is important for physicians as well as for legal and insurance purposes.

Isokinetic devices have some disadvantages. They are large, noisy, cumbersome, and costly and can only be operated by staff trained in positioning the patient, managing the computer and its software, and training and testing procedures for various body parts.

Kinetic chain exercises

Kinetic chain exercises are divided into open chain and closed chain exercises. "Chains" can be thought of as links of body parts, such as the foot, ankle, knee, and hip as they interact during walking. Because open and closed kinetic chain exercises provide somewhat different benefits, all exercise programs should include some combination of open and closed kinetic chain exercises.

Open kinetic chain exercises

Open kinetic chain exercises utilize isometric, isotonic (concentric), or eccentric muscle contractions or a combination thereof. Limb motion is usually in a single plane. The distal segment of the limb can move freely, as in standing shoulder flexion with

WALL SLIDE EXERCISE

In this example of a closed kinetic chain exercise for the lower extremities, the patient places his back against a wall. His feet remain fixed on the floor as he slowly slides down into a sitting position.

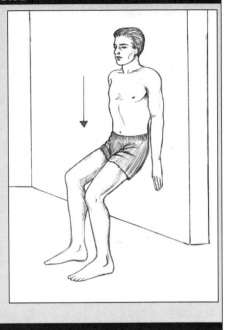

wrist weights or a supine straight leg raise with weights on the ankle. In these examples, resistance is applied to the upper extremity at the wrist and to the lower extremity at the ankle, while the hand and ankle remain relatively free to move. (See *Open kinetic chain exercise*.)

In these exercises, the patient uses the muscles in a nonfunctional manner, particularly with lower extremity exercises where weight bearing is usually one of the goals. Loading and stabilization of the extremity aren't normal because of the lack of compression at joints and lack of synergistic muscle activity. However, open kinetic chain exercises may be the only type of exercise available to a patient if he can't use weights because of fracture or surgery.

Closed kinetic chain exercises

In closed kinetic chain exercises, movement is performed while the distal segment is fixed and the extremity can move in three planes of motion rather than one. All weight-bearing exercises, such as walking and squatting, are closed kinetic chain exercises. A wall slide exercise used to strengthen the quadriceps, hamstrings, and gluteal muscles is an example of such an exercise for the lower extremities. (See *Wall slide exercise*.)

Closed kinetic chain exercises are better than open chain exercises for balance, coordination, and stability, particularly for the lower extremities. However, the upper extremities can also be trained in a closed kinetic chain manner. An example would be the chair push up because the distal segment, the hands, are fixed on the

CHAIR PUSH-UP EXERCISE

In this example of a closed kinetic chain exercise for the upper extremities, the patient keeps his hands fixed on the edge of the seat as he performs a chair push-up.

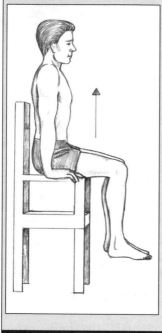

chair. The patient depresses his shoulders to lift his body from the chair. (See *Chair push-up exercise*.) The movement is usually functional. (The patient rises from a chair.) Synergistic muscle activity occurs because the distal segment, which is fixed and stable, allows the proximal segments to move. The synergistic muscle activity provides good stabilization and normal feedback through a normal weight-bearing load.

Conditioning exercises

Conditioning exercises are low-intensity, high-repetition exercises of large muscle groups that enhance overall cardiopulmonary fitness. These exercises increase the patient's ability to perform activities of daily living and to tolerate a sustained level of functional activity, such as walking and stair climbing.

Aerobic exercise

The most common type of conditioning exercise, aerobic exercise encompasses muscle strengthening and cardiopulmonary endurance. Using the overload principle, large muscle groups (arms and legs) are exercised rhythmically and continuously to slowly increase oxygen consumption. Aerobic exercises may include cycling, walking, calisthenics, swimming, rowing, and aquatic exercises. All aerobic exercises should be controlled and progressive, with warm-up and cool-down periods. The intensity of aerobic exercise is measured by heart rate or perceived exertion level. (See chapter 8, Cardiac rehabilitation.)

ALERT Guidelines that emphasize lengthy periods of exercise are geared toward adults and aren't suitable for children. Children older than age 6 should engage in 30 to 60 minutes of age-appropriate physical activity nearly every day.

The advantages of aerobic exercise in a therapeutic exercise program include:
• increased endurance
• decreased heart rate at rest and submaximal effort
• increase coronary blood flow

- decrease exercise recovery time
- increased blood cortisol level
- increased high-density lipoproteins and decreased low-density lipoproteins and triglycerides
- enhanced blood flow to limbs and organs
- possibly enhanced weight control.

Proper aerobic technique is required to optimize benefits and prevent injuries.

 WOMEN'S HEALTH Adolescent girls may notice an increase in body fat when the body begins to produce estrogen. For such patients, aerobic exercises (such as walking, swimming, and dancing) are better than "crash diets" for maintaining ideal body weight.

Relaxation exercises

Relaxation exercises are performed to induce a relaxation response. They can be used alone or in combination with other kinds of exercises. Relaxation exercises include controlled breathing, progressive muscle relaxation, dissociative visualization, and autogenic relaxation training.

Relaxation exercises induce beneficial physiologic changes, including reduced oxygen consumption, respiration rate, heart rate, and blood pressure as well as reduced anxiety and muscle tension and increased brain alpha waves. These exercises also relieve pain.

 WOMEN'S HEALTH Relaxation exercises may help control menstrual pain. However, other sources of pain should be ruled out during a gynecologic examination.

Plyometric exercises

Plyometric exercises are a form of power exercises. This system of exercises was developed in Europe and was originally called jump training or shock training. The plyometric exercise program takes advantage of two useful physiologic factors in the body — the stretch reflex and the elasticity of muscle. The muscle undergoes a cycle of stretching (eccentric contraction) followed by a quick shortening (concentric contraction). In classic plyometric exercises, the patient executes a series of rapid, repetitive jumps for height or distance. Alternatively, the patient jumps off a stool or platform then jumps from the floor for vertical height or linear distance.

The primary use of plyometrics is to bridge the gap between speed and strength. Many activities of daily living, such as walking, utilize the stretch-shortening muscle cycle. Plyometric exercises are designed to improve strength, power, endurance, neuromuscular coordination, speed, and balance. The outcome is a more efficient musculoskeletal system and a more responsive neurologic system. The patient will be better prepared to react, manage, and withstand the rapid and ballistic activities, such as sports and ADLs, that the physical therapist is attempting to approximate.

Plyometric exercise regimen

Plyometric exercise training is a high-velocity program normally employed during the later stages of rehabilitation. A thorough orthopedic screening by the physical therapist is needed to determine the level of plyometric training consonant with the patient's safety.

ALERT Elderly patients may not be suited to plyometric training because of the risk of fracture or other injury, especially if they have such conditions as osteoarthritis and osteoporosis. Likewise, young children (under age 12) with incompletely developed bones and growth plates may be susceptible to injury or fracture.

The patient must wear good supportive sneakers or training shoes, and the floor surface must be safe and resilient. He should be advised to use good form and technique during the course of the training, because poor technique can lead to injury. He should warm up first to enhance blood flow, increase heart rate, and raise core body temperature prior to stretching the appropriate muscles. The patient must maintain appropriate strength for the activity. A 1 repetitive maximum, consisting of a weight approximately 1.5 to 2 times the patient's body weight, is usually appropriate for initial training of the lower extremities.

The therapist should teach the patient the landing component of the regimen prior to incorporating the concentric muscle activity of jumping. This will help to determine the patient's ability to maintain balance and absorb the shock and loading of landing.

Screening tests for plyometric exercises

Before beginning the exercise program, some simple tests can be used to determine the patient's ability to perform plyometric training. The first is a single leg stance with the trunk, hip, and knee slightly flexed. In this preliminary test, the patient stands on one leg with the knee slightly flexed and the other foot elevated. He holds this position for 10 to 30 seconds while the physical therapist assesses his ability to keep his balance. Patients who have proprioception or balance problems may fail this test and will be at risk for injury. The patient can also perform the more difficult single-leg squat with the hip, knee, and trunk flexed to the lowest point possible without lateral deviation or loss of balance and hold that position for 10 to 30 seconds.

Dynamic tests can also evaluate the patient's ability to absorb shock and forces developed during repeated jumping and landing. The *jump test* helps to determine the patient's ability to land in a stable and controlled manner on the involved lower extremity. It also gives an indication of how well the patient can absorb the shock of landing. For example, in the single-leg *hop-down test* the patient hops or jumps off a stool or platform 12″ to 16″ high and attempts a smooth, controlled landing.

The *hop for distance test* evaluates linear distance and stability on landing. The patient stands on one leg behind a line, hops forward as far as possible for maximum linear distance, and must land in an upright stable position on the same leg. The position on landing must be held and controlled for a few seconds to allow the therapist to determine stability of the lower extremity.

The final test is the *repetitive jumps test*. The patient stands on one leg and performs a series of jumps while lifting the knees high. The landing must be controlled and stable with each jump. The therapist observes the concentric to eccentric muscle action during each jump. This test gives a baseline for balance, coordination, stability, and fatigue for future exercises. It can also be performed using both legs, if appropriate.

Lower extremity plyometric drills

Some examples of lower extremity plyometrics are *standing jumps* that can be performed in the same manner as the repetitive jumps in the preliminary dynamic tests. Standing jumps can be vertical for height or linear for distance.

In *multiple response jumps,* the patient jumps from one platform to another, or he can jump from the platform to the floor and then back up on the platform. Multiple response jumps can be performed by repetitive jumping up and down but can include change of direction for speed, agility, power, and endurance.

In another lower-extremity drill, called *in-depth jumps,* the patient jumps from one surface height to another (usually different) surface height. The patient can jump from a low to a high surface or vice-versa. Varying the routine, such as jumping from a soft, high surface and landing on a hard, low surface, enhances the patient's ability to negotiate uneven terrain.

Upper extremity plyometric drills

Plyometric drills for the upper extremity can use weighted balls, a medicine ball, or elastic tubing. One common upper extremity drill is the *two-hand overhead soccer throw,* which develops speed, power, and endurance of the trunk and upper extremities. The patient lifts a medicine ball overhead with both hands and tosses it to a partner or against a wall. The weight of the ball stretches and loads the upper extremities and trunk as the ball is brought back to the overhead position. The ball is then tossed quickly using both hands.

Another upper extremity drill is the *two-hand chest pass* with a

weighted ball. Each partner tosses the ball with both hands back and forth, employing the eccentric (catching) and concentric (tossing) phases of muscle movement.

Final considerations

Here are some final points to consider for a therapeutic exercise program.
• The program should begin with small components of complete movements to ensure that the patient is competent at each level and with all the exercises. The latter can be expanded to larger and more complex movements as the patient's competency improves.
• Muscles should be trained in functional patterns and, if appropriate, activities should be included that will increase power and endurance.
• Ensure the patient's safety by encouraging good form and technique for all components of the exercise. Discontinue an exercise when the technique is poor or when the patient compensates due to fatigue. Keep in mind that smaller muscle groups fatigue more quickly than larger muscle groups.
• Determining the number of repetitions for a particular exercise is largely an educated guess. Use the concept of a *repetition maximum* to assist in the initial stages and modify this by continued reassessment of the patient's performance after each session and on successive days.
• Move the patient through a progression, gradually increasing weight and decreasing repetitions. As the patient gets stronger, first, increase the repetitions; then increase the weight and decrease the repetitions.
• Therapeutic exercise sessions should occur at least two or three times weekly for most maintenance

programs. Alternating days allows muscle recovery and healing from delayed-onset muscle soreness. If appropriate, alternate upper and lower extremity exercises each session for the patient who likes to train daily.

• Advise the patient of the appropriate exercises to perform and the progression of repetitions and sets that can be increased or altered for each exercise. Be sure to obtain medical clearance from a doctor before starting any patient on a therapeutic exercise program — especially cardiovascular conditioning and aerobic exercises.

• Therapeutic exercise can and should be enjoyable for patients; however, patients may have difficulty perceiving any progress if they have a chronic or painful disease or other preexisting condition. Positive feedback is always important but it's especially so in these instances.

• Include activities the patient enjoys to help him take an active role in rehabilitation. For example, the patient may not see his golf or tennis swing improving, but videotaping the sessions may allow him to see the changes from one week to the next.

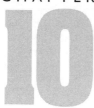

Gait anatomy and physiology

Phases of the gait cycle

Gait can be defined as a particular manner of walking from one place to another. To execute normal gait, the patient must possess adequate range of motion, strength, coordination, sensation, and balance as well as the ability to adapt to various environ- mental and task demands, such as uneven surfaces, obstacles, and the concurrent use of the upper extremities. If the patient loses part or all of his ability to walk as a result of disease, pathology, or injury, he may not be able to perform activities of daily living, and may be severely restricted in his work, social, and leisure activities. Regaining proper gait and walking skills is often of primary concern for patients and their caregivers.

Lower-limb movement in gait is inherently reciprocal, involving repet-

PHASES OF THE GAIT CYCLE

This chart shows the different periods and phases of the gait cycle.

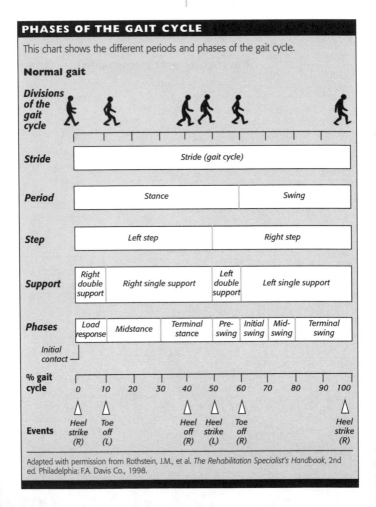

Adapted with permission from Rothstein, J.M., et al. *The Rehabilitation Specialist's Handbook*, 2nd ed. Philadelphia: F.A. Davis Co., 1998.

MEASURES OF STEP AND STRIDE

The illustration below shows a spatial comparison of gait step and stride.

itive and alternating movements of the lower limbs. The gait cycle — the interval from initial contact of one foot to initial contact of the same foot — is divided into a stance period and a swing period. The *stance period* covers the period that a foot is in contact with the ground; this constitutes 60% of the gait cycle. During the *swing period*, the remaining 40% of the gait cycle, the foot is in motion. (See *Phases of the gait cycle*.)

For assessment purposes, the two major periods of the normal gait cycle are subdivided into eight phases.

Stance period
• *Initial contact phase* — the moment a foot first touches the floor
• *Load response phase* — the period between initial contact and the point at which the contralateral leg is lifted for swing
• *Midstance phase* — begins as the contralateral foot is lifted and continues until the body is directly over the supporting leg
• *Terminal stance phase* — begins as the heel rises and continues until the contralateral foot hits the ground
• *Preswing phase* — begins with the next initial contact of the contralateral foot and ends with toe-off of the ipsilateral foot

Swing period
• *Initial swing phase* — begins at the end of foot contact with the floor

and ends with maximal knee flexion in the swinging leg
• *Midswing phase* — begins with maximal knee flexion in the swinging leg and ends when the tibia is perpendicular to the ground
• *Terminal swing phase* — begins with the tibia perpendicular to the ground and ends with the foot's initial contact

During the initial contact and loading phases of the normal gait cycle, body weight must be transferred from the weight-bearing leg to the opposite leg, without interrupting forward progression. The midstance and terminal stance phases require single-leg support and ongoing progression of the body over the supporting leg. As weight is transferred to the contralateral foot, the body positions the ipsilateral leg for swing. During the swing phase, the swing leg is advanced and the foot clears the floor.

Spatial and distance factors in gait

Additional elements of the gait cycle have diagnostic significance. These include spatial measures of *stride* (the period between initial contact of one foot and initial contact of the same foot) and *step* (the period between initial contact of one foot and initial contact of the other foot). (See *Measures of step and stride*.) They

CHANGES IN GAIT PARAMETERS BY AGE

This chart shows developmental changes in the parameters related to walking.

Time and distance parameters	1 year	3 years	7 years
Single limb stance (% of cycle)	32	35	38
Step length (centimeters)	22	33	48
Cadence (steps/minute)	176	154	144
Walking velocity (meters/minute)	38.4	51.6	68.4

also include the temporal measures of *cadence* (the number of steps per unit of time) and *walking velocity* (the distance walked per unit of time).

The average walking velocity and cadence for adults is 3.26 miles per hour, or 110 steps per minute for men or 115 steps per minute for women. Greater walking velocity can be achieved by increasing the step length or cadence. As speed increases, the percentage of time spent in the stance period decreases in relation to the time spent in the swing period. During running, the stance phase represents 40% of the gait cycle and the swing phase 60%.

A number of changes in the duration of single-limb stance, walking velocity, cadence, and step length occur as children develop mature walking patterns. For example, the length of time spent in single-leg stance increases with maturity and is evidence of increasing stability and muscular control. Similarly, as a child's legs grow longer, step length also increases. Walking velocity increases and cadence decreases throughout childhood. (See *Changes in gait parameters by age.*)

Joint range of motion and muscle activity

Progressing through the phases of gait requires the coordinated use of many muscles and joints. To become independent in functional ambulation, the patient must have adequate strength and range of motion (ROM). Researchers have developed a set of optimal ROM values for all aspects of normal gait. The first table gives ROM values in normal gait for the hip, knee, and ankle joints. (See *Total ROM requirements for normal gait.*)

The additional tables give specific ROM values and muscle actions for the hip, knee, and ankle joints in each phase of gait. (See *ROM and muscle activity during gait,* pages 286 to 288.)

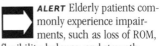 **ALERT** Elderly patients commonly experience impairments, such as loss of ROM, flexibility, balance, and strength, which may alter the normal gait cycle. These changes include:
• mild rigidity
• decreased cadence
• shorter step length
• wider stride width and decreased swing to stance ratio with more time in double stance
• decreased toe-to-floor clearance
• decreased velocity of limb motions.

TOTAL R.O.M. REQUIREMENTS FOR NORMAL GAIT

This table lists the total sagittal plane range-of-motion (ROM) values that are needed for normal gait.

Joint	Stance period	Swing period
Hip	0° to 30° of flexion 0° to 10° or 20° of hyperextension	20° to 30° of flexion
Knee	0° to 40° of flexion	0° to 60° of flexion
Ankle	0° to 10° of dorsiflexion 0° to 20° of plantar flexion	0° to 10° of plantar flexion

Correcting gait abnormalities

Gait analysis

Such methods as observation, camera systems, measurement of ground reaction forces by means of force plates, and electromyography may be used to examine a patient's gait pattern and performance. Gait analysis aims to distinguish normal gait from abnormal gait, classify the degree of disability, assess the efficacy of treatment, enhance performance, and identify underlying mechanisms.

Observational gait analysis

Observational gait analysis (OGA) is the most common method of analysis and identification of gait problems in a clinical setting. In this approach, critical gait parameters are identified through visual observation. OGA requires little investment of equipment, time, or expense. However, this method is subjective and depends on the therapist's skill level, which may produce inconsistent results from one rater to another. The reliability of OGA may be improved by using videotaped recordings, so that the same sequence of gait may be viewed repeatedly and at slower speeds. In addition, ROM at various joints can be examined by taking goniometric measurements from the screen.

Implementation

Important procedural considerations in OGA include:
• identifying an open and unobstructed area for the examination
• observing the patient from the front or back
• observing the gait pattern as an entire process and then examining each joint segment throughout the gait cycle, beginning with the foot and ankle and progressing upward
• determining visually if the patient's performance is significantly different from normal gait for each observed segment and gait cycle phase.

Calculating temporal and spatial variables

Besides OGA, clinical gait analysis may include an assessment of the patient's need for physical assistance and assistive devices. It may also include measurement of temporal and spatial variables. For example, by asking a patient to walk a measured distance (d) and timing the walk (t), you can determine average walking velocity, using the formula: $v = d/t$.

Similarly, if you count the number of steps taken (n) during this walk and divide it by the time, you can de-
(Text continues on page 288.)

R.O.M. AND MUSCLE ACTIVITY DURING GAIT

Joint	Motion	Muscle action
From initial contact to the end of the loading response		
Hip	• Remaining at 30° of flexion • Medial rotation of the femur on the pelvis	• Gluteus maximus, hamstrings, and adductor magnus contract eccentrically to counteract the hip flexion moment.
Knee	• Extending from 0° to 15° of flexion • Medial rotation of the tibia	• Quadriceps initially contracts isometrically to hold the knee in extension and then eccentrically to counteract flexion moment. • Long head of biceps femoris controls medial rotation of the tibia.
Ankle	• Extending from 0° to 15° of plantar flexion • Subtalar joint pronation reaching a maximum at the end of the loading response, thus allowing the foot to adapt to the supporting surface	• Tibialis anterior, extensor digitorum longus, and extensor hallucis longus contract eccentrically to control the lowering of the foot to the ground.
From the end of loading response to the end of midstance		
Hip	• Extending from 30° to 0° of flexion • Medial rotation of the femur on the pelvis continuing to a neutral position at midstance • Adduction moment continuing throughout single support	• Gluteus maximus contracts concentrically into extension. • Hip abductors are active to prevent excessive lateral tilting.
Knee	• Extending from 15° to 5° of flexion • Tibia beginning to rotate laterally	• Quadriceps contracts concentrically into extension.
Ankle	• Moving from 15° of plantar flexion to 5° to 10° of dorsiflexion • Foot beginning to move in the direction of supination from its pronated position at the end of loading response • Foot reaching a neutral position at midstance	• Soleus, gastrocnemius, and plantar flexors contract eccentrically to control the advancement of the tibia over the foot.

R.O.M. AND MUSCLE ACTIVITY DURING GAIT *(continued)*

Joint	Motion	Muscle action
Middle of midstance to prior to end of terminal stance		
Hip	• Extending from 0° to 10° to 20° of extension • Lateral rotation of the femur and adduction	• Hip flexors contract eccentrically. • Hip abductors are active to prevent excessive lateral tilting.
Knee	• Extending from 5° to 0° of flexion • Lateral rotation of the tibia	• No activity is present.
Ankle	• Plantar flexing from 5° to 0° of dorsiflexion • Increasing supination of subtalar joint	• Soleus and plantar flexors contract eccentrically and then concentrically.
End of terminal stance to end of preswing		
Hip	• Flexing from 20° to 0° of extension • Abduction occurring as the weight is shifted onto the opposite extremity • Lateral rotation of the femur	• Iliopsoas, adductor magnus, and adductor longus contract concentrically to flex the hip. • Hip adductors control eccentrically.
Knee	• Moving from 0° to 30° of flexion	• Quadriceps contracts eccentrically or not at all.
Ankle	• Moving from 0° to 20° of plantar flexion • Supination of subtalar joint	• Gastrocnemius, soleus, peroneus brevis, peroneus longus, and flexor hallucis longus contract concentrically or not at all.
Initial swing through midswing		
Hip	• Moving from 0° to 30° of flexion • Rotation from lateral to medial rotation	• Iliopsoas, gracilis, and sartorius contract concentrically.
Knee	• Moving from 30° to 60° of flexion	• Biceps femoris, sartorius, and gracilis contract concentrically.
Ankle	• 20° of plantar flexion to neutral • Unweighted subtalar joint returns to slight supination	• Tibialis anterior, extensor digitorum longus, and extensor hallucis longus contract concentrically.

(continued)

R.O.M. AND MUSCLE ACTIVITY DURING GAIT *(continued)*

Joint	Motion	Muscle action
Terminal swing		
Hip	• Remaining at 30° of flexion • Pelvis rotating forward to increase step length	• Gluteus maximus contracts eccentrically.
Knee	• Extending from 30° to 0° of flexion	• Hamstrings contract eccentrically to counteract the momentum of the swing extremity while full knee extension is ensured by a brief concentric contraction of the quadriceps.
Ankle	• Remaining in neutral position	• Tibialis anterior, extensor digitorum longus, and extensor hallucis longus contract isometrically.

termine cadence (c) using the formula: $c = n/t$.

To find the average step length (l), divide the distance walked by the number of steps taken: $l = d/n$.

Walkway marking methods, such as chalked shoes, absorbent paper, and carbon paper, will help you measure spatial variables. You can use a ruler or tape measure to identify variables, such as the patient's stride length, step length, foot angle, and base of support.

Gait deviations

Gait deviations are observed variations from the normal gait pattern. They may occur after a variety of neuromusculoskeletal injuries and diseases. These disorders may result in such impairments as decreased ROM, weakness, loss of sensation, pain, abnormal muscle tone, impaired motor control (including impaired balance and coordination), and limb length difference. In turn, these impairments may contribute to difficulties with postural control, balance, and gait.

From a biomechanical perspective, gait deviations can be classified in terms of kinematics (related to gait

motion) and kinetic segmental variations (related to alterations in gait forces) at specific points during the gait cycle. For example, the deviation known as "foot slap" occurs at initial contact and can be described as an ankle-foot deviation that results in the forefoot slapping to the ground. For a review of common gait deviations, possible causes, and potential treatment approaches for the ankle, foot, knee, and hip throughout the phases of the gait cycle, see *Common gait problems*.

Gait training

After examining a patient's gait pattern, you may decide to institute a gait training program. Such a program may be useful for teaching the patient about the use of appropriate assistive devices as well as identifying and treating underlying impairments that may contribute to his gait deviations or walking difficulties.

Assistive devices

Assistive devices are prescribed to improve balance and stability, reduce lower limb pain, provide sensory
(Text continues on page 292.)

COMMON GAIT PROBLEMS

Deviation and description	Possible causes	Possible treatment approaches
Ankle and foot		
Initial contact • Foot slap: At initial contact, the forefoot slaps the ground.	• Flaccid or weak dorsiflexors	• Strengthening of weak musculature through exercise, functional retraining, and neuromuscular electrical stimulation • Use of an ankle-foot orthosis
• Toes first: The toes contact the ground instead of the heel; the tiptoe posture may be maintained throughout the phase or the heel may contact the ground.	• Leg length discrepancy • Plantar flexor contracture • Spasticity of plantar flexors • Flaccidity of dorsiflexors • Painful heel	• Lift or orthotic to address leg length discrepancy • Stretching and modalities to increase dorsiflexion ROM • Spasticity reduction techniques • Strengthening of weak dorsiflexors • Treatment of painful heel
• Foot flat: The entire foot contacts the ground at heel strike.	• Excessive fixed plantar flexion • Flaccid or weak dorsiflexors	• Stretching and modalities to increase plantar flexion ROM • Strengthening of weak dorsiflexors
Midstance • Excessive positional plantar flexion: The tibia doesn't advance to neutral from 10° of plantar flexion.	• Excessive fixed plantar flexion • Flaccid or weak dorsiflexors • Spasticity of the plantar flexors	• Stretching and modalities to increase dorsiflexion ROM • Strengthening of weak dorsiflexors • Spasticity reduction techniques
• Heel lift in midstance: The heel doesn't contact the ground in midstance.	• Excessive fixed plantar flexion • Spasticity of the plantar flexors	• Stretching and modalities to increase plantar flexion ROM • Spasticity reduction techniques
• Excessive positional dorsiflexion: The tibia advances too rapidly over the foot, creating a greater than normal amount of dorsiflexion.	• Inability of weak plantar flexors to eccentrically control advancement of the tibia • Knee or hip flexion contractures	• Strengthening of plantar flexors • Stretching and modalities to increase knee and hip flexion ROM
• Toe clawing: Toes flex and "grab" the floor.	• Positive supporting reflex • Spastic toe flexors	• Reflex integration techniques • Spasticity reduction techniques

(continued)

COMMON GAIT PROBLEMS (continued)

Deviation and description	Possible causes	Possible treatment approaches
Ankle and foot (continued)		
Terminal stance to preswing • No roll-off: There is an insufficient transfer of weight from lateral heel to medial forefoot.	• Mechanical fixation of ankle and foot • Flaccidity of plantar flexors • Pain in forefoot	• Strengthening of plantar flexors • Treatment of painful forefoot
Swing • Toe drag: There is an insufficient dorsiflexion (and toe extension) so that forefoot and toes don't clear the floor.	• Flaccidity or weakness of dorsiflexors and toe extensors • Inadequate knee or hip flexion due to weakness or loss of range of motion (ROM)	• Strengthening of weak musculature through exercise, functional retraining, and neuromuscular electrical stimulation • Stretching and modalities to increase knee and hip flexion ROM
• Varus: The foot is excessively inverted.	• Spasticity of the invertors • Flaccid or weak dorsiflexors	• Spasticity reduction techniques • Strengthening of dorsiflexors
Knee		
Initial contact • Excessive knee flexion: Knee flexes or "buckles" rather than extends as the foot contacts the ground.	• Painful knee • Spasticity of knee flexors • Flaccid or weak quadriceps	• Treatment of painful knee • Spasticity reduction techniques • Strengthening of quadriceps through exercise, functional retraining, and neuromuscular electrical stimulation
Loading response to midstance • Knee hyperextension: There is a greater than normal extension at the knee; the ankle may be plantar flexed as body weight moves over the foot.	• Flaccid or weak quadriceps and soleus compensated for by pull of gluteus maximus • Spasticity of quadriceps • Accommodation to a fixed ankle plantar flexion deformity	• Strengthening of weak quadriceps • Stretching and modalities to increase dorsiflexion ROM • Spasticity reduction techniques
Terminal phase to preswing • Excessive knee flexion: The knee flexes to more than 40° during preswing.	• Rigid trunk • Knee or hip flexion contractures • Dominance of flexion synergy	• Stretching and modalities to increase trunk, knee, and hip ROM • Neurotherapeutic treatment approaches to encourage integration of flexion synergy

COMMON GAIT PROBLEMS *(continued)*

Deviation and description	Possible causes	Possible treatment approaches
Knee *(continued)*		

Initial phase to midswing

• Limited knee flexion: The knee doesn't flex to 65°.	• Pain in knee • Diminished knee ROM • Extensor spasticity	• Treatment of painful knee • Stretching and modalities to increase knee ROM • Spasticity reduction techniques

Hip

Initial contact to loading response

• Excessive hip flexion: Hip flexion exceeds 30°.	• Hip or knee flexion contractures • Hypertonicity of hip flexors	• Stretching and modalities to increase hip and knee ROM • Spasticity reduction techniques
• Limited hip flexion: Hip flexion doesn't attain 30°.	• Weakness of hip flexors • Limited ROM of hip flexion	• Strengthening of hip flexors • Stretching and modalities to increase hip ROM

Loading response to midstance

• Limited hip extension: The hip doesn't attain a neutral position.	• Hip flexion contractures • Spasticity of the hip flexors	• Stretching and modalities to increase hip ROM • Spasticity reduction techniques
• Hip internal rotation: There is an internally rotated position of the extremity.	• Spasticity of internal rotators • Weakness of external rotators	• Spasticity reduction techniques • Strengthening of the external rotators
• Hip adduction: There is an adducted position of the lower extremity.	• Spasticity of the hip flexors and adductors	• Spasticity reduction techniques • Strengthening of the hip abductors

Swing

• Circumduction: There is a lateral circular movement of the entire lower extremity, consisting of abduction, external rotation, adduction, and internal rotation.	• A compensation for weak hip flexors • A compensation for the inability to shorten the leg so that it can clear the floor	• Strengthening of the hip flexors • Stretching and modalities to increase dorsiflexion ROM • Strengthening of weak dorsiflexors • Spasticity reduction techniques
• Hip hiking: There is a shortening of the swing leg by action of the quadratus lumborum.	• A compensation for lack of knee flexion or ankle dorsiflexion • A compensation for extensor spasticity of swing leg	• Stretching and modalities to increase knee and ankle ROM • Spasticity reduction techniques

TYPES OF CRUTCHES

Different types of crutches are shown below

Axillary crutches

Adjustable axillary crutch	Axillary crutch with platform	Ortho crutch	Telescoping underarm aluminum crutch
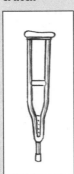	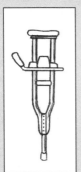	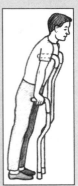	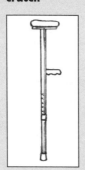
Made of wood or tubular aluminum and can be adjusted for length	For patients who can't bear weight through the hand	More comfortable than standard axillary crutches for some patients	Offers more adjustability

feedback, and assist acceleration during locomotion. Some common assistive devices are crutches, canes, and walkers.

A particular assistive device and gait pattern need to be tailored to the patient's functional status, his ability to maintain an erect body posture, and the amount of weight-bearing and balance assistance needed. Walkers provide the greatest stability, crutches provide moderate stability, and canes provide the least amount of stability.

Using crutches

Crutches remove weight from one or both legs, enabling the patient to support himself with his hands and arms. These functions allow crutches to be used to accommodate lower-limb weakness or abnormal motor control and to improve balance. Crutch selection and walking gait depend on the patient's condition. Many crutch designs are available to answer a variety of therapeutic needs.

Axillary crutches include an axillary bar that rests 1″ to 2″ below the axilla to provide better trunk support than nonaxillary crutches. Axillary crutches, such as standard crutches and single-upright crutches (telescoping and ortho-crutches), are prescribed for short-term use by patients with good balance and coordination.

Forearm or arm crutches are nonaxillary crutches that provide support for the forearm. They're prescribed for long-term use by patients with good balance and confidence in ambulation. This group includes Canadian or Lofstrand crutches (the most popular type), platform crutches,

Non-axillary crutches

Triceps crutch (Canadian Elbow Extensor Crutches)	Forearm crutch with closed cuff	Adjustable forearm crutch	Platform crutch or forearm support crutch

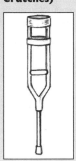 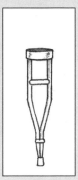 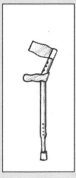 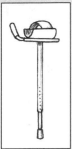

Has two cuffs, one above and one below the elbow, for patients with triceps weakness

For patients who have less hand control or who wish to fill hands without dropping the crutches

Most popular nonaxillary crutch; allows patient to free hand without dropping crutch

Often used by arthritic patients with flexion contracture of the elbow

forearm crutches with closed cuff, and triceps crutches. (See *Types of crutches.*)

Equipment preparation

For proper use, crutches should be adjusted to fit the individual patient. Crutches should fall approximately two finger widths below the axilla when the patient is standing. The hand piece should provide for 20 to 30 degrees of elbow flexion. With the elbow extended, this can be estimated by lining up the hand piece with the patient's wrist. The crutch tips should fall 2″ lateral and 6″ anterior to the patient's foot. (See *Fitting a patient for a crutch,* page 294.)

Gait training with crutches can incorporate a number of different ambulation patterns. These patterns include:

• *Two-point gait* — In two-point gait, the patient advances one crutch and the contralateral leg. Then he advances the ipsilateral leg. (See *Using a two-point gait,* page 295.)
• *Three-point gait* — This gait pattern is used when one leg must be maintained in a non-weight-bearing position. The patient advances the crutches first and then advances the non-involved leg. (See *Using a three-point gait,* pages 296 and 297.)
• *Four-point gait* — In this pattern, the patient first advances the left crutch, then the right leg. Then he advances the right crutch followed by the left leg. (See *Using a four-point gait,* page 298.)
• *Swing-to and swing-through gait* — These patterns are often used when a patient has bilateral lower-limb involvement, as in paraplegia.

FITTING A PATIENT FOR A CRUTCH

Position the crutch so that it extends from a point 4″ to 6″ (10 to 15 cm) to the side and 4″ to 6″ in front of the patient's feet to 1½″ to 2″ (4 to 5 cm) below the axillae (about the width of two fingers). Then adjust the handgrips so that the patient's elbows are flexed at a 15-degree angle when he's standing with the crutches in the resting position.

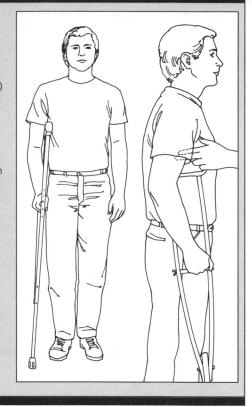

In these patterns, the patient advances both crutches and then swings both legs simultaneously, either *to* the crutches or *through* the crutches.

Essential steps

• To teach the patient who uses crutches how to get up from a chair:
—Instruct him first to slide his hips forward in the chair.
—Next, have him place the foot of the uninvolved (stronger) leg slightly behind the involved (weaker) leg.
—If the patient can't bend the knee, advise sliding the heel forward prior to standing.

—Next, tell the patient to hold the crutches on the same side as the involved leg.
—Then tell the patient to lean on the crutches and the armrest of the chair, lean forward, and push up to a standing position.
—When the patient is standing, tell him to transfer one crutch to his free hand, and he's ready to walk.
• To sit down, the patient should reverse the process.
—Tell the patient to begin to turn in the direction of the uninvolved leg and to back up until both legs are touching the chair.
—Then have him hold both crutches on the side of the involved leg and

USING A TWO-POINT GAIT

If your patient can't support her full weight on both legs but has good coordination and arm strength, you or the doctor may choose the two-point gait for her. This is a natural gait that mimics walking with alternating swings of the arms and legs. To use this gait, following these steps.

Moving the left crutch and the right foot

Have the patient stand with her weight evenly distributed between both legs and the crutches. To take a step, tell her to shift her weight to the right crutch and her left foot as she moves the left crutch (A) and her right foot (B) about 8" forward.

Moving the right crutch and the left foot

Have the patient shift her weight to the left crutch and her right foot. At the same time, tell her to move the right crutch (C) and her left foot (D) about 8" forward. Have her repeat these steps until she feels she has mastered the gait.

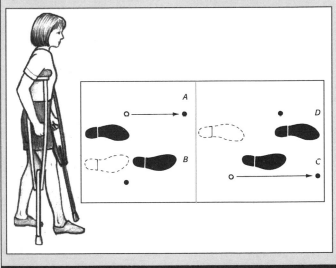

reach back for the armrest of the chair with the other arm.
— Tell the patient to use arm support along with the strength in the uninvolved leg to help lower himself into the chair.

Special considerations
• During crutch walking, the patient should support his body weight by the hands and not the axillary region. Instruct him to maintain an erect posture with head facing forward.
• When initially instructing a patient in a particular gait pattern, use a gait belt for patient safety. Stand close to and slightly behind the patient on the side of the involved leg.

Documentation
When documenting a program of crutch walking, include the type of crutches used, the gait pattern, weight-bearing restrictions, assistance required, and the distance and frequency of ambulation.

Using a cane
Canes provide less support than other assistive devices. However, they may

USING A THREE-POINT GAIT

If your patient can't support her weight on one leg but has normal use of her arms, upper body, and other leg, you or the doctor may choose the three-point gait for her. To use this gait, follow these steps for an injured left leg; reverse the steps if the patient has an injured right leg.

Positioning
Have the patient stand with her weight distributed between her right leg and the crutches. Tell her to keep her left foot off the floor and her left knee slightly flexed, and to try to relax her shoulders.

Shifting weight
Tell the patient to lean slightly forward, supporting her weight on her right leg and the crutches. Next, have her shift her weight to her right leg and move both crutches forward (A). Then, tell her to swing her left leg forward, remembering not to put weight on it.

Moving forward
Have your patient balance her weight on both crutches as she swings her right leg forward (B). Next, have her

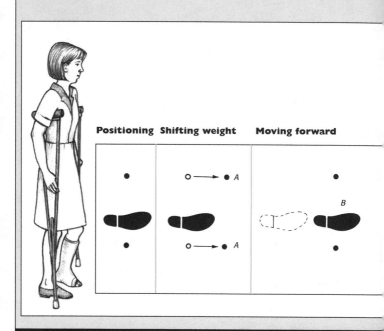

Positioning   Shifting weight   Moving forward

be appropriate for patients who need only partial weight relief or support. As with crutches, canes come in a number of types.

Standard canes are made of wood or aluminum, have a variety of handle styles, and can be adjusted or cut to the appropriate length. *Quad* canes, with four small feet, provide additional stability if needed. *Hemiwalkers* combine the features of a walker and a quad cane. They're foldable and provide a wider base of support and better lateral support than a quad cane. They're used by hemiplegic patients who aren't ready return her weight to her right leg, using the crutches to maintain balance. Then, tell her to move both crutches and her left leg forward to repeat the procedure.

Using a swing-through three-point gait

When your patient has mastered the three-point gait and her balance and strength improve, you or the doctor may recommend the swing-through three-point gait for her. To use this gait, have the patient first move her right leg beyond the crutches (A). Then, tell her to advance both crutches (B) and swing her right leg past the crutches (C). Have her repeat this sequence until she feels she has mastered the gait.

Starting a swing-through three-point gait

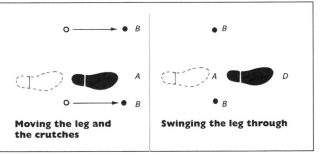

Moving the leg and the crutches

Swinging the leg through

to use a quad cane. (See *Types of canes*, page 299.)

Equipment preparation

To measure a patient for a cane, use the greater trochanter as a landmark for the top of the cane. In addition, as with crutches, the patient's elbow should be flexed 20 to 30 degrees when the hand is resting on the cane.

Essential steps

• Canes should be held in the hand opposite the involved leg.

(Text continues on page 300.)

USING A FOUR-POINT GAIT

If your patient can't support his full weight on both legs, you or the doctor may choose the four-point gait for him. Although this is the safest gait, it calls for greater coordination than the others because the patient must constantly shift his weight. To use this gait, follow these steps.

Moving the left crutch
Have the patient stand with his weight evenly distributed between both legs and the crutches. Then tell him to move the left crutch about 8" forward (A). As he does so, tell him to shift his weight so it's evenly distributed between the right crutch and both legs.

Moving the right foot
Next, have the patient move his right foot about 8" forward (B), making it even with the left crutch.

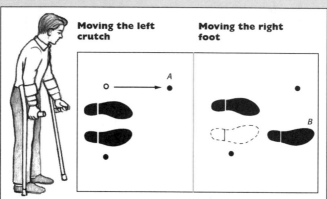

Moving the left crutch

Moving the right foot

Moving the right crutch
Now, have the patient move the right crutch about 8" forward (C). At the same time, tell him to shift his weight onto the left crutch and both legs.

Moving the left foot
Next, tell the patient to move his left foot 8" forward (D), making it even with the right crutch. Have him repeat this sequence — left crutch, right foot, right crutch, left foot — until he feels he has mastered the gait. Suggest that the patient try counting to help develop rhythm and tell him to make sure each step is the same length.

Moving the right crutch

Moving the left foot

TYPES OF CANES

The illustrations below show different types of canes.

C-handle wooden straight cane

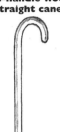

C-handle adjustable aluminum straight cane

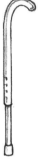

Ortho-cane (offset cane)

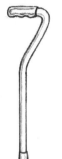

Narrow-based quadruped cane

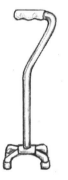

Forearm quad cane

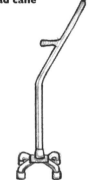

Wide-based quadruped cane

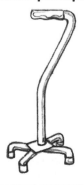

Hemiwalker

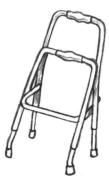

TYPES OF WALKERS

Different types of walkers are illustrated below.

Nonfolding standard walker

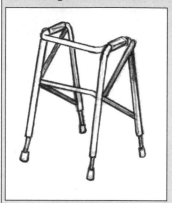

Rolling or gliding walker

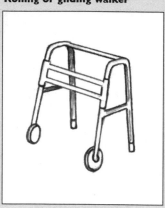

Bilateral platform walker

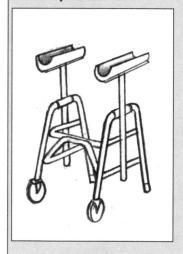

Rolling triceps walker

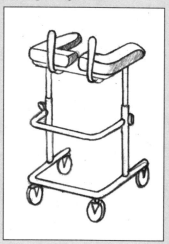

• To teach a patient who uses a cane to get up from a chair:
−Advise him to slide his hips forward in the chair.
−Have him place the foot of the un-involved leg slightly behind the in-volved leg.

−Next, tell him to push on the chair's armrest and the cane while leaning forward to stand.
• When walking with a cane, patients can use one of two common gait patterns:

Stair-climbing walker

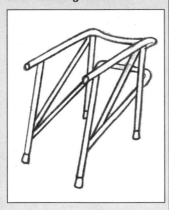

Reverse rollator or posture-control walker

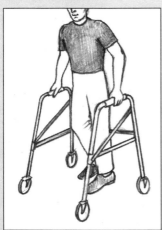

As the patient progresses, increase the degree of independence you allow.
• To teach the patient how to sit:
– Tell the patient to approach the chair, turn in the direction of the uninvolved leg, and back up until both legs are touching the chair.
– Then have him reach back for the chair arm, using his free hand (on the uninvolved side).
– Finally, tell the patient to slowly settle down into the chair with support from the armrest and the cane.

Special considerations
Of all the available assistive devices, canes provide the least amount of stability. Although hemiwalkers are the most stable canes, they can be difficult to maneuver in tight spaces.

Documentation
When documenting gait training with a cane, note the type of cane, gait pattern, level of assistance required, distance, and frequency of ambulation.

Using a walker
Of all of the assistive devices available for gait training, walkers provide the most stability and support. They're effective devices for patients who need to maintain a restricted weight-bearing status, those with balance difficulties, and those with lower-limb weakness or general debilitation. (See *Types of walkers.*)

One disadvantage of walkers is that they're more difficult than other devices to maneuver in narrow spaces.

Various types of walkers are available. Many are adjustable and can be folded for storage.

Standard walkers require good balance, arm strength, and sufficient hand strength and ROM. *Rolling walkers* have wheels on the front legs to assist walker movement for patients who can't lift the device due to

– First advancing the involved leg and the cane simultaneously, and then advancing the uninvolved leg
– First advancing the cane, followed by the involved leg, and then the uninvolved leg.
• As with other forms of gait training, use a gait belt for patient safety.

lack of coordination or lack of strength in the arms and trunk. *Platform walkers* provide forearm support for patients who have flexion contracture of the elbow or pain or deformities of the wrist and hand.

Rolling triceps walkers are used by patients with limited arm strength and ROM. Their padded platforms and four wheels allow the patient to push the walker forward without lifting. *Reciprocal walkers* have swivel joints that allow reciprocal action (each side of the walker moves alternatively). They're commonly used by patients recuperating from hip replacements.

Reverse walkers, which can be fitted with wheels if desired, are used mostly by pediatric patients to encourage a more extended posture during gait. Finally, *stair-climbing walkers* provide stability in stair climbing and are used by motivated patients who have good balance and superior strength in their arms.

Equipment preparation

To measure a patient for a walker, use the greater trochanter as a landmark for the top of the walker. The patient's elbows should be flexed 20 to 30 degrees when his hands are resting on the walker.

Essential steps

To teach the patient how to stand:
• Tell the patient to place the walker directly in front of him and to slide his hips forward in the chair.
• Then have him place the foot of the uninvolved leg slightly behind the involved leg.
• Next, tell him to push on the armrests of the chair while leaning forward to stand up. Warn him not to pull on the walker because it may tip and cause a fall.
• When the patient is standing, instruct him to move the walker forward first, then the involved leg, and then the uninvolved leg.

To teach the patient how to sit:
• Tell him to approach the chair, turn in the direction of the uninvolved leg, and back up until both legs are touching the chair.
• Then have him reach back for the armrests of the chair with both hands and slowly settle down into the chair.

Documentation

Documenting gait training with a walker is similar to documentation for other assistive devices. Note the type of walker, gait pattern, level of assistance, distance, and frequency of ambulation.

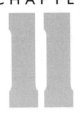

Prostheses and orthoses

Ensuring fit and function

Patients who suffer limb loss or musculoskeletal malformations require correctional therapy and training in the use of prosthetic or orthotic devices. *Prostheses* are artificial limbs and *orthoses* are orthopedic supports (braces). Both types of devices are prescribed by doctors and are usually fabricated and fit by prosthetists and orthotists, who are trained in evaluating, fabricating, fitting, and adjusting prosthetic and orthotic devices. These specialists are members of the health care team and work with other team members and the patient to provide a highly specialized service.

Prostheses and orthoses should be lightweight, durable, and cosmetically acceptable. Proper fit, function, and care are essential to obtain maximal function from these devices. This chapter reviews amputation and congenital deformities as well as the fitting, patient training, and care of prosthetics and orthoses.

Orthotic and prosthetic devices are an integral part of medical care today. They are used for a wide variety of medical conditions. Many health care professionals are involved in the process of evaluation, prescription, delivery, training, and follow-up, and it's important that all team members communicate with one another and with the patient regarding the treatment. When this occurs, the patient receives the maximum benefit of the device and achieves the highest functional level and outcome.

Using prosthetic devices

Causes of amputation

Loss of body parts may result from traumatic injury, disease, or congenital anomalies. Traumatic amputations can occur following such occurrences as train accidents (the most common cause of multiple limb amputations), motor vehicle or farm-related accidents, severe burns, severe fracture or crush injuries, gunshot or knife wounds, and firecracker detonations.

Disease-related causes for amputation include tumors, complications of diabetes or peripheral vascular disease, paralysis, gangrene, and osteomyelitis. Amputations secondary to tumor usually result in higher-level upper and lower extremity amputations, such as hip and shoulder disarticulation and hemipelvectomy. In congenital amputations, the patient lacks one or more limbs or limb segments at birth. These can occur alone or be associated with other anomalies.

A higher level of amputation means a greater functional loss of the limb and the more the patient must depend on the prosthesis for function and cosmetic appearance. (See *Amputation levels.*)

Preparing the residual limb

After amputation, the residual limb isn't usually ready for prosthetic fitting unless a temporary device was applied immediately after surgery. The surgical incision must be kept clean and dry until the sutures or staples are removed, and the residual limb must heal properly and completely. The limb is usually placed in a soft dressing. In a transtibial (below-knee) amputation, the limb may also be placed in a rigid plaster cast. This helps protect and shape the residual limb, control swelling, and avoid knee flexion contractures. Typically, a drain is in place after the operation for the first 24 hours.

During this time, the residual limb and the entire extremity are positioned properly to avoid joint con-

AMPUTATION LEVELS

The illustrations below show levels of upper- and lower-limb amputations. Typically, a higher level of amputation means a more complex prosthesis and more associated training are necessary. The percentages indicate the relative incidence of these amputations.

Transhumeral amputations

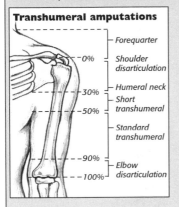

- Forequarter
- 0% — Shoulder disarticulation
- Humeral neck
- 30%
- Short transhumeral
- 50%
- Standard transhumeral
- 90% — Elbow disarticulation
- 100%

Transradial amputations

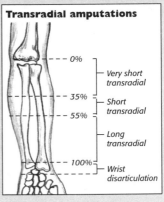

- 0%
- Very short transradial
- 35%
- Short transradial
- 55%
- Long transradial
- 100% — Wrist disarticulation

Transfemoral amputations

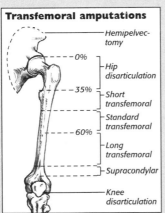

- Hemipelvectomy
- 0% — Hip disarticulation
- 35%
- Short transfemoral
- Standard transfemoral
- 60%
- Long transfemoral
- Supracondylar
- Knee disarticulation

Transtibial amputations

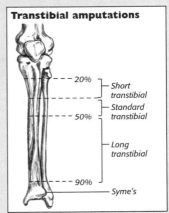

- 20% — Short transtibial
- Standard transtibial
- 50%
- Long transtibial
- 90% — Syme's

Partial foot amputations

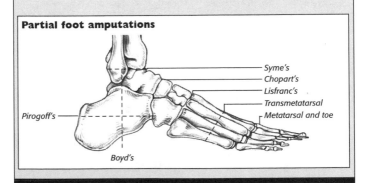

- Syme's
- Chopart's
- Lisfranc's
- Transmetatarsal
- Metatarsal and toe
- Pirogoff's
- Boyd's

tractures. Knee flexion contractures are common with transtibial amputations; hip flexion contractures are common with transfemoral (above-knee) amputations. Proper positioning doesn't include the use of pillows, towel rolls, or cushions because they may contribute to joint contractures. Ideally, the patient maintains a prone position as often as possible to help stretch the hip and the knee and uses a board under a transtibial amputation during prolonged sitting to maintain knee extension.

Gentle range-of-motion (ROM) exercises with both the affected limb and the unaffected limb maintain muscle tone, increase muscle strength, and help avoid contractures and weakness. ROM exercises progress to resistive and strengthening exercises.

Limb shaping

The residual limb is ready for shaping as soon as the drain is removed. Shaping helps desensitize the limb and prepares it for prosthetic fitting. Ideally, the transtibial residual limb has a conical shape and the transfemoral residual limb is cylindrical. This is usually accomplished with elastic bandage wraps that are applied almost immediately or after the drain is removed. The patient wears these bandages at all times except for dressing changes; they're reapplied several times a day because they lose their elasticity and pressure over time. Patients and caregivers must learn proper wrapping techniques. (See *Wrapping the residual limb*.)

If appropriate, elastic "shrinkers" may be used instead of elastic bandage wraps. Shrinkers come in various pressure gradients, sizes, and lengths; usually, the prosthetist provides them after measuring the length and circumference of the residual limb. Shrinkers are usually

easier than bandage wraps for the patient to use (especially with transfemoral residual limbs), but they tend to stretch out and can't be as easily adjusted to accommodate significant changes in limb size, shape, and volume.

The residual limb remains wrapped throughout the postoperative and rehabilitation periods and even after the initial prosthetic fitting. The patient wears the wrap whenever he takes off the prosthesis and during the night. Wrapping usually continues until the residual limb shape and volume have stabilized, which usually takes 6 to 12 months.

Preprosthetic activities

In addition to the positioning and shaping of the residual limb, the patient must begin to prepare for using the prosthesis. This involves transfer training, learning to ambulate with crutches or a walker, residual limb strengthening, and strengthening of the unaffected extremities. During this phase, it's critical to avoid falls and injuries to the residual limb. Teaching must emphasize and reinforce safety and awareness with the patient and caregiver.

Quadriceps strengthening, along with overall hip musculature, is especially important with the transtibial amputee. Hip flexor, extensor, abductor, adductor, and gluteal strengthening are important with the transfemoral amputee. Traditional physical therapy exercise programs and techniques can be used with slight modification at the amputation site. For example, the patient can use bolsters, towel rolls, or cuff weight extenders to protect the residual limb when force is applied to it during strengthening exercises.

WRAPPING THE RESIDUAL LIMB

The first set of illustrations depicts the correct way to wrap a transtibial amputation using a modified figure-eight technique. The second set illustrates a figure-eight wrap for a transfemoral amputation.

Transtibial amputation

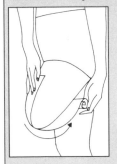 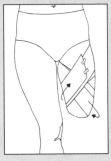 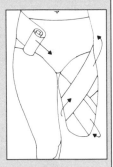

Center the end of a 4″ elastic bandage at the top of the patient's thigh. Unroll the bandage downward over the stump and up the back of the leg.

Make three figure-eight turns to adequately cover the end of the stump.

Use the second 4″ bandage to anchor the first bandage around the waist. Secure the bandage with clips, safety pins, or adhesive tape.

Transfemoral amputation

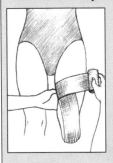 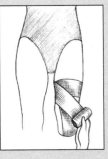 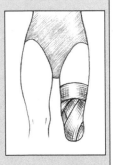

Using only one 4″ elastic bandage, center the end over the top of the patient's thigh.

Make enough figure-eight turns to adequately cover the end of the stump.

Finish by wrapping the bandage around the thigh. Secure the bandage with clips, safety pins, or adhesive tape.

TYPES OF TRANSTIBIAL PROSTHESIS

Three examples of transtibial prosthesis are shown below.

Transtibial prosthesis with thigh corset, knee joints, and hyperextension strap

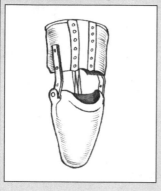

Exoskeletal transtibial prosthesis with a supracondylar suspension cuff and pelite liner

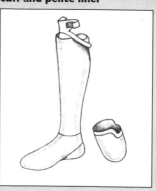

Prosthetic evaluation

After the surgeon has determined that adequate healing, shaping, and strengthening have occurred, the patient is ready for prosthetic evaluation. This is typically done by a prosthetic team composed of the doctor (usually a physiatrist [a doctor certified in physical medicine and rehabilitation] or surgeon), a physical therapist, a prosthetist, and other rehabilitation team members. The team meets with the patient and evaluates such factors as past medical history, bodily strength, range of motion, and ability to ambulate. They also talk with the patient about his goals, employment, hobbies, and other personal areas.

The team recommends a prosthesis with components appropriate for the patient's individual needs, goals, and abilities. Many types of prostheses are available, and the technology is always changing. Prosthetists are usually knowledgeable in this area

and can help keep the entire team updated on new designs, components, and technology.

The prosthetic team also recommends a rehabilitation plan for fitting, training, and follow-up. The plan lends itself to inpatient, outpatient, or the home setting according to the patient's amputation level, overall physical condition, personal preference, transportation needs, and medical insurance coverage.

Prosthetic fitting

After the prosthetic team determines a prescription, the prosthetist takes a cast of the patient's residual limb or measures it for the prosthesis. The prosthetist then fabricates the device and fits it to the patient, who may need several visits to achieve the optimal fit. The socket, the hollow container that accepts the residual limb, must fit properly for maximum comfort and function. Proper prosthetic

Endoskeletal transtibial prosthesis without cosmetic cover

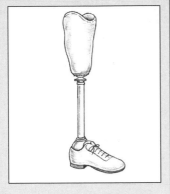

socket management is also an important part of patient teaching.

The patient usually begins physical therapy with the prosthesis immediately after being fitted. The prosthetist works closely with the patient and physical therapist — especially during the early stages of rehabilitation when the most adjustments need to be made on the residual limb, which is still fragile and changing in shape and volume. This is also the time when a patient with a lower-limb amputation experiences the most changes in gait. Prosthetic use changes as the patient progresses, and all of these factors affect the alignment of the prosthesis. After the prosthesis is fitted and properly functioning, the prosthetist becomes much less involved and may only see the patient for routine follow-ups and further adjustments.

Transtibial prostheses

A transtibial amputation and a Syme's amputation (an amputation of the foot at the ankle joint) are treated prosthetically in the same manner. The most common socket design for a transtibial prosthesis is the patella tendon–bearing (PTB) socket. The PTB socket is designed to relieve pressure on the bony prominences of the residual limb (such as the tibial tuberosity, fibular head, and anterior distal tibia) and to apply pressure on pressure-tolerant areas of the residual limb (such as the patella tendon, gastrocnemius, and interosseous membrane of the tibia and fibula). The socket is attached to a shin section, which may have an exoskeletal design (a rigid hard shell) or an endoskeletal design (a pipe with a soft cover), and is shaped to match the unaffected shin. The shin is then attached to the prosthetic foot.

PTB sockets often have an inner liner that cushions the residual limb from the hard outer socket. The liner decreases the effect of sheer forces on the residual limb during ambulation and improves prosthesis comfort and fit. (See *Types of transtibial prosthesis.*)

Several types of suspension systems are available for a transtibial prosthesis. The device can be suspended with a waist belt and strap, with a PTB cuff, or with silicone suspension. The socket itself can also be modified to "self-suspend" the prosthesis; these modifications change the socket from a traditional PTB to a supracondylar patella tendon socket (PTS) or a supracondylar-suprapatellar socket (SC-SP).

The suspension occurs with a more proximal trimline with a wedge medially just above the femoral condyles. The wedge helps hold the prosthesis in place by applying pressure above the medial condyle of the femur. Both the supracondylar PTS and SC-SP PTS provide greater stability of the knee from side to side; the SC-SP PTS also helps control hyperextension of the knee. If the knee requires greater stability and control, external knee joints can be added with a thigh corset.

Prosthetic devices for partial foot amputations vary according to the degree of amputation. Toe amputations don't usually require a complex prosthesis. Toe fillers and partial foot prostheses are used to support and protect the rest of the foot and to fill a shoe cosmetically. Many kinds of prosthetic feet are available, such as solid ankle cushioned heel, dynamic, and energy-storing designs. The prosthetic foot prescribed depends on the patient's weight, activity level, and functional potential.

Transfemoral prosthetics

There are two basic designs of transfemoral prosthetic sockets — the quadrilateral socket and the ischial containment socket. The *quadrilateral socket* is rectangular in shape and more narrow in the anterior-posterior dimension compared to the medial-lateral dimension. The ischial tuberosity rests on the posterior socket wall. The *ischial containment socket* is oval-shaped and more narrow in the medial-lateral dimension than the anterior-posterior dimension. The ischial tuberosity is contained within the socket. Either socket can be made of thermoplastic material or laminated with resin.

The socket is attached to the prosthetic knee. Selection of the appropriate prosthetic knee design depends on the length of the residual limb, its strength, and the patient's weight and activity level. Prosthetic knees vary greatly in design and function, ranging from a manually locked knee (for maximal stability in stance) to hydraulic and pneumatic knees, which adjust for variable cadences. In appearance, the transfemoral prosthesis is identical to the transtibial prosthesis below the knee, with

the same shin, foot, and ankle components.

Suspension of a transfemoral prosthesis can be achieved with a suction device, belts, or a pelvic band and hip joint. The type of suspension depends on the residual limb, the ability of the patient to put on and remove the prosthesis easily, and the amount of control needed to use the prosthesis. (See *Types of transfemoral prosthesis*.)

Prosthetic training

Prosthetic training begins at the initial fitting with the prosthetist and continues with the physical therapist throughout the physical therapy and rehabilitation phases. Patients must first learn how to properly put on and remove the prosthesis. Ambulation training usually begins in the parallel bars with a mirror placed at one end for maximal assistance, security, and visual feedback.

Gait training with a transtibial prosthesis is much easier than with a transfemoral prosthesis. This is because the anatomical knee is controlling stability at initial contact with the floor in stance and foot clearance during swing phases of gait. Patients must learn to ambulate on various surfaces, uneven terrain, and up and down stairs and inclines. They must also learn how to safely lower and raise themselves from the floor and from a sitting position, walk at various cadences, and perform higher physical activities, such as running, jogging, biking, and golfing. (See chapter 10, Gait problems.)

Early stages of training usually require assistive devices; the type of device changes as rehabilitation progresses. If the patient is capable, the ultimate goal is to ambulate independently and unassisted. Patients must work to avoid developing bad

TYPES OF TRANSFEMORAL PROSTHESIS

Two examples of transfemoral prosthesis are shown below.

Endoskeletal prosthesis
The cosmetic cover is removed. Note the modular design foot with single axis. The knee has an extension assist.

Exoskeletal prosthesis
This cutaway drawing shows the single axis knee and solid shin with solid ankle and cushioned heel foot.

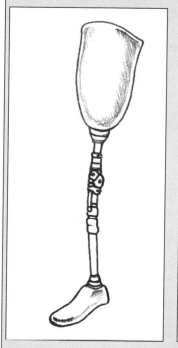

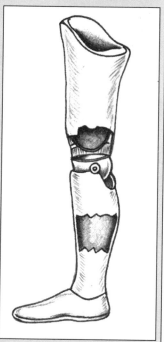

habits and gait deviations (such as vaulting and circumduction) early in the training because such habits are very difficult to correct. Too often, treatment focuses on only the prosthesis and the involved extremity; however, this can lead to significant weakness and gait deviations. Training must not neglect the unaffected limb and the trunk, which must remain strong to achieve as normal a gait pattern as possible.

The frequency of therapy usually decreases as the amputee becomes familiar with the prosthesis. After he achieves all of the treatment goals, therapy can be scaled down to a home exercise program. Ideally, patients continue to improve after therapy is discontinued; they become their own teachers and are able to cope with situations that arise in their daily lives.

Follow-up care

Prostheses don't automatically adjust to changes in the user's weight, shape, and overall health. For example, as a pediatric amputee or congenital amputee grows and develops, his leg length changes. Therefore, prosthetic components and supplies need repair and replacement to keep pace with growth. A prosthetic patient needs to develop a positive relationship with the prosthetist and see this specialist regularly for routine maintenance and follow-up care.

Using orthotic devices

Lower-limb orthoses

The goal of a lower-limb orthosis or orthopedic support is to protect, support, and assist the limb. Orthoses are used in rehabilitation related to a wide variety of diseases and conditions, such as cerebrovascular accident, spinal cord injury, fracture, sports injury, arthritis, postpolio syndrome, and diabetes. As with prostheses, most orthotic devices are prescribed by a doctor and are assembled, fitted, and delivered by orthotists.

Orthoses can be custom made or custom fitted to suit the patient's size and individual needs. Lower-extremity orthoses are named according to the joints that they control, protect, or support. This section reviews transtibial orthoses (foot orthoses and ankle-foot orthoses) and transfemoral orthoses (knee-ankle-foot orthoses and hip-knee-ankle-foot orthoses).

Foot orthoses

Foot orthoses (FOs) are prefabricated or custom-made devices that fit into shoes. They're primarily used to help support and protect the foot in a wide variety of foot-related problems, such as foot pain, diabetic ulcerations, and sports injuries. FOs usually include one or more components, such as

metatarsal pads, longitudinal arch pads, heel pads, and heel cups. Most FOs require a breaking-in period. They're worn for several hours each day, and the wear time is gradually increased over 5 to 7 days until the patient is able to wear the orthosis 8 hours a day. FOs don't always fit into every shoe, especially dress shoes and high-fashion shoes; they may need modifications to obtain optimum fit and function. FOs are prescribed by doctors and can be provided by orthotists, physical therapists, and podiatrists; some can also be readily obtained at shoe stores, pharmacies, and health care equipment suppliers.

Ankle-foot orthoses

Ankle-foot orthoses (AFOs) control and assist the foot and ankle. Prescribed by a doctor and usually provided by orthotists, they're most commonly used to correct footdrop. The goals of AFOs are to keep the foot from slapping at heel strike and to assist with foot clearance at a 90-degree angle in swing period.

AFOs can be custom-made to fit measurements or a patient model, and can be fitted with a variety of ankle joints, such as fixed, limited range of motion (ROM), planter flexion, dorsiflexion assist, or free motion joints. The ankle joint selected depends on the patient's strength, ROM, diagnosis, and orthotic and functional goals.

Traditional AFOs are made of metal and leather and attach to a shoe. They include a leather-clad metal calf band attached to metal uprights that contour the calf. The metal uprights attach to ankle joints, which then attach to a metal stirrup mounted to the sole of a shoe. Newer designs are made from thermoplastic materials, which are in total contact with the back of the calf and foot and fit into shoes. The type of plastic,

TYPES OF ANKLE-FOOT ORTHOSIS

Three types of ankle-foot orthosis (AFOs) are shown below.

Posterior leaf spring AFO
This is used in footdrop with no instability in the ankle from side to side.

Solid AFO with adjustable hinge
The adjustable hinge can be set to the desired range of ankle dorsiflexion or plantar flexion.

AFO with free-motion ankle joint
This assists weak dorsiflexors in the swing phase of the gait.

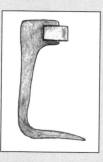
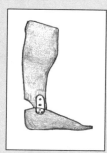
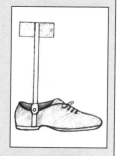

thickness, and trimlines of the orthosis depend on the patient's weight, diagnosis, medical history, and other orthotic needs.

The more anterior the trimlines of the orthosis, the more control it provides. For example, a posterior leaf spring AFO has minimal trimlines (posterior to the malleoli) and controls only weakness of the dorsiflexors. A rigid AFO with moderate trimlines (bisecting the malleoli) controls stability of the ankle, inversion, and eversion as well as prevents plantar flexion.

An AFO offers some support for knee stability. When set in slight dorsiflexion, it helps minimize knee recurvatum (hyperextension); when set in slight plantar flexion, it helps minimize knee buckling. If an AFO doesn't provide enough stability at the knee, a knee-ankle-foot orthosis may be needed. (See *Types of ankle-foot orthosis.*)

Knee-ankle-foot orthoses

Knee-ankle-foot orthoses (KAFOs) control and assist the knee as well as the ankle and the foot. The transtibial components are identical to the AFO; knee joints and a thigh section have been added. Knee joints for KAFOs vary in design and style and come with or without locks and with adjustable ROM. The choice of knee joint is determined by the patient's individual needs. Free knee joints are usually used when increased side-to-side stability is required, for excessive varus (bowing of the leg) and valgus (knock knees), and posteriorly with recurvatum. Locked knee joints are commonly used when anterior stability is required to counteract excessive knee flexion (buckling) at heel strike and throughout stance. The drop locks are released just before or immediately after sitting and engaged before or just after standing.

As with the AFO, the KAFO can be fabricated by the orthotist in metal

TYPES OF KNEE-ANKLE-FOOT ORTHOSIS

Two examples of knee-ankle-foot orthosis (KAFOs) are shown below.

Double-upright metal KAFO
This KAFO has drop-lock locks and leather cuffs to provide maximal knee stability in gait.

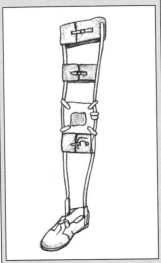

KAFO with plastic and metal joints
This KAFO has free joints, which help stabilize the knee from side to side.

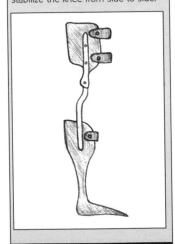

and leather or in thermoplastic materials. The KAFO can be easily changed to an AFO if the patient's condition and needs change, especially with the newer modular components currently available. (See *Types of knee-ankle-foot orthosis*.)

Hip-knee-ankle-foot orthoses

A hip-knee-ankle-foot orthosis (HKAFO) controls and stabilizes the hip as well as the knee and foot. This device is identical to the KAFO with the addition of a pelvic band, belt, and hip joint. The pelvic band wraps around the pelvis and secures with a leather belt. The metal hip joint attaches to the knee joint upright on the lateral side. A free hip joint promotes stability and restricts abduction and adduction of the hip and entire lower limb while allowing free hip flexion and extension to neutral position. It also helps improve a reciprocal gait pattern. The addition of drop locks, which prevent all hip motion, promotes maximum stability in stance. These locks are released before sitting and engaged immediately after standing.

Ambulation with an HKAFO requires a great deal of energy and effort. HKAFOs are commonly used in thoracic and lumbar spinal cord injuries and in pediatric patients with spina bifida and other spinal cord related diagnoses. (See *Hip-knee-ankle-foot orthosis*.)

Lower-limb orthotic evaluation

A lower-extremity orthosis may be needed for a short period of time or indefinitely. In any case, the device must be adaptable to the patient's needs over time as his physical and functional ability improves or, in some cases, declines. Selection depends on the patient's diagnosis, treatment goals, and home situation. Overbracing a patient is sometimes easy to do and must be avoided. A good way to prevent this is to first try some ready-made diagnostic orthoses with the patient. Commonly available in physical therapy departments, these diagnostic devices aren't as comfortable or functional as custom-made or fitted orthoses, but they can give the rehabilitation team and the patient a good idea of what the appropriate orthosis can provide.

The orthosis is a mechanical device that must be maintained carefully to work properly and provide maximum assistance. The patient and caregiver must be instructed in its proper care and use; this may require written, verbal, and illustrated instructions as well as formal patient and family training. Throughout the treatment period, the patient should maintain contact with the orthotist.

Spinal orthoses

Spinal orthoses are primarily used to support and protect the spinal column during treatment for injury or disease as well as after surgery. These devices may be simple elastic supports that are custom-made to fit measurements or complex constructions that provide total-contact multisegment immobilization, which are custom-made to patient models. Spinal orthoses are named according to the levels of the spine that they help immobilize. For instance, a collar for the cervical spine is called a cervical orthosis (CO) and a corset for the thoracic and lumbar spine is called a thoracolumbosacral orthosis (TLSO).

HIP-KNEE-ANKLE-FOOT ORTHOSIS

The illustration shows a typical hip-knee-ankle-foot orthosis (HKAFO) with a pelvic band and belt.

Conventional HKAFO

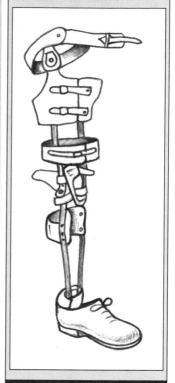

Cervical orthoses

COs are primarily custom-fit to the cervical spine and neck. They're designed to hold the neck straight with the chin slightly elevated to promote healing and prevent reinjury. They range from simple, soft foam collars to rigid, molded devices such as the two-piece Philadelphia collar. COs don't completely immobilize, but they limit range of motion, especially in the flexion and extension ranges.

COMMON CERVICAL ORTHOSIS

This illustration shows a typical hard cervical orthosis, commonly known as the Philadelphia collar. Made of rigid plastic, this collar holds the patient's neck firmly, keeping it straight with the chin slightly elevated and tucked in.

Hard (Philadelphia) collar

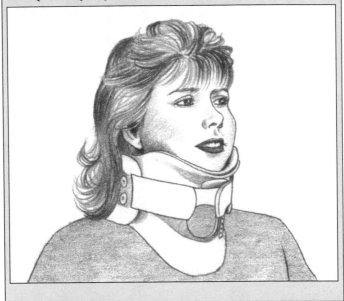

COs can be worn for brief periods or 24 hours per day, depending on the patient's diagnosis and orthotic treatment goals. For maximum benefit, they must be worn properly; they're frequently worn too loose. They must also be kept clean and dry to prevent skin breakdown and irritation, especially under the chin and at the base of the skull. A liner made of lambs' wool, rather than synthetic liner material, should be used to prevent chafing and irritation. (See *Common cervical orthosis.*)

Cervical thoracic orthoses

Cervical thoracic orthoses (CTOs) are similar to cervical orthoses, but they provide additional support to the cervical and upper thoracic spine. Some examples of CTOs are the sternal occipital mandibular immobilizer, Minerva, and Yale orthoses. They limit rotation and side bending of the neck and upper spine in addition to flexion and extension. CTOs may be used postoperatively to help stabilize a fusion or fracture or following the removal of a Halo traction device. (See *Common cervical thoracic orthosis.*)

Thoracolumbosacral orthoses

Thoracolumbosacral orthoses (TLSOs) are designed to immobilize

The illustrations show a typical cervical thoracic orthosis. This design is the sternal occipital mandibular immobilizer (SOMI).

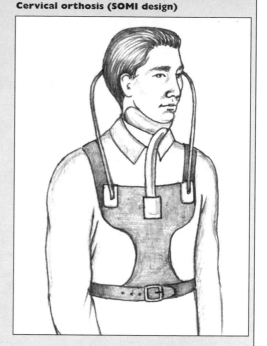

the thoracic, lumbar, and sacral vertebrae. They limit flexion, extension, rotation, and side bending of the trunk and are used to treat back pain, compression fractures, preoperative and postoperative trauma, and scoliosis. The patient's diagnosis dictates which TLSO design the doctor prescribes. The material, design, and trimlines of the individual orthosis determines the amount of motion that is limited and controlled.

Lumbosacral orthoses

Lumbosacral orthoses (LSOs) are similar to TLSOs except that only the lumbar and sacral vertebrae are immobilized. LSOs are used to treat the lower spine for diseases and injuries. As with TLSOs, they range from custom-fit corsets and "warm-n-form" (supports molded to fit in a pocket in the corset's posterior section) to rigid plastic custom styles. Materials, care, and use remain important, but these vary according to the orthotic goals. (See *Common lumbosacral orthosis,* page 318.)

Orthotic evaluation for scoliosis

Scoliosis is a spinal deformity that occurs idiopathically or as a result of a neuromuscular disease. It causes lateral curvature and changes in the spine and may be found in the thoracic, lumbar, or thoracolumbar

COMMON LUMBOSACRAL ORTHOSIS

These pictures show a patient wearing a thoracic lumbosacral orthosis (TLSO). This design controls flexion, extension, rotation, and lateral motion of the thoracic, lumbar, and sacral spine.

Posterior view

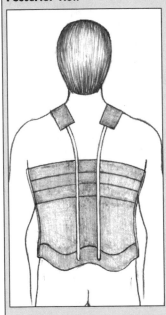

Lateral view

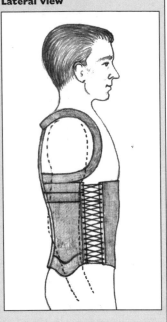

spinal segments. Curves are usually designated as primary or compensatory (secondary) curves. Scoliosis occurs in the adolescent years and is more common in girls than boys. Early diagnosis, which may occur during a school health screening, is key to preventing severe curves that can cause greater deformity later in life, possibly requiring surgical correction. Children with this disorder are usually referred to an orthopedist specializing in scoliosis. X-rays and other diagnostic tests determine the amount and location of curvature.

Minimal curves in the spine are closely monitored during growth until the patient reaches skeletal maturity, at which time scoliosis curvature usually stops. Orthotic treatment is indicated if curvature continues to increase during puberty, increases at a rapid rate, or if the angle of curvature is greater than 20 degrees. A 20-degree curve is an indication for bracing. Curves of 50 degrees or more have been shown to progress after apophyseal closure and to predispose the patient to cardiopulmonary complications. (See *Cobb method for measuring angle of curvature*.) A curve of 50 degrees or greater is difficult to brace and is usually corrected surgically with internal fixation using a Harrington rod and fusion. A traditional thoracolumbosacral orthosis (TLSO) is typically required postoperatively until the fusion is solid.

Although exercises alone won't stop progressive curvature in a growing child, they help to maintain spinal flexibility and improve posture. Children placed in a Milwaukee brace, or another similar device, must perform exercises while wearing the brace and when not wearing it. Orthotic treatment varies with the type, location, and severity of the curvature as well as the age and skeletal maturity of the child.

Orthotic treatment for scoliosis

The most common orthosis for treating scoliosis is the low-profile design of a TLSO. The Boston and Providence braces and the Charleston Bending Brace are examples of low-profile thoracolumbosacral-type scoliosis orthoses. The Milwaukee brace is a high-profile orthosis. The device is usually made by an orthotist from measurements and a model of the patient. It's made of thermoplastic material and has a padded lining. The Milwaukee brace has metal attachments. The trimlines of the device are determined by the location and direction of the curve. The patient is usually X-rayed while wearing the orthosis to determine its effectiveness.

Some orthoses are worn 23 hours per day (with the 1 hour off for bathing and exercise). Others are worn only at bedtime. Most devices are used until skeletal maturity is achieved. The child is gradually weaned from the device at this time until it's no longer required. The goal of any scoliosis orthosis is to hold spinal curvature to the degree present at diagnosis. Although curvature often improves while the patient wears the orthosis, the curve generally returns to its prebracing magnitude af-

COBB METHOD FOR MEASURING ANGLE OF CURVATURE

The Cobb method measures the angle of curvature in scoliosis. The top vertebra in the curve (T6 in the illustration) is the uppermost vertebra whose upper face tilts toward the curve's concave side. The bottom vertebra in the curve (T12) is the lowest vertebra whose lower face tilts toward the curve's concave side. The angle at which perpendicular lines drawn from the upper face of the top vertebra and the lower face of the bottom vertebra intersect is the angle of the curve.

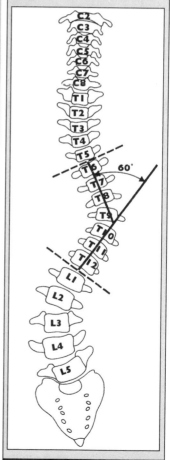

Shown below are two thoracolumbosacral braces for scoliosis: the Boston brace (left) and the Milwaukee brace (right).

Boston brace

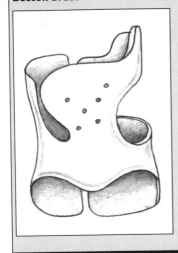

Milwaukee brace

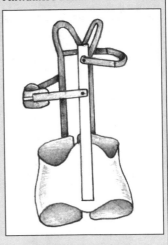

ter weaning. The orthosis will frequently need to be repaired, adjusted, and remade to adjust for the patient's growth and changes in the scoliosis curve.

The prescribing doctor determines the specific orthosis and the exact wearing schedule. During the entire orthotic phase of treatment, the doctor, physical therapist, patient, family, and orthotist must work closely together. (See *Types of scoliosis brace*.)

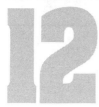

CHAPTER

Wheelchair fit
Matching the patient's needs

Understanding equipment choices

Manual and powered wheelchairs

Illness or injury can severely limit a patient's ability to move around, perform activities of daily living and self-care, and interact in social or job situations. Wheelchairs provide an efficient, comfortable way to provide postural support and alignment and restore mobility to help patients move about independently. Patients with limited mobility may be candidates for manual or powered wheelchairs, depending upon their needs.

Proper fit and function are crucial. A patient who obtains a wheelchair without being properly assessed and fitted by a knowledgeable and skilled practitioner risks loss of function as well as additional physical and physiologic problems. Selecting wheelchairs with appropriate seating and positioning systems is a necessarily complex and important part of your clinical practice. This chapter discusses aspects of chair components, selection, and fitting.

A wheelchair consists of a frame, a seat and back, four wheels, and a combination of other wheelchair components. Wheelchairs may be manual or powered. Most manual wheelchairs are designed with small front wheels and large rear wheels that have hand rims to allow a patient to mechanically control the wheelchair with his own body power. Manual wheelchairs can be propelled with both arms, both legs, or one arm and one leg.

Power wheelchairs help patients who are unable to propel a manual wheelchair due to physical weakness or lack of endurance or those who re-quire constant movement all day. All types of power wheelchairs consist of a wheelchair frame or power base, a power source (motor and batteries) to move the wheels, associated electronics, and a control device. The user operates the control device, which electronically signals the motor to move the wheelchair forward, backward, left, or right. In some power wheelchairs, the wheelchair control can give commands to devices that tilt or receive the wheelchair, move the legrests, and control communications devices. In addition to traditional power wheelchairs, powered mobility also comes from scooters and power add-on units, which create power via an attachment to the wheels of a manual wheelchair or underneath the seat.

Wheelchair components

When selecting a wheelchair, there is a variety of components from which to choose. This section describes different options available for each wheelchair component and lists advantages and disadvantages of each. (See *Wheelchair components*.)

Wheelchair frame configurations

Generally, manual and power wheelchairs are available with either folding or rigid frames. Folding-frame wheelchairs have a collapsible cross brace that connects the two side frames. Rigid-frame wheelchairs lack this folding cross brace; however, they frequently have a back that folds down and wheels that are easily removed. Folding-frame wheelchairs fold vertically. Rigid-frame wheelchairs fold into a box shape.

Both manual and power wheelchairs come in a number of configu-

WHEELCHAIR COMPONENTS

This diagram shows the various components of a manual wheelchair.

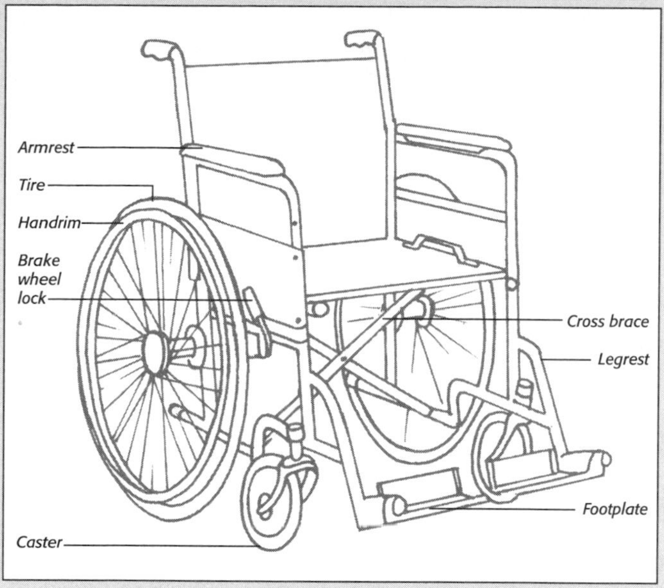

Armrest

Tire

Handrim

Brake wheel lock

Cross brace

Legrest

Footplate

Caster

---

rations to allow for positioning of the patient and for optimal function. *Tilt-in-space* wheelchairs have a seat frame that can be oriented backward from the frame of the wheelchair while maintaining the patient's body alignment and seat-to-back angle. *Recliner* wheelchairs consist of a back that reclines away from the seat, allowing the patient's head and trunk to be lowered while opening up the seat-to-back (hip) angle. Tilt-in-space and recliner wheelchairs are available on power or manual wheelchairs. *One-arm-drive* wheelchairs allow a patient to propel a manual wheelchair with only one arm, using a push handle or a specially designed pushrim that controls a lever attached to both wheels. A *companion* wheelchair is designed with four equally sized small wheels to provide maneuverability in limited indoor spaces such as nursing homes.

Stroller-type wheelchair frames are used for some children and smaller adults. One-arm drive, companion, and stroller wheelchairs are available only on manual frames. (See *Comparing wheelchair frames,* page 324.)

Wheelchair frames also come in different heights. Standard height wheelchairs are typically 19½″ from seat to floor, but frames vary among manufacturers. Hemiheight wheelchairs have lower seat-to-floor heights that allow for propulsion and control with one or both legs. These are typically 17½″ or lower. Many lightweight and ultralightweight wheelchairs are available with several seat height options on one wheelchair or an adjustable axle plate that allows for multiple seat height and center of gravity changes.

The height of the wheelchair ordered is determined by the patient's

COMPARING WHEELCHAIR FRAMES

The table below compares advantages and disadvantages of each type of wheelchair as listed in this table.

Frame type	Advantages	Disadvantages
Rigid frame	• Increased durability and strength due to frame design and fewer removable parts • May decrease overall chair length due to tighter front riggings • Smooth ride on level terrain • More responsive • Lightweight	• May be more difficult to transport secondary to bulky shape • Less smooth ride on uneven terrain
Folding frame	• Easily transportable • Folds narrowly without removing parts	• Increased maintenance required secondary to number of moving parts • May not be durable enough for very active user • Less responsive than a rigid frame
Recliner	• Allows patient to change position and rest during day • Gravity assists with positioning • Allows for pressure redistribution	• Not conducive to changes in position with custom backs secondary to poor alignment • May trigger spasticity • Difficult to self-propel due to rear wheel position • Shear created at back during recline • Long frame
Tilt-in-space	• Allows patient to maintain position • Allows pressure relief without shear • Gravity assists with positioning	• Maintains one posture for less mobile patients, thereby contributing to contractures • Can be difficult to self-propel • Increases overall wheelchair depth and usually height • Difficult to transport
One-arm-drive	• Allows more independence with manual wheelchair use, if only one upper extremity is available	• Adds weight to wheelchair • Requires good strength and coordination
Companion or travel	• Narrow width allows increased accessibility in tight areas • Good for limited dependent use (transportation)	• Patient unable to self-propel with upper extremities • Limited seating options available

height, method of propulsion, arm length, trunk length, transfer status, and other variables. In general, the more adjustable a wheelchair is and the more options available, the more expensive the wheelchair.

Manual wheelchair weight categories

Manual wheelchairs come in four basic weights: heavy duty, standard weight, lightweight, and ultralightweight. Because they are made of

COMPARING WHEELCHAIR WEIGHTS

The table below lists factors to consider when selecting a wheelchair based on weight.

Wheelchair weight	Advantages	Disadvantages
Heavy duty	• Necessary for overweight (over 250 lb) users because it includes reinforced frame and crossbrace	• Extremely heavy • May not go through most doorways • May not fold for transport • Increased expense
Standard weight • Institutional wheelchair • Standard manual	• Can be less expensive than lightweight and ultralightweight • More durable in an institutional setting • Easy to repair • Model less likely to change significantly over the years	• Cumbersome and heavy (greater than 36 lb without riggings) to move in and out of small places • Frame more likely to rust
Lightweight	• Made of stainless steel or aluminum (weight less than 36 lb without riggings) • Doesn't rust and more durable than a standard wheelchair • Easier to load in and out of cars and small places than a standard wheelchair • Easier to propel than a standard wheelchair • Readily available	• Much less maneuverable than an ultralightweight wheelchair
Ultralightweight	• Made of aluminum alloys, titanium, or composite materials (weight less than 30 pounds without riggings) • Moldable composites, which results in a more attractive frame that is very strong and comfortable for the very active user • Good for users with very weak upper body who will self-propel • Best maneuverability for very active users	• Frequent changes to products so parts aren't always available • Repair challenges due to special welding • Most expensive

more expensive materials, lighter weight chairs cost more. (See Comparing wheelchair weights.)

Power wheelchair basics

Power wheelchairs may be driven by direct drive, in which motors are connected directly to the drive wheels; belt drive, in which drive wheel axles are controlled by a belt attached to the motors; and chain drive, in which the motor is connected to the wheel axles via chain gears. Though belt- and chain-driven wheelchairs are still made, direct drive is favored for its better responsiveness and control.

Drive wheels can be in the front, middle, or rear of the frame. The position of the drive wheel determines the wheelchair's maneuverability and turning radius. Front-wheel-drive wheelchairs can turn sharp corners easily but may be difficult to steer at

COMPARING WHEELCHAIR ARMRESTS

This table describes common types of armrests along with their advantages and disadvantages.

Armrest and description	Advantages	Disadvantages
Full length • Armrest extends almost the full length of the seat (approximately 14″).	• Good surface for sit-to-stand transfers • More postural support • Able to use lap board	• Limited access to pull up to tables
Desk length • Armpad extends partially down the length of the seat (approximately 10″).	• Allows wheelchair to pull up to tables	• Unable to adequately support lap boards • Sit-to-stand transfers more difficult
Fixed height • Armrest height can't be adjusted.	• Decreased cost • Increased durability • Decreased weight	• Doesn't allow good positioning for clients requiring upper extremity support
Adjustable height • Height of armpad can be changed within a preset range via a mechanism on the armrest.	• Allows for proper upper extremity positioning	• Moving parts can break down or get lost • Heavier • Increased cost
Nonremovable • Armrests are welded or screwed in place.	• Low maintenance	• Makes transfers more difficult
Removable • Armrests can be removed from side of wheelchair using several mechanisms; some can only be flipped backward.	• Removable for transfers	• Easily lost or broken parts
Space-saver or wraparound • Armrests are set in behind seat rails, not beside them.	• Decreased overall width of wheelchair	• Limited room for overflow items such as clothing

higher speeds. Mid-wheel-drive wheelchairs have a smaller turning radius but aren't as stable on uneven terrain or in quick stops. Rear-wheel-drive wheelchairs don't maneuver as well in small areas, but they do well outdoors and at higher speeds.

Power wheelchairs can be controlled by the user in several ways: by a joystick operated with the arm, chin, head, or foot; by head control,

by a pneumatic (sip and puff) switch; or by other types of switches.

Armrests

Wheelchair armrests, which help the patient with balance, posture, control, and alignment, come in many configurations of length, height adjustment, and removability. Most armrests are padded for comfort as

COMPARING WHEELCHAIR LEGRESTS

This table compares advantages and disadvantages of various options for wheelchair legrests.

Footrest description	Advantages	Disadvantages
Rigid, fixed nonremovable • Front rigging welded to frame of wheelchair • May have flip-up footplates or footplate	• Decreased cost • Increased durability • Lighter weight	• May make transfers more difficult due to decreased proximity to transfer surface and feet not necessarily touching floor
Removable swingaway footrests • Footrests with flip-up footplates that swing out of the way • Optional angle-adjustable footplates	• May allow for easier transfers (The patient can get closer to the surface and get both feet on the floor.) • When removed, decreases overall length of wheelchair for tight spots	• Adds weight to wheelchair • Decreased durability due to more moving parts
Elevating legrests with calf pad and footplate • Elevate lower extremities from a dependent position	• May help decrease swelling • Helps prevent contractures and maintain joint flexibility	• Heavy • Less durable due to more moving parts • Increases length of wheelchair

well, with the padding extending the length of the armrest. (See *Comparing wheelchair armrests.*)

Front rigging

The front rigging of the wheelchair consists of footrests or legrests and footplates. Footrests may be rigid (fixed) or swingaway and removable, and they may have flip-up foot plates. Elevating legrests are equipped with calf pads. (See *Comparing wheelchair legrests.*)

Wheels

All conventional manual wheelchairs come equipped with four wheels. Rear wheels are available in different sizes, can be attached to the wheelchair in different ways, and can be mounted at different angles and in different positions. The smaller front wheels are called casters. The large rear wheels are wire-spoked or made of solid-spoked "mag" construction. Wire-spoked wheels are lighter and provide more shock absorption than the solid mag types, but they require more maintenance.

Conventional wheelchairs usually have a 24″-diameter large wheel. Other sizes may be chosen to alter the seat-to-floor height or change the efficiency of the patient's stroke when propelling the wheelchair. The standard drive wheel size for power wheelchairs is 14″, but other sizes of drive wheels and casters are available. Many power wheelchairs have four small (8″ to 20″ diameter) balloon-type tires.

Wheelchair wheels are also fixed or removable. Fixed wheels are bolted to the wheelchair frame; removable wheels are disengaged from the wheelchair by means of quick-release axles, which makes it easier to transport a rigid wheelchair.

Camber refers to the angle from a perpendicular line at which the wheels are mounted to the wheelchair. Most factory wheels are set at 0 or 3 degrees of camber. The greater the camber, the greater the stability and the lower the center of gravity of the wheelchair. With increased camber, the wheels are closer together at the top and further apart at the bottom, thereby increasing overall wheelchair width.

Large wheels can be fitted with a variety of handrims. Handrims with projections may make propulsion easier for a patient with weak arms, but they increase the overall width of the wheelchair and require good timing. Handrims with plastic coating may also make propulsion easier, but they nick easily and may burn the user's hands.

Casters may be 3″ to 8″ in diameter on manual wheelchairs and 8″ to 10″ on power wheelchairs. Smaller casters may provide a smoother ride on hard surfaces and make a wheelchair more maneuverable, but they tend to get caught in cracks and sink in soft surfaces. Larger casters are less likely to sink into surfaces but increase the wheelchair's turning radius, making it hard to turn in confined spaces.

Tires

Wheelchair tires are available in different widths. Narrow tires have less rolling resistance and are appropriate for hard, flat, indoor surfaces but need more force to propel over uneven surfaces. They aren't suited for outdoor use. Wide tires are easier to propel on uneven outdoor surfaces, but have greater rolling resistance. Several types of tires are available. (See *Comparing wheelchair tires.*)

Other options and accessories

There are many options and accessories than can greatly enhance wheelchair safety and performance.
• *Wheel locks* — can be push-lock or pull-to-lock to secure the wheel from rolling (They can be fitted with brake extensions to increase lever arm length, making brake locking easier.)
• *Amputee attachment or axle* — to change the chair's center of gravity to prevent posterior tipping if the patient's body mass shifts
• *Positioning belt* — available for the lap and chest to ensure patient safety and maintain positioning
• *Backpacks or carrying bags* — for carrying medical supplies and other items
• *Antitippers* — extensions of the lower rail installed in the rear of the wheelchair to prevent at-risk patients from tipping backward

Seating and positioning

Use of proper seating and positioning products gives the patient maximum benefit from a wheelchair. Maintaining proper seating and positioning allows optimal biomechanical alignment of the trunk, head, neck, spine, and extremities; allows maximal respiratory and swallowing function; prevents orthopedic deformity; and provides comfort, skin protection, and pressure relief. It also gives the patient maximal ability to function and

COMPARING WHEELCHAIR TIRES

Options for wheelchair tires include solid, pneumatic, and semipneumatic or air-less inserts. Advantages and disadvantages of each are listed below.

Tire and description	Advantages	Disadvantages
Solid rubber • Solid tire glued to wheel rim • May or may not have tread	• Requires no maintenance • Doesn't puncture • Long wearing • Effective on smooth indoor surfaces • Less expensive	• Difficult to propel on uneven terrain • Higher rolling resistance • Poor shock absorption compared to pneumatic
Pneumatic • Air-filled tire that requires a tube • Comes in many sizes with a variety of tread types for different activities	• Provides smooth ride with good shock absorption • Works well on uneven terrain if tread is present • Lightest option	• Punctures easily • Requires regular maintenance to keep appropriate amount of air
Semipneumatic or airless inserts • Hard rubber tire with air-filled inner core or pneumatic tire with foam insert	• Better shock absorption than solid rubber • Low maintenance	• Heavier than ordinary pneumatic tires • Inserts may be twisted by very active user

interact visually with the surrounding environment.

The patient requires a thorough postural evaluation so that appropriate products can be selected. This section discusses the seating and positioning systems that are available.

Cushions and backs

Seating and positioning systems include wheelchair cushions, backs, and a variety of accessories. There are three general types of cushions and backs.

• *Planar* products consist of flat, noncontoured surfaces for cushions and backs and are available custom made or in standard sizes. Without accessories, they provide minimal postural control.

• *Contoured* seats and backs provide more support than planar products. Because they're manufactured in standard preset sizes to more closely

match body contours, these products help maintain proper alignment and distribute pressure from the patient's weight.

• *Custom-contoured* or *molded* products provide the most bodily contact and thereby provide maximal support. However, they allow only limited mobility while sitting and may hinder patient transfers.

Most seating systems work best with a solid seat insert to provide a stable base of support from which the rest of the body can be aligned.

Materials for wheelchair cushions and backs include foam, air, gel, fluid, or any combination of these. The patient's specific needs and circumstances determine the type of material used. Air and gel media have traditionally provided the best pressure relief, while foam provides a sturdy base.

Accessories for wheelchair cushions include abductor and adductor

(See *Working with ADA specifications.*)

WORKING WITH ADA SPECIFICATIONS

The Americans with Disabilities Act (ADA) provides basic dimensional guidelines for providing wheelchair accessibility in buildings, parking areas, and other public spaces. According to the ADA, specifications for new construction should include these minimum dimensions.

Passageways
• Clear hallway width for a wheelchair: 36″
• Clear turning diameter for a wheelchair: 60″
• Clear floor space for a wheelchair: 30″ × 48″
• Width of clear openings for doors and passages: 32″
• Beveling at thresholds, level changes maximum slope: 1 to 2 ratio
• Toilet stalls: standard 60″ wide and 56″ deep

Heights
• Maximum height for door handles, pulls, latches, locks, and other operating devices: 48″
• Mounting height to operable parts of switches, handles, dispensers, and controls for forward reach: 15″ to 48″
• Height of table and countertops: 28″ to 34″
• Height of clear knee space: 27″
• Toilet height: 17″ to 19″ to top of toilet seat
• Sink height: 34″ maximum to rim or countertop

Parking and ramps
• Parking spot dimensions: 8′ wide with 5′-wide access aisle (8′ × 8′ for a van)
• Accessible parking maximum slope: 1 to 50 ratio
• Path of travel maximum slope: 1 to 20 ratio
• Maximum slope of ramps and curb cuts: 1 to 12 ratio
• Minimum width for curb ramps: 36″

guides to hold the lower extremities in a neutral position, pelvic guides, wedges, and lap belts. Accessories for backs include lateral and lumbar supports, chest belts, harnesses, and headrests. These accessories must be carefully chosen with reference to the patient's function and mobility needs.

Selecting the proper system

Evaluating the patient's environment

It's a good idea for the physical therapist to visit with the patient to assess the suitability for wheelchair use of the home and community environments. During this assessment, measure all pertinent dimensions, including entrances, exits, and access to individual rooms (especially the kitchen, bathroom, and bedroom). Discuss with the patient where he goes each day (neighborhood, shopping, job location) so you can evaluate those areas as well. Careful assessment of the environment also helps you make the most beneficial wheelchair recommendations for the patient. (See *Working with ADA specifications.*)

Measuring the patient

To ensure proper fit of the wheelchair and seating system, wheelchair dimensions must be based on actual physical measurement and assessment of the patient. For accurate measurements, position the patient on a firm surface, with the thighs well supported and parallel to the floor, and the feet firmly supported on the floor or on a stool. The best position is normal sitting posture and alignment. Failure to provide equipment of the appropriate dimensions may result in altered function and physiologic problems for the patient.

You may need to adjust measurements for patients with significant musculoskeletal abnormalities, such as severe scoliosis and joint contractures, and other special needs. For example, patients who propel with their legs or have a large-angle front rigging may require a shorter seat depth. Patients with excessive soft tissue in their legs and a narrow trunk may be able to use a narrower seat without skin compromise (See *Proper wheelchair dimensions*, pages 332 and 333.)

Matching the equipment to the patient

Determining the appropriate wheelchair and seating systems for a patient is a complex process. They should be chosen together to ensure that all parts of the patient- or power-driven mobility system are successful. Before selecting the equipment, conduct a thorough physical therapy evaluation, including an interview with the patient and caregiver. Their comments are an essential part of the decision-making process.

Generally, the procedure for prescribing and ordering wheelchair equipment includes these steps.

• Interview the patient, caregiver, and other members of the rehabilitation team.

• Complete a physical, perceptual, and cognitive assessment of the patient.

• Discuss transportation and housing issues.

• Establish goals for seating and mobility.

• Measure the patient for the equipment.

• Make recommendations and try out the equipment.

• Collaborate with the patient to complete the equipment order.

• Work with funding sources and vendors to get approval for the equipment.

• Receive equipment, fit the patient, and complete the training of the patient and caregiver.

Special considerations

These considerations aid in selecting an appropriate wheelchair and seating system.

• *Diagnosis and history:* What is the diagnosis? Does the patient have a progressive disorder? Will his status improve, remain static, or worsen? Does he have endurance limitations? If the patient previously used a wheelchair, what worked and didn't work? Will he use the wheelchair part- or full-time?

• *Patient and family goals:* What degree of independence is desired or attainable? What are the specific accessibility issues?

• *Neurologic status:* Does the patient have high, low, or normal muscle tone? Is trunk, head, or neck support needed, and how does this need impact the patient's respiratory and swallowing status?

• *Orthopedic status:* Does the patient have any musculoskeletal deformities? Are they fixed or flexible? Should they be corrected or accommodated? Is the patient still growing? Is he gaining or losing weight? What is his body type?

• *Sensation:* Does the patient have sensation? Has he had pressure sores in the past? How will he perform pressure reliefs?

• *Functional status:* Can the patient propel a manual wheelchair? If so, what is the best method? If not, is power indicated and by what drive method? How will the patient transfer

PROPER WHEELCHAIR DIMENSIONS

Use the diagrams and table below to measure your patient and determine appropriate wheelchair dimensions.

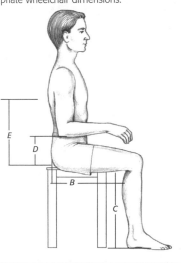
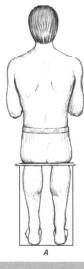

Key:
A = seat width
B = seat depth
C = seat height and leg length
D = armrest height
E = back height

Measurement	Appropriate wheelchair dimension	Possible dimensional problems and consequences
Seat width (A) • Measure the widest point of the patient's lower extremities between the buttocks and the knees.	• Add 1″ to 2″ to measurement A.	Seat too narrow: • Skin breakdown Seat too wide: • Decreased balance and stability • Difficulty with propulsion • Decreased accessibility
Seat depth (B) • Measure from the back of the buttocks to a pen firmly placed in the popliteal fossa.	• Subtract 1½″ to 2″ from measurement B.	Seat or cushion too long: • Decreased circulation at popliteal fossa • Inability to maintain neutral pelvic position with subsequent postural and skin problems • Difficulty propelling with feet Seat or cushion too short: • Poor distribution of pressure throughout lower extremities, resulting in increased pressure through buttocks • Altered center of gravity
Legrest and footrest length (C) • Measure from a pen firmly placed in the popliteal fossa to the bottom of the heel. (Consider the type of shoes the client wears.)	• Subtract the height of the cushion that will be used from the anatomical measurement.	Footrest too short: • Increased pressure through buttocks • Poor sitting posture Footrest too long: • Increased pressure on distal posterior thighs • Poor sitting posture

PROPER WHEELCHAIR DIMENSIONS *(continued)*

Measurement	Appropriate wheelchair dimension	Possible dimensional problems and consequences
Seat to floor height (C) • Measure from a pen firmly placed in the popliteal fossa to the bottom of the heel. (Consider the type of shoes client wears.)	• Add 2" to the desired footrest length (as determined above) to allow for clearance of the footplates (for foot propellers, subtract ½" from the desired footrest length).	Seat too high: • Difficulty scooting back in wheelchair • Difficulty transferring Seat too low: • Poor foot clearance • Difficulty performing sit-to-stand transfers
Armrest height (D) • Measure from sitting surface to the bottom of 90-degree bent elbow.	• Add the height of the wheelchair cushion to be used.	Armrest too low: • Poor glenohumeral support • Difficulty maintaining upright position Armrest too high: • Elevated shoulders • Increased risk of skin breakdown on elbows
Back height (E) • Measure from the bottom of the buttocks to the inferior angle of the scapula.	• For clients who don't need scapular support, add the height of the cushion. • For clients who require scapular support, add the height of the cushion plus approximately 3".	Back height too low: • Poor balance and trunk support Back height too high: • Difficulty using upper extremities for functional tasks such as propelling wheelchairs

in and out of the chair? Does the patient need a specific seat or head height?

• *Cognition and perception:* Are the patient's vision and perception sufficient to operate the chair safely? Is his judgment good enough to move away from dangerous situations? How likely is he to use the chair as a weapon?

• *Environment:* How will the chair be used? Indoors or out? At school or work? Is the home, work, or school environment accessible?

• *Transportation:* How will the chair be transported? Will the patient sit in it to drive a van? Is it suitable for public transportation?

• *Funding:* Who will pay for the chair and for repairs? Should the patient rent or purchase?

Any prescription for wheelchair and seating systems submitted to a third-party payer must include justification for all components. In managed care, available resources may be a big factor in what is ultimately prescribed. To keep costs down, you may need to request standard sizes, rather than customized equipment, or lower-priced items and fewer options.

Use and care considerations

Whether your patient is using a standard or power wheelchair, a number of factors influence propulsion or control of the wheelchair. For a manual wheelchair, these factors include the wheel configuration, axle location, frame design, and chair weight. Wheel size and handrim size should provide optimal arm positioning and force generation. Patients with long arms may prefer smaller handrims, while larger handrims work best for patients with short arms.

The location of the large wheel axle also affects propulsion control. A patient may be able to manually propel the chair more easily if the axle is mounted just forward of the angle where the seat and back meet. However, forward-mounted wheels may make the chair tip backward more easily.

Because a wheelchair's path is seldom straight and smooth, the patient and caregiver must learn to safely handle the wheelchair indoors and out. It's important that they train together in a safe setting that allows for gradual skill progression, so they can learn to apply their skills to any environment.

Important considerations for wheelchair propulsion are:
• surface grade and smoothness
• predictability of surface and overall environment
• patient skill
• caregiver skill
• axle placement on the wheelchair and how the chair tips in response to inclined surfaces

• camber of wheels (manual wheelchair only)
• relationship of patient's arm length to rim diameter to allow for force generation (manual wheelchair only)
• type of frame, components, and tires
• ability to stop quickly using the control (power wheelchair)
• visual acuity (power wheelchair)
• patient's cognition and safety awareness (power wheelchair).

In addition to these points, wheelchair management training should include such topics as assembly and disassembly; moving the (manual) wheelchair up and down stairs, ramps, and curbs; correct use of seating and positioning systems; and basic maintenance and repairs.

In transporting or storing an unused wheelchair, weight is an important factor. A heavy wheelchair shouldn't be lifted into a car or other storage area if it puts the lifter at risk for injury. Instead, a lift should be used, and a mode of transportation that lifts the patient and wheelchair on board may be advisable. Lightweight or ultralightweight wheelchairs may be transported and stored with relative ease; many fold easily and have wheels that pop off to allow easier storage.

Choosing a wheelchair is a major decision and should include input from many sources, including the patient and caregiver, clinicians, and medical supply companies. This rapidly changing technology requires you to keep your knowledge up-to-date. Your involvement as a knowledgeable and skilled physical therapist ensures that patients are provided with equipment appropriate for their treatment and circumstances.

Common modalities

Focusing physical energy on healing

Selected procedures

Anthropometric measurements

Anthropometry is the study of body dimensions, including measurements of standing height and weight (body mass index [BMI]), girth, waist-to-hip ratio, and skin-fold measurements. These data provide relatively accurate estimates of body composition and fat distribution patterns and are used to assess a patient's weight, body composition, and associated health risk as well as monitor changes in body fat composition over time.

BMI is used to evaluate body mass and can be found by dividing body weight in kilograms by height in meters squared (kg/m^2). Increases in BMI are associated with increased mortality from heart disease, diabetes, and cancer. However, BMI can be misleading because it doesn't measure proportional composition of the body or the percentage of fat; a person who is lean but has an extremely large muscle mass might have an unusually high BMI.

Girths are circumferential measurements taken at standard anatomic sites on the body. Girths are a good measure of proportionality and are useful for determining fat distribution in obese patients as well as for monitoring changes in fat distribution during weight loss or strength training. The accuracy of girth measurements depends on the tester's ability to maintain constant, even tension on the tape and to use the exact anatomic sites. Girths and skinfold measurements give a clearer picture of changes in muscle and fat composition and distribution.

Waist-to-hip ratio is a simple method for assessing body fat distribution and for assessing and monitoring changes in body composition. This ratio is significant because a high waist-to-hip ratio is associated with an increased risk of morbidity and mortality. Specifically, persons with more fat around their abdomen are at increased risk for hypertension, diabetes, and heart disease.

Skin-fold measurements are made using special calipers and are effective for estimating body fat. Data developed from this procedure are based on regression equations that have been validated using hydrodensitometry, and are based on the subject's age, gender, and activity level.

Equipment

BMI
Scale ✧ calculator ✧ pen ✧ paper

Girth measurements
Tape measure ✧ pen ✧ paper

Waist-to-hip ratio
Tape measure ✧ pen ✧ paper

Skin-fold measurements
Skin-fold calipers ✧ calculator ✧ pen ✧ paper

Preparation of equipment

For skin-fold measurements, calipers should be calibrated to zero and should exert a pressure of 10 g/mm^2 of surface area.

Essential steps

BMI
• Weigh and measure the patient.
• Apply measurements to the formula:
BMI = weight (in kilograms) ÷ height (in meters) squared
• Compare findings to the recognized standard. (See *BMI classification system*.)

B.M.I. CLASSIFICATION SYSTEM

The Panel on Energy, Obesity, and Body Weight Standards recommends the following classification system for BMI values.

BMI values	Index grade
20 to 24.9 kg/m²	Desirable (adult men and women)
25 to 29.9 kg/m²	Grade 1 obesity
30 to 40 kg/m²	Grade 2 obesity
> 40 kg/m²	Grade 3 obesity (morbid obesity)

Girth measurements
• Ask the patient to stand relaxed, with feet slightly apart and arms hanging down but slightly away from the trunk, with forearms supinated.
• Measure the circumference of the following body parts (on the right side of the body where appropriate) with a tape measure:
– abdomen: at the level of the umbilicus
– hip: at the maximal protrusion of the buttocks
– thigh: at the maximal girth site of the upper thigh, just below the gluteal fold
– calf: at the maximal girth site between the ankle and the knee
– upper arm: at the midpoint between the elbow and the shoulder
– forearm: at the maximal circumference site just distal to the elbow.
• Pull the tape measure to proper tension, being careful not to pinch the skin.
• Take three measurements at each site and then average these measurements. Retest if the three measurements don't agree within 7 mm.

Waist-to-hip ratio
• Measure the abdominal circumference halfway between the lowest lateral portion of the rib cage and the iliac crest.

• Measure the hip circumference at the level of the maximal protrusion of the gluteal muscle.
• Divide the abdominal circumference by the hip circumference. A waist-to-hip ratio greater than 0.86 in women and 0.95 in men may indicate excess abdominal adipose tissue, associated with an increased risk of morbidity and mortality.

Skin-fold measurements
• Measure the skin-fold thickness by grasping the patient's skin between the thumb and forefinger at the following locations:
– *triceps:* vertical fold; posterior surface of the upper arm, halfway between the elbow and the shoulder on the nondominant arm
– *abdomen:* vertical fold; ¾″ (2 cm) to the right of the umbilicus
– *suprailiac:* diagonal fold; just superior to the iliac crest, running angle of crest, at the anterior axillary line
– *thigh:* vertical fold; middle of the anterior thigh halfway between the superior border of the patella and the inguinal crease
– *chest:* diagonal fold; one-third the distance between the anterior axillary line and the nipple (for women) or one-half the distance between the anterior axillary line and the nipple (for men)

TAKING SKIN-FOLD MEASUREMENTS

Skin-fold thickness is measured in several different areas, including the triceps, abdomen, suprailiac, thigh, chest, midaxillary, and subscapular. Measuring triceps skin-fold thickness is illustrated below.

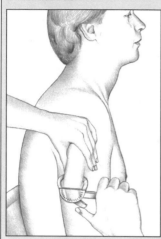

After measuring the various areas, apply one of the following prediction equations for body density and percent body fat.

Seven-site formula
In this formula, measurements are taken from the triceps, abdominal, suprailiac, thigh, chest, midaxillary, and subscapular areas.

Men
Body density = 1.112 – ([0.00043499] [sum of the 7 skinfold measures]) + ([0.00000055] [sum of the 7 skin-fold measures]^2) – [0.00028826] [age])

Women
Body density = 1.097 – ([0.00046971] [sum of the 7 skin-fold measures]) + ([0.00000056] [sum of the 7 skin-fold measures]^2) – ([0.00012828] [age])

Three-site formula
In this formula, measurements are taken from the triceps, abdominal, and suprailiac areas.

Men
Percent body fat = (0.39287) (sum of the 3 skin-fold measures) – ([0.00105] [sum of the 3 skin-fold measures]^2) + ([0.15772] [age]) – ([5.18845] [sum of the 3 skin-fold measures])

Women
Percent body fat = (0.41563) (sum of the 3 skin-fold measures) – ([0.00112] [sum of the 3 skin-fold measures]^2) + 0.03661(age) + 4.03653 (sum of the 3 skin-fold measures)

– *midaxillary:* vertical fold; on the midaxillary line at the level of the xiphoid process
– *subscapular:* diagonal fold; about ⅜″ to ¾″ (1 to 2 cm) below the inferior angle of the right scapula
• At each location, hold the calipers at the midpoint and squeeze for about 3 seconds.
• Record each measurement registered on the handle gauge to the nearest 0.5 mm.
• Take two or more readings at each site and average them to compensate for any errors. (See *Taking skin-fold measurements.*)

Bed mobility

Bed mobility is the ability to turn over in bed; to scoot up, down, or toward either edge of the bed; and to come to a sitting position at the edge of the bed. If the patient lacks sufficient strength and motor-planning skills to perform these movements independently, you'll need to assist with these tasks.

Rolling the patient

A lifting sheet allows regular position changes with minimum strain on the patient and therapist. Usually performed by two persons, this procedure is commonly used for a patient who can't or is forbidden to roll himself. After the lifting sheet is in place, one person may be able to reposition the patient depending on the patient's size.

Equipment

Bed ✧ lifting sheet ✧ pillows

Preparation of equipment

• Ensure that the bed rail on the side to which the patient is rolling is in the upright position and that the bed brakes are set.
• Raise the bed to a comfortable working height.

Essential steps

• Stand at the side of the bed opposite the side the patient is turning to so that as rolling is completed you're standing behind the patient.
• Stand close to the bed and place one foot slightly in front of the other.
• Grasp the corners of the lift sheet firmly and pull the patient toward you.
• Give the lift sheet a firm upward tug causing the patient to roll away from you.
• Place pillows behind the patient, underneath the lift sheet, to maintain the patient's position and place a pillow between his knees.

Special considerations

• Patients who have had total-hip or knee replacement surgery shouldn't be rolled to the involved side; roll them toward the uninvolved side.

• Place pillows or a foam abduction wedge in between the legs of patients who have had total-hip or knee replacement surgery before attempting to roll them.
• Patients with feeding tubes, closed head injury, and postoperative neurologic conditions can be rolled, but the head of the bed should be elevated to 30 degrees.
• Patients with compromised respiration who are lying on one side should also have a pillow placed under the topmost arm to allow clearance for chest expansion.

Pulling the patient up in bed

When a patient is ill, disabled, or recovering from surgery, he may need assistance in moving his body toward the head of the bed.

Equipment

Bed ✧ lifting sheet ✧ pillow

Preparation of equipment

• Lower the bed rails and ensure that the bed brakes are on.
• Place a pillow flat against the headboard of the bed.

Essential steps
One-person assist

• Roll the bed far enough away from the wall to allow you to move behind the headboard.
• Position the head of the bed flat or, if there are no contraindications, lower the head of the bed (Trendelenburg's position) so that gravity can assist the maneuver.
• Flex the patient's knees if his diagnosis permits. (If the patient can't voluntarily maintain the flexed position and the lower extremities fall to one side, the patient will still be more compact.)
• Press your thighs firmly against the headboard, grasp the top corners of

the lift sheet, and pull. The patient should slide toward you on the sheet.
• Place the pillow that was padding the headboard under the patient's head and assist the patient with repositioning his legs.
• Return the bed rails to the up position.

Two-person assist
• Flex the patient's knees if his diagnosis permits.
• Position each team member on opposite sides of the bed.
• Each person should stand close to the bed at the patient's hip level, with one foot placed slightly in front of the other and pointed toward the headboard.
• Grab the corners of the pullsheet and, on the count of three, lift in unison and step toward the headboard with the leg closest to the headboard. The patient should slide smoothly toward the headboard.
• Replace the pillow under the patient's head and assist the patient with repositioning his legs.

Special considerations
• Certain diagnoses require that the patient not be placed in a recumbent position with the lower extremities higher than the head (Trendelenburg's position). This includes patients with feeding tubes, closed head injuries, postoperative neurologic conditions, and respiratory compromise. In these cases, a two-person assist will be needed to pull these patients up in bed. Patients with unilateral lower-extremity involvement can be moved up in bed by one person by flexing the uninvolved lower extremity. If flexing is contraindicated, two persons are needed.

Helping the patient sit up

Patients may need to be helped to reach a sitting position on the side of

the bed. This can be done if the patient has adequate hip and knee extension as well as good sitting balance.

Equipment
Bed

Preparation of equipment
• Lower the bed rail on the side to which the patient is moving, and ensure that the bed brakes are on.

Essential steps
• Position yourself directly on the side of the patient to which he is going to move, using your body to block his torso.
• Raise the head of the bed.
• Guide the patient's shoulders into an upright position while simultaneously lowering his legs over the side of the bed.
• Support the patient until he has ascertained that his sitting balance is adequate to permit unassisted sitting.

Transfer from bed to wheelchair

For the patient with little or no lower-body sensation, one-sided weakness, immobility, or injury, transfer from bed to wheelchair may require partial support to full assistance — initially by at least two persons. Subsequent transfer of the patient with generalized weakness may be performed by one person.

Equipment

Wheelchair with brakes (or a sturdy chair) ✦ shoes or slippers with nonslip soles ✦ towel ✦ gait belt

Preparation of equipment

One-person assist pivot transfer

• Position the wheelchair at a 45-degree angle at the head of the bed and on the patient's "good" side.
• Make sure the brakes on the wheelchair and the bed are locked.
• Make sure that all invasive lines and tubes have enough room to move with the patient without becoming dislodged.

Two-person lift

• Position the wheelchair parallel to the bed.
• Make sure the brakes on the wheelchair and the bed are locked.
• Remove the wheelchair armrest closest to the bed to provide easier access.
• Make sure that all invasive lines and tubes have enough room to move with the patient without becoming dislodged.
• Raise the head of the bed 35 to 40 degrees.

Essential steps

One-person assist pivot transfer

• Help the patient to sit up, as described in the previous section.
• Place the gait belt around the patient's waist, if not contraindicated.
• Position the patient's feet flat on the floor with the knees bent at a 90-degree or greater angle, if possible.
• Stand in front of the patient, blocking his toes with your feet and his knees with yours, to prevent his knees from buckling.
• Flex your knees slightly toward the back, and grasp the gait belt at the sides. Ask the patient to place his hands on the edge of the bed or

around your waist. Never permit him to place his hands around your neck. Avoid bending at your waist to prevent back strain.
• Instruct the patient to push himself off the bed and to support as much of his own weight as possible. At the same time, straighten your knees and hips, raising the patient as you straighten your body.
• Supporting the patient as needed, pivot toward the wheelchair, keeping your knees next to his.
• Help the patient lower himself into the wheelchair by flexing your hips and knees but not your back. Instruct him to reach back and grasp the other wheelchair armrest as he sits, to avoid abrupt contact with the seat.
• If the patient can't position himself correctly, help him move his buttocks against the back of the chair so that the ischial tuberosities, not the sacrum, provide the base of support.

Two-person lift

• The therapist should stand behind the wheelchair and next to the patient's head.
• The second person should stand facing the bed at the level of the patient's knees.
• The therapist reaches under the patient's axilla and grasps the patient's forearms, folding them against his chest.
• The second person slides his forearms, palms up, under the patient's thighs and calves. (Avoid placing either forearm behind the knee because this may cause the patient to jackknife.)
• On the count of three, the therapist should step sideways with her lateral leg and the second person should step backward, gently lowering the patient into the wheelchair.

Special considerations

One-person assist pivot transfer

• If the wheelchair can't be placed at the head of the bed and on the patient's "good" side because of space limitations, place the wheelchair at the foot of the bed so that the patient can still move toward their "good" side.

• If possible, remove the armrest closest to the patient from the wheelchair to permit easier access for larger, heavier patients.

• A transfer board or folded towel placed over the gap between the wheelchair and the bed alleviates anxiety by eliminating the void between the bed and the wheelchair.

• A gait belt is contraindicated with certain diagnoses, such as pregnancy, fractured ribs, abdominal surgery, and burns or other wounds to the torso. In these cases, you should wear the gait belt and allow the patient to grasp the belt.

• Feeding tubes should be disconnected and flushed before the transfer. They can be reconnected after the transfer is completed.

Two-person lift

• It's helpful to have the taller person at the head of the patient because tall people generally have the longest reach.

• For a particularly heavy patient, this transfer can be modified by having a third team member place his hands under the ischial tuberosities to assist the lift.

Transfer from bed to stretcher

Transfer from bed to stretcher is a common patient transfer that can require the help of one or more persons, depending on the patient's size and condition.

Equipment

Stretcher ✧ slide board or lift sheet

Essential steps

• Adjust the bed to the same height as the stretcher.

• Place the stretcher parallel to the bed and lock the wheels of the stretcher and the bed.

• The tallest team member should stand facing the patient at his head, the second team member should stand at the patient's hips, and the third team member should stand below the patient's knees.

• The tallest team member should spread his legs and grasp both sides of the lift sheet at the patient's head. The second team member should slide his arms, with elbows extended and palms facing up, under the lift sheet, supporting the patient's ischial tuberosities. The third team member should grasp both sides of the lift sheet from his position below the patient's knees.

• On the count of three, everyone lifts simultaneously and pulls the patient toward the stretcher and slides his arms out from under him.

Special considerations

• For the return lift to the bed, or with an especially heavy patient, the second team member may find it helpful to kneel on the stretcher or the bed, a maneuver best accomplished by the most flexible person in the group.

Trigger point identification

Trigger points are tender spots or muscle hardenings located in different skeletal muscles, fasciae, tendons, ligaments, or the periosteum and pericapsular areas. When a trigger point is involved, it may radiate pain into a specific area or zone of referred pain. (See *Trigger point locations*.) The trigger point can be activated by pressure, by piercing with a needle, during activity, or even spontaneously during rest. Contributing factors can include sports- or work-related injuries, strains, sprains, repetitive injuries, arthritis, or muscle tension. Myofascial pain syndromes, fibromyalgia, electrolyte disorders, vitamin deficiencies, and chronic infections may also demonstrate trigger point involvement.

Trigger point therapy may be carried out using injections, electrical stimulation, topical coolants coupled with therapeutic exercises, and other techniques. It should be used as part of an overall treatment plan that involves correction of other factors, such as poor body mechanics or posture, stress, vitamin deficiency, and hypothyroidism.

Equipment

Drape or towel

Essential steps

• Explain the procedure to the patient and tell the patient what kind of sensations to expect.
• Ask the patient to remove all jewelry and clothing from the area to be examined.
• Position the patient for comfort and modesty.
• Palpate the various muscle groups to locate the trigger point and corresponding area of pain reference.

TRIGGER POINT LOCATIONS

Common trigger points are shown in the anterior and posterior views below. Trigger points tend to be located over sliding surfaces and moving body parts.

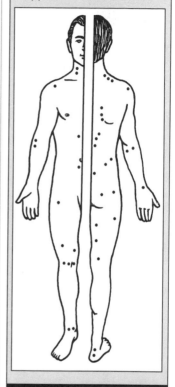

Selected physical modalities

Biofeedback, electromyographic

Biofeedback is a training technique that allows a patient to recognize and exert control over physiologic processes such as muscle tension. In surface electromyographic biofeedback (EMGBF), the most commonly used form, electrodes are placed on the skin overlying the muscle to monitor the muscle's electrical activity (action potential) as it's contracting and transmit a visual or auditory output signal to the patient. The patient cortically integrates the signal and makes voluntary adjustments to the muscular contraction.

To allow the patient to achieve voluntary self-correction, the biofeedback signal must be accurate, relevant, and timed to the physiologic process being altered. If the goal is to increase the output signal, the feedback is considered positive; if the goal is to decrease the signal, the feedback is considered negative.

In EMGBF, positive feedback is used to assist muscles with weak muscular contraction due to uppermotoneuron problems, such as cerebrovascular accident, traumatic brain and spinal cord injuries, cerebral palsy, and multiple sclerosis. This form of feedback can also reeducate skeletal and pelvic floor muscles weakened by peripheral nerve injury, surgical repair, pain, postural habit, or disuse.

Negative feedback is used to decrease contraction in muscles with spasticity due to upper-motoneuron problems, poor postural habit, local injury or pain, and tension headaches. It's also used to promote total body muscle relaxation.

Although there are no contraindications for EMGBF, the technique should be used cautiously in patients with impaired cognition and in those with hypotension or diabetes, where deep relaxation may affect body homeostasis. Because EMGBF depends on the transmission of muscle electrical activity through body tissues to the skin interface, patients with thickened skin due to scarring or with excessive adipose tissue may be poor candidates for this therapy.

Equipment

EMGBF unit ✧ two sensor electrodes and one reference electrode (size appropriate to muscle size) ✧ electrode lead wires ✧ Velcro straps or tape to secure electrodes and wires ✧ electrode gel ✧ alcohol pads

Preparation of equipment

• Set variables of the EMGBF unit: gain (sensitivity) and output signal (these settings vary with the patient and procedure).
• Apply a small amount of electrode gel to all the electrodes before applying them to the patient.

Essential steps

• Explain the procedure and treatment goals to the patient. Ascertain the patient's understanding and answer any questions.
• Make sure the patient signs a consent form.
• Place the patient in a quiet area and position the body part comfortably, allowing for proper movement.
• Determine if the patient is allergic to electrode gel, and inspect the skin for broken areas.
• Clean oil and dirt from the skin with an alcohol pad to enhance signal conduction.
• Palpate the muscle to be monitored. The electrode must be placed accurately to ensure proper muscle monitoring.
• Place sensor electrodes along the longitudinal axis of the muscle belly, and apply the reference electrode to a nearby bony prominence. Apply the electrodes firmly to the skin, and fix them with Velcro or tape to ensure good signal detection and output signal quality.
• Turn on the unit.
• Ask the patient to actively contract or relax the muscle to increase or de-

crease the output signal based on the goals and type of feedback of the treatment desired. Sessions may be 10 to 20 minutes long. Eventually, the patient should be able to perform the activity without input from the EMGBF unit.

• Turn off the unit, remove the electrodes, and clean the skin.

• Assess the patient's response to the treatment.

• Document unit settings, patient performance, and response.

Cryotherapy

In cryotherapy, cold is used to reduce pain and swelling. It works by causing vasoconstriction of superficial blood vessels and reducing blood flow to the affected area. Cold also reduces nerve conduction velocity, decreasing neural input to muscles. Depending on the treatment, cryotherapy can reduce tissue temperatures to a depth of 1⅝″ (4 cm). Deeper tissues are unaffected because of the insulating effect of body fat. The most common forms of cryotherapy include cold packs and ice massage.

With proper instruction from a physical therapist (PT) or a PT assistant, cold pack and ice massage treatments can be performed by the patient or with the help of a caregiver at home. In the clinical setting, cryotherapy is most often performed by a PT or a PT assistant.

Cryotherapy is indicated in many acute, subacute, and chronic conditions for reducing edema, pain, inflammation, muscle spasms, and muscle facilitation (with quick icing). It's also indicated for the acute management of burns and hemorrhage.

It's contraindicated for:

• patients with particular cold sensitivities, such as cold urticaria, Ray-

naud's disease, cryoglobulinemia, and paroxysmal cold hemoglobinuria

• patients with uncontrolled angina pectoris or other unstable cardiac dysfunction

• patients with severe arterial insufficiency

• patients with lack of sensation in the area to be treated

• areas where peripheral nerves may be regenerating

• open wounds after 48 to 72 hours (prolonged vasoconstriction may lend to poor healing).

 ALERT Use cryotherapy cautiously in older adults and young children, who may have poor thermoregulation, as well as in those with hypertension.

Equipment

Cold pack

Cold packs in a variety of shapes and sizes ✧ freezer unit ✧ towels or pillowcases ✧ timer ✧ call bell or other alerting device

Ice massage

Small foam plastic or paper cup containing ice ✧ freezer unit ✧ towels ✧ tongue depressor (optional)

Essential steps

Cold pack

• If appropriate, prepare a private or semiprivate area for treating the patient.

• Explain the treatment and procedure, and tell the patient what sensations to expect.

• Check the patient for intact temperature sensation and skin integrity.

• Have the patient remove all clothing and jewelry from the area to be treated.

• Position the patient for comfort and modesty. Make sure that the rest of the patient's body is kept warm.

• Cover the area to be treated with a warm, damp towel to decrease the initial shock of the cold pack and enhance heat exchange between the cold pack and the patient.

• Place a cold pack of an appropriate size over the area to be treated and secure the pack well. Place a dry towel over the pack to insulate it.

• Provide the patient with a bell or another alerting device to use if your assistance is needed during the treatment.

• Leave the cold pack in place 10 to 20 minutes.

• Remove the pack and dry the treated area with a towel.

• Inspect the skin in the treated area. Mild redness is normal; however, other reactions, such as wheals and rash, are abnormal and should be investigated before further cold treatments are given.

Ice massage

• If appropriate, prepare a private or semiprivate area for treating the patient.

• Explain the treatment and procedure, and tell the patient what sensations to expect.

• Check the patient for intact temperature sensation and skin integrity.

• Have the patient remove all clothing and jewelry from the area to be treated.

• Position the patient for comfort and modesty.

• Place towels around the area to be treated to absorb any dripping water.

• Tear off an area of the foam plastic cup to expose the ice. Smooth any rough edges on the cup by rubbing your warm hand or a towel over the edges.

• Rub the ice over the treatment area using small circular or overlapping motions. Wipe away any residual moisture.

• Continue the ice massage through all three stages of the cold experi-

ence: cold, painful, and numb. This usually takes 5 to 10 minutes, depending on the patient and the size of the area to be treated.

• When the treatment is finished, dry the area and inspect the skin. A normal response to treatment may include reddening of the skin. Wheals and a rash aren't normal responses; if they occur, the cause should be investigated before any further application of cold.

Special considerations

• Cryotherapy treatments are uncomfortable and patients may tolerate them poorly. Conversing with the patient during the treatment often reduces anxiety, distracts from the cold sensation, and may help patients better tolerate the procedure.

• If appropriate, decrease the intensity of the cold in a cold pack by replacing the damp, warm cloth with a thin pillowcase. To reduce it further, use a towel. These measures reduce the efficiency of heat exchange but may allow better tolerance of the treatment.

Diathermy

Diathermy uses moderate- to high-frequency electromagnetic waves to generate heat in some part of the body. It's considered a "deep" heating agent, meaning it's able to increase tissue temperature to depths of $1\frac{1}{8}''$ to $2''$ (3 to 5 cm). Diathermy is most often performed using shortwave diathermy (SWD) equipment. Microwave diathermy units are used less often. The energy is delivered in continuous or pulsed modes by means of coils or plates applied to the body part.

Continuous SWD is used in subacute and chronic conditions to increase tissue extensibility, control pain, and decrease muscle spasm. Pulsed SWD is used to improve wound healing, control pain and edema, and enhance peripheral nerve and bone healing.

The effectiveness of pulsed SWD in these conditions may be specific to the utilization of a capacitance or inductance method of application. In a *capacitance* application (electrical field application), current passes through the patient and generally concentrates in more of the superficial tissues, but it can penetrate more deeply if there's little tissue of high resistance in the area, such as fat or cartilage. In an *inductance* application (magnetic field application), the current does not pass through the patient but is delivered via magnetically induced electric eddy currents, which mostly affect highly conductive tissues like blood and muscle. This allows more heating of deeper tissues and less heating of superficial tissues. (See *Types of shortwave diathermy application,* page 348.)

Diathermy is contraindicated in patients with acute inflammatory conditions, malignancies, cardiac insufficiency, active bleeding, lack of sensation in the treatment area, unreliable thermoregulation, fever, peripheral vascular disease, metal in or near the treatment site, pacemakers or implantable cardioverter-defibrillators, pregnancy, over growing epiphyses, and devitalized tissues. In addition, diathermy shouldn't be applied over the eyes or testes.

Equipment

SWD unit appropriate for desired results (inductive or capacitance type unit) ✧ a wood treatment table with no metal parts ✧ towels or sheet ✧ call bell or other alerting device ✧ timer

Preparation of equipment

• Select the appropriate diathermy device based on your evaluation of the patient's condition.
• Tune the device if needed. Some recent diathermy units do this automatically. The unit may require a brief warm-up period before tuning.
• Select the appropriate treatment parameters based on the desired therapeutic results.
• Provide the patient with a bell or another alerting device to use if your assistance is needed during the treatment.

Essential steps

• Provide a private or semiprivate treatment area.
• Instruct the patient about the treatment and explain any sensory changes that may occur.
• Remove the patient's watch and all other metal jewelry as well as any clothing containing metal fasteners, such as zippers and grommets, from the electromagnetic field around the area to be treated.
• Check the patient for intact temperature sensation and skin integrity.
• Position the patient for comfort and modesty.
• If applying continuous diathermy, place a towel around or over the area to be treated to absorb any perspiration that may accumulate.
• Position the diathermy device for a safe and effective application.
• After 5 minutes, check on the patient to make sure that the unit is providing the appropriate amount of heat.
• Diathermy treatments typically last 15 to 30 minutes. When the treatment is complete, turn all dials or digital readouts back to zero. Remove the applicator and dry any perspiration from the patient.

TYPES OF SHORTWAVE DIATHERMY APPLICATION

Several methods of applying shortwave diathermy are illustrated below.

Cable-type inductive application

For a cable-type inductive applicator, wrap the limb to be treated with a towel. Then wrap the cable around the towel. The coils of the cable should be at least 1" (2.5 cm) apart.

An alternative for larger, flatter surfaces (such as the lumbar region) is to coil the cable into a flat spiral the size of the area to be treated. The spirals should be about 2" (5 cm) apart and placed over the area to be treated on top of six to eight layers of toweling.

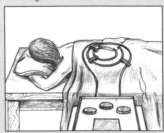

Drum-type inductive application

Some diathermy devices use a drum instead of cables. Place the drum directly over the area to be treated. Move the drum as close as possible to the patient without allowing it to touch the patient. Advise the patient to move as little as possible but allow room for slight motion (such as a cough). Keep the surface of the drum parallel to the surface to be treated. Place a single layer of toweling between the drum and the patient's body to absorb perspiration.

Capacitive application

When using a capacitive diathermy device, place the two air-spaced plates an equal distance (1" to 3" [2.5 to 7.6 cm]) from the patient on either side of the area to be treated. Wider spacing will allow for deeper energy penetration and, therefore, deeper heating. However, if plates are spaced more than 3" from the body, the unit may not operate. Equal placement is important to avoid uneven distribution of the electromagnetic field and uneven heating of the tissues within the field. Keep both plates parallel to the surface being treated.

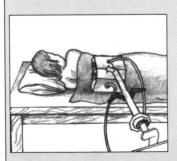

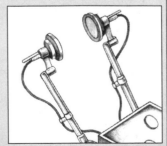

• Check the treated area. A normal response may include reddening of the skin. Mottling and rashes aren't normal responses and the causes should be investigated before another application is performed.
• Return all materials for use during the next treatment.

Special considerations

• Because adipose tissue has high electrical resistance, an obese patient may experience excessive superficial tissue heating.
• Intrauterine devices (IUDs) contain a small amount of metal (copper) that may become heated. However, in vivo measurements have shown only slight temperature changes in the region with application of therapeutic levels of SWD. Use cautiously in women who have IUDs.

Electrical stimulation, neuromuscular

Many forms of electrical stimulation are used in physical therapy. The practicing therapist requires fundamental knowledge of the principles of electricity and its physiologic effects on the body.

Neuromuscular electrical stimulation (NMES) for innervated and denervated tissue is used to excite nerve fibers to cause a muscle contraction. It aims to improve the force output and strength of muscles, increase muscular endurance, facilitate muscle fiber recruitment, reduce muscle guarding, reduce spasticity, increase range of motion, and indirectly improve circulation and reduce edema.

The effects of electrical stimulation depend on the specific therapeutic parameter of the device and the condition of the tissue being treated. For example, a method that causes a muscle to contract in a person with full motor control and capabilities won't do so in a person whose muscle is denervated.

NMES is delivered via alternating current (AC) to innervated muscles to cause a contraction. It's delivered to denervated muscle via direct current (DC), which applies current in one direction for a longer period. In denervated muscles, which lack adequate nerve innervation due to injury, the DC current acts directly on the muscle by bypassing the neural pathways.

Many patients become independent with the operation of a portable NMES unit and pain control units, but all initial applications of portable units as well as operation of all clinical units should be performed by a physical therapist (PT) or a PT assistant.

NMES is contraindicated in patients with demand-type pacemakers and uncontrolled cardiac conditions; over areas of indwelling phrenic nerve or urinary bladder stimulators; over the abdominal, lumbosacral, or pelvic regions during pregnancy (except the use of transcutaneous electrical stimulation during labor and delivery); in areas with venous or arterial thrombosis or thrombophlebitis; and over the carotid sinus, laryngeal or pharyngeal muscles, eyes, and mucosal membranes.

Equipment

NMES for innervated tissue
Electrical stimulation unit with all applicable lead wires (Machines often used include portable and clinical NMES units and high-voltage pulsed galvanic stimulators ✧ electrodes (self-adhesive or manufacturer-acceptable reusable type) ✧ conductive gel (if using reusable electrodes) ✧ nylon wraps or transpore or micropore tape to secure electrodes to skin ✧ alcohol wipes or $2'' \times 2''$ gauze

pads soaked in alcohol ✧ bell or other alerting device ✧ private or semi-private treatment area if necessary

Electrical stimulation for denervated tissue

DC electrical stimulation unit with applicable lead wires or probes ✧ electrodes (self-adhesive or manufacturer-acceptable reusable type) ✧ conductive gel (if using electrodes) ✧ 2″ × 2″ gauze pads or manufacturer-approved sponge covers (if using probes) ✧ rubber bands (if using 2″ × 2″ gauze) ✧ cup of water (if using probes) ✧ private or semiprivate treatment area if necessary

Essential steps

Innervated tissue

• Explain to the patient what you are planning to do and the expectations of the treatment, including what he should expect to feel. Electrical stimulation is a very unusual sensation, and the patient should be well prepared for the expected sensation.
• Inspect the area for possible skin irritation, and check the level of sensation in the area to be treated.
• Ask the patient to remove any jewelry from the area to be treated.
• Clean and abrade the local treatment area with alcohol wipes or rubbing alcohol and gauze.
• Position the patient for comfort or function. Initially, a patient receives electrical stimulation for improved muscle performance in a relaxed position to allow the stimulation to perform much of the work. If using the stimulation as an adjunct to normal functional activity, position the patient for that activity.
• Position the stimulation unit so that it doesn't interfere with the anticipated motion from the muscle contraction.

• Select an appropriately sized electrode. The electrode shouldn't be larger than the targeted tissue.
• Prepare the electrode if necessary. Self-adhesive types are provided with conductive gel, but may require a small amount of water to make them more conductive. Reusable electrodes should only be used with a conductive gel or with wet sponges as an interface.
• Apply the electrodes to the designated muscle or muscle groups; set them no closer than one electrode width apart to facilitate longitudinal current flow. (See *Unipolar and bipolar application techniques.*)
• If the electrodes are placed too close together, current flow may be too shallow; if they're too far apart, the current penetrates more deeply but may cause an undesirable contraction of other muscles. One electrode should be placed over or near a motor point, which is the point over a muscle where a contraction may be elicited by a minimal intensity, short-duration electrical stimulus. This point corresponds to the location of the terminal portion of the motor nerve fibers. (See *Motor point locations*, pages 352 and 353.)
• More than two electrodes can be used to stimulate a muscle if necessary. Some stimulation units use four electrodes of equal size with one larger dispersive electrode to stimulate back muscles.
• Make sure that the electrodes are well-adhered or well-taped to the treatment area so that they don't move during the treatment.
• Set the parameters for polarity, frequency, phase duration, on-off duty cycle, and modulation appropriate to the patient's condition. (See *Recommended NMES parameter settings for strength and endurance,* page 354.)
• Turn the unit on and slowly increase the amplitude (intensity). Ask

UNIPOLAR AND BIPOLAR APPLICATION TECHNIQUES

Use one of the following techniques to apply the electrodes to the designated muscle or muscle groups when performing neuromuscular electrical stimulation.

Unipolar

The unipolar method uses electrodes of two different sizes, one larger than the other. The smaller electrode is considered the "active" electrode; although both electrodes carry the same amount of electric current, the smaller electrode will have a more concentrated flow of current, which means it has a larger current density for its size. The larger electrode is considered the "dispersive" electrode.

The active electrode is usually placed over the muscle being stimulated (on or near the motor point) and the dispersive electrode is placed at a distance away from the motor point. Unipolar application is typically used to isolate smaller muscles. It's also utilized when using a probe to isolate a muscle. The probe is considered the active electrode and a larger pad is used as the dispersive electrode.

Bipolar

In bipolar electrode placement, both electrodes are of equal size and carry equal amounts of current. One is placed over the motor point and the other over the nerve corresponding distally to the muscle. This form of electrode placement is typically used to stimulate larger muscles or muscle groups, especially when electrical stimulation is used while performing functional tasks.

---

the patient to indicate when he begins to feel the electric current. This is a good sign that you are nearing the amplitude needed to elicit a contraction.

ALERT Most NMES units can be set to provide a continuous flow of current while you adjust the unit. This control option should be used while setting up the amplitude for the first time. If your unit doesn't have this option, be aware that you only have a set amount of time until the unit goes into the "off" cycle. Don't continue to turn up the amplitude during the "off" cycle. This could raise the amplitude too sharply, risking injury to the patient.

• When the patient indicates that current can be felt, continue to increase the amplitude until a muscle contraction is reached. If the patient becomes intolerant of the current before you have achieved a visible contraction, turn the amplitude down

and adjust the other parameters or the position of the electrodes. Sometimes increasing the frequency or adjusting the ramp and fall time resolves the problem. After you have accomplished a strong muscle contraction, switch the controls to run the on-off cycle. Total treatment time is usually 20 to 30 minutes.

• At the end of the treatment, return the amplitude control to zero and remove the equipment from the patient. Dry or clean any areas that have residue from the conductive medium.

• Assess skin condition and the patient's response to treatment.

Essential steps

Denervated tissue

• Explain the procedure to the patient and tell the patient what kind of sensations he should expect to feel during treatment.

(Text continues on page 354.)

MOTOR POINT LOCATIONS

Motor points are sites on the skin surface where the underlying muscle can be more easily stimulated to contract by electrical means. The figures below show approximate locations of motor points for major muscle groups.

Anterior motor points

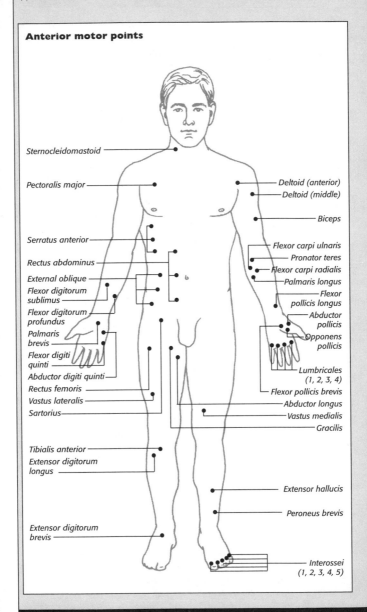

Posterior motor points

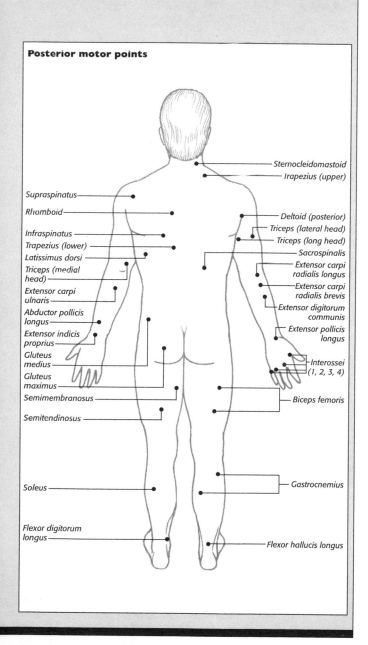

RECOMMENDED N.M.E.S. PARAMETER SETTINGS FOR STRENGTH AND ENDURANCE

Parameter	Setting
Current type	Biphasic pulsed, alternating current, high-voltage pulsed galvanic stimulators
Polarity	None or negative
Frequency	30 to 50 Hz (pps)
Phase duration	200 to 300 microseconds
On-off duty cycle	1:5 or 1:6 (lower as the patient works on endurance of the muscle)
Modulation	None or surged
Ramp and fall time	1 to 2 seconds
Amplitude (intensity)	To muscle contraction
Electrode configuration	Bipolar (larger muscle) or monopolar (smaller muscles)
Treatment time	20 to 30 minutes (possibly less time at the beginning, depending on the patient's condition)

• Inspect the area for possible skin irritation, and check the level of sensation in the area to be treated.

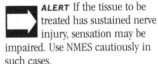 **ALERT** If the tissue to be treated has sustained nerve injury, sensation may be impaired. Use NMES cautiously in such cases.

• Ask the patient to remove any jewelry from the area to be treated.

• Clean and abrade the local treatment area with rubbing alcohol and gauze.

• Position the patient comfortably. Functional activities aren't usually replicated with DC stimulation, because the patient doesn't have the ability to assist with the activity.

• Position the unit or machine so that it doesn't interfere with the anticipated motion from the muscle contraction.

• Select the appropriate size probe for the targeted muscle. (If using electrodes, choose the appropriate size and follow the instruction for electrode application in the previous section on application for innervated tissue.)

• Prepare the probe by placing a sponge wrap over it (usually provided with the machine), or by placing two or three 2″ × 2″ gauze pads over the probe, being sure to cover the entire contact surface. Secure the gauze with a rubber band.

• Wet the sponge- or gauze-covered probe with water. Keep a cup of water handy to wet the probe during the treatment period, if necessary.

• A dispersive pad, larger than the size of your selected probe, should be placed on the extremity remote to where the probe will be applied. Prepare the dispersive pad with some type of conductive gel. Often, the patient will rest his arm on the dispersive pad, which is quite suitable for most facial and upper extremity application. For a lower-extremity application, the patient can place the pad under his thigh.

• Set the parameters for polarity, frequency, phase duration, and on-off

RECOMMENDED N.M.E.S. PARAMETER SETTINGS FOR DENERVATED MUSCLE

Parameter	Setting
Current type	Direct current
Polarity	Negative
Frequency	None
Phase duration	1 second
On-off duty cycle	5 to 10 seconds (on), 1 second or more (off)
Amplitude (intensity)	To muscle contraction
Electrode configuration	Monopolar probe application
Treatment time	6 to 10 contractions

duty cycle. (See *Recommended NMES parameter settings for denervated muscle.*)

• Place the probe over or near the motor point of the muscle to be stimulated. Most probes will have a contact switch, which allows delivery of the current through the probe. The current will only run through the probe when this switch is pressed. Turn up the amplitude control slightly and press the probe switch. Watch for a muscle contraction. If there is no contraction, turn up the amplitude and try again until you see a muscle contraction. You may also want to adjust the position of the probe if you aren't certain that you're over the motor point of the muscle.

• Contract the muscle 6 to 10 times with at least a 1-minute rest period between each contraction.

• When the treatment is complete, check the patient's skin for any irritation. Because DC can cause some chemical changes in the cutaneous tissue layer, it isn't unusual to see mild reddening of the skin in the area of the active electrode.

Special considerations

• Current literature indicates that the most comfortable waveform with which to deliver NMES is the symmetrical biphasic waveform found on pulsed current units. Many units offer the option to use "Russian" current setting, a type of alternating current delivered in bursts, or a symmetrical biphasic current. Most patients will be more comfortable with a symmetrical biphasic current setting, and it will be able produce the same amount of force during the muscle contraction as the "Russian" current setting.

• Use NMES cautiously in tissues vulnerable to hemorrhage or hematoma; in areas of skin irritation, severe edema, or sensory loss; and in areas where superficial metal is present (for example, embedded shrapnel, which may become heated, causing a burning sensation). Also use NMES cautiously in patients who are obese or who have osteoporosis.

• For treating denervated tissue, DC electrical stimulation is most often used during the rehabilitation stage of a nerve injury. This is primarily to prevent or slow atrophy of the muscle while the nerve is healing. Some animal studies suggest that electrical stimulation may impede nerve regeneration by inhibiting axonal sprouting of the partially innervated nerve. However, it should be noted that the parameters used in one influential study weren't typical of those used in most rehabilitation programs.

• As the nerve regenerates, the patient is often able to assist with the muscle contraction. At this time the therapist may want to consider switching to an AC or pulsed-current applicator, which would be more comfortable for the patient.

Electrical stimulation for pain control

Electrical stimulation is believed to help control pain by stimulating nerve fibers to block the transmission of pain impulses to the brain. Another theory is that electrical stimulation can promote the release of endogenous opiates, which then bind to receptor sites in the central and peripheral nervous system that block transmission of the painful sensation.

The most common electrical stimulation device used for pain control is the transcutaneous electrical nerve stimulation (TENS) unit. Many clinical stimulation units can produce the same parameters as TENS units, but the latter are more compact and portable and can be taken home and worn for many hours at a time by the patient.

There are many strategies for electrode placement when using electrical stimulation for pain control. They can be placed along a myotomal or dermatomal path or along the path of a peripheral nerve if that appears to be the cause of the pain. Selection of a strategy for electrode placement is very specific to the dysfunction or pathology found during the patient's evaluation.

Another type of applicator often used in the clinical setting is the interferential current (IFC) unit. In IFC, the therapeutic effects derive from the crossing of two current pathways in the treatment field. One current pathway flows at one frequency (such as 4,000 Hz) while the other flows at a slightly different frequency (4,100 Hz). When these two currents intersect, they create an "interfering" frequency. Advantages of this type of current are that it can create a deep flow of current into the tissue and it's better at preventing accommodation to the electric current.

TENS and IFC are used to treat a variety of acute or chronic pain conditions. Other indications specific to IFC include increasing blood flow and muscle relaxation.

TENS and IFC treatments are contraindicated in patients with demand-type pacemakers and uncontrolled cardiac conditions; over areas of indwelling phrenic nerve or urinary bladder stimulators; over the abdominal, lumbosacral, or pelvic regions during pregnancy (except the use of TENS during labor and delivery); in areas with venous or arterial thrombosis or thrombophlebitis; and over the carotid sinus, laryngeal or pharyngeal muscles, eyes, and mucosal membranes.

IFC should always be applied by a physical therapist (PT) or PT assistant, and a TENS unit should always be set up initially by a PT or a PT assistant until the patient learns to use it properly without supervision.

Equipment

For TENS application
TENS unit with lead wires ✧ self-adhesive electrodes ✧ tape ✧ alcohol wipes or 2″ × 2″ gauze pads soaked in alcohol

RECOMMENDED PARAMETER SETTINGS FOR CONVENTIONAL AND NOXIOUS-LEVEL T.E.N.S.

Parameter	Setting
Current type	Biphasic pulsed or alternating current
Polarity	None or negative
Frequency	100 Hz (pps) conventional, 1 to 5 Hz (pps) noxious-level
Phase duration	20 to 100 microseconds (conventional), as high as possible (noxious-level)
On-off duty cycle	Continuous
Modulation	Modulate amplitude, frequency, or phase duration per patient comfort for conventional transcutaneous electrical nerve stimulation (TENS) only
Amplitude (intensity)	Sensory (conventional), strong rhythmic muscle contraction (noxious-level)
Electrode configuration	Bipolar following dermatome, myotome, or path of peripheral nerve
Treatment time	Varies depending on condition being treated

For IFC application

IFC unit with lead wires ✧ various sizes of reusable or self-adhesive electrodes ✧ electrode gel for reusable electrodes ✧ nylon wraps or transpore or micropore tape to secure electrodes ✧ alcohol wipes or 2″ × 2″ gauze pads soaked in alcohol ✧ towels or sheet ✧ alerting device

Equipment preparation

• Preset the parameters for frequency, phase duration, and modulation.

Essential steps

• Explain the procedure to the patient and tell the patient what kind of sensations will be felt during the treatment.
• Inspect the area for possible skin irritation, and check for the level of sensation.
• Ask the patient to remove all jewelry from the treatment area.

• Clean and abrade the local treatment area with an alcohol wipe.

For TENS application

• Plug the lead wires into the unit and into the electrodes.
• Place the electrodes on the treatment area. TENS usually utilizes a bipolar electrode placement.
• Turn the unit on and slowly increase the amplitude to a sensory level. Continue to increase the amplitude until the patient has reached the strongest stimulation level tolerated and then decrease the amplitude slightly. This should allow for the most intense treatment at a tolerable level. If a "noxious-level" stimulation is desired, the amplitude should be turned up until there is a strong, rhythmic muscle contraction. (See *Recommended parameter settings for conventional and noxious-level TENS.*)

ELECTRODE PLACEMENT FOR AN I.F.C. UNIT

To use interferential current (IFC) effectively, it's necessary to place four electrodes oriented diagonally across the area to be treated at an even interval, as shown in the diagram.

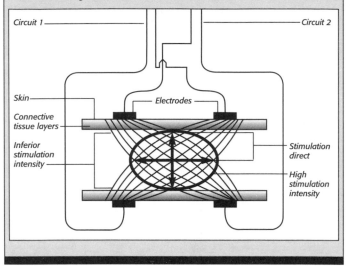

For IFC application

• Position and drape the patient for comfort.

• Determine the electrode placement scheme. (See *Electrode placement for an IFC unit*.)

• Prepare the electrodes. Self-adhesive types are provided with conductive gel, but they may require a small amount of water to make them more conductive. Reusable electrodes should only be used with a conductive gel or wet sponges as an interface.

• Apply the electrodes per your placement scheme, being sure to cross them on a diagonal. Use nylon wraps or tape to keep the electrodes in place.

• Set the parameters for polarity, frequency, beat frequency, phase duration, and modulation appropriate to the problem. (See *Recommended parameter settings for interferential current*.)

• Turn on the unit and begin to turn up the amplitude of one channel. When the patient reports a strong sensation of current flow, begin to turn up the other circuit. After both circuits are turned up, the patient should feel the majority of the current flow in the targeted area.

• Some units come with a targeting device that allows the therapist to slightly move the area of perceived stimulation. This is done through a modulation. Use this if the patient doesn't feel that the current is targeting the correct tissues.

• Most IFC treatments last for 20 to 30 minutes.

• At the end of the treatment, turn off the unit and return all controls to the zero position.

• Remove the electrodes, clean the skin area under the electrodes, and inspect the patient for any possible skin irritation.

RECOMMENDED PARAMETER SETTINGS FOR INTERFERENTIAL CURRENT

Parameter	Setting
Polarity	None or negative
Frequency	Preset into the machine, usually 4,000 to 5,000 Hz
"Beat" frequency	1 to 10 Hz (chronic conditions), 100 to 150 Hz (acute conditions)
Phase duration	200 to 300 microseconds
On-off duty cycle	Continuous
Modulation	None; amplitude modulation for patient comfort
Amplitude (intensity)	Strong sensory
Electrode configuration	Crossing bipolar (quadrapolar)
Treatment time	20 to 30 minutes (possibly less time at the beginning, depending on the patient's condition)

Special considerations

• If preparing a patient to take a TENS unit home, make sure that he understands how to attach the electrodes to his body.

• Advise periodic reevaluation of the need for the machine, especially when the patient contemplates using a TENS unit for hours at a time. In some cases, patients use the unit even when their pain has subsided; this may cause increased accommodation to the electric current when the patient needs to use the machine for increasing pain levels. Many treatment times are for only 20 to 30 minutes, especially in "noxious-level" stimulation.

Electrical stimulation for wound healing

Electrical stimulation has been shown to be highly effective in improving the healing rate of slowly healing wounds and for providing bactericidal effects in infected wounds. Most of these effects are attributed to the polarity used and net charges formed with direct current (DC) or monophasic, pulsed current. The current is dispersed to the wound bed via a piece of saline-soaked gauze placed on the wound and connected to an alligator-type electrode clip. This avoids irritating the tissues surrounding the wound.

Many patients can be apprehensive about having electric current flow through their wound, so the procedure should be well explained to the patient before the actual treatment.

This treatment is indicated for infected or slowly healing wounds. Contraindications are the same as for neuromuscular electrical stimulation and other electrical stimulation therapies.

Equipment

DC or a monophasic pulsed current unit (often referred to as high-voltage pulsed galvanic stimulator [HVPGS]) with applicable lead wires ✧ alligator clip ✧ gauze pads of appropriate size

RECOMMENDED PARAMETER SETTINGS FOR ELECTRICAL STIMULATION

Parameter	Setting
Current Type	Direct current (DC) or high-voltage pulsed galvanic stimulator (HVPGS)
Polarity	Negative on days 1 to 4 and positive after day 4 for infected wound
Frequency	None (DC), 50+ for patient comfort (HVPGS)
Pulse duration	None (DC), 20 to 100 microseconds (HVPGD)
On-off duty cycle	Continuous
Modulation	None
Amplitude (intensity)	Sensory
Electrode configuration	Monopolar with active electrode over the wound
Treatment time	30 minutes to 2 hours depending on the size and condition of the wound

✧ normal saline solution ✧ alerting device ✧ private or semiprivate treatment area

Essential steps

• Explain the procedure to the patient and tell him what kind of sensations he will feel during the treatment.
• Remove dressings from the wound.
• Place enough saline-soaked gauze in the wound site to fill it completely.
• Apply the electrodes. A unipolar electrode placement must be used to obtain the polarity effects necessary to enhance wound healing. The smaller, active electrode will be placed over the wound, and the dispersive electrode will be placed remote from the wound. The active electrode should be an alligator clip. Attach the alligator clip to the gauze so that the clip itself doesn't come in contact with the patient.
• Preset the parameters for polarity, frequency, pulse duration, and modulation. (See *Recommended parameter settings for electrical stimulation*.)
• Turn on the unit and begin to increase the amplitude. Continue to increase the amplitude until a strong sensory level is achieved.
• Treatment times last from 30 minutes to 2 hours, depending on the size and condition of the wound and the patient's tolerance of the procedure.
• When the treatment is complete, turn off the machine and return all amplitude controls to zero.
• Carefully remove the alligator clip from the gauze.
• Remove the gauze from the wound site for reassessment.
• Apply fresh wound dressing as appropriate for that type of wound.

Special considerations

• Another well-used application of DC stimulation is a treatment known as *iontophoresis*. In this type of treatment, a prescribed topical medication is driven into the skin with DC. The polarity of the current is chosen based on the polarity of the medication. Several units designed to provide this type of stimulation are available. These units are highly recommended for performing iontophoresis and the manufacturer's instructions are usually specific to their unit. These instructions are usually adequate to help the physical therapist with a successful application.

Hydrotherapy

Hydrotherapy, or the use of water as a therapeutic agent, is one of the oldest methods used to treat disease and injuries. Water is an excellent medium in which to exercise, because it provides either assistance to or resistance against the motion of the exercise. Most commonly used for its mechanical effects to treat burns and other serious wounds, hydrotherapy is also used to increase or decrease tissue temperature, to promote increased circulation, to facilitate relaxation, and for analgesia.

Indications for hydrotherapy include joint stiffness, musculoskeletal strains or sprains, arthritis, and some types of peripheral vascular disease. It's also used to promote strengthening in various neurologic and musculoskeletal disorders and to promote gait training in instances where the patient needs decreased joint weight bearing. Although hydrotherapy usually involves immersing the patient in a tub of water ("tubbing"), other water spray techniques may replace this method in some facilities.

Contraindications for hydrotherapy include bowel and bladder incontinence, skin infections, unstable blood pressure, uncontrolled seizure disorder, active tuberculosis, acute fever, fear of water, and any condition where exposure to water is contraindicated (such as when a cast is pre-

sent). Any patient who is unable to give the physical therapist accurate feedback regarding water temperature and general well-being during treatment is a poor candidate for hydrotherapy.

Equipment

Appropriate style whirlpool, such as a "highboy" for upper-extremity or deep immersion, a "lowboy" for lower-extremity immersion, and a Hubbard tank for full-body immersion ✧ chemical additives as appropriate for wound care ✧ an elevated chair, plinth, or other seat to position the patient in the tub ✧ a safety belt for use with lift chair assemblies and Hubbard tank stretchers ✧ personal protective equipment, such as gloves, gowns, goggles, and masks, which may be clean or sterile depending on patient need and the facility's infection-control policy ✧ clean towels ✧ a sterile barrier ✧ debridement instruments and dressing supplies as needed for wound care ✧ bath blankets ✧ clean sheets ✧ a noncorrosive commercial disinfectant ✧ scrub brush

 ALERT Full-body immersion and exercise in a Hubbard tank places a greater demand on the body's ability to dissipate heat and raises core body temperature. For patients without cardiorespiratory compromise, immersion time shouldn't exceed 20 minutes. For elderly and compromised patients, it's best to start with 10 minutes and gradually increase immersion time according to patient tolerance. Use caution with patients who have pulmonary diagnoses and a vital capacity less than 1,000 cc. All patients with cardiopulmonary dysfunction need to have their vital signs monitored throughout the treatment.

Preparation of equipment

• Keep the whirlpool area at a higher temperature than the general treatment area to prevent patients from getting cold during and after the treatment.

• Provide adequate ventilation to clear away the odors of any chemical additives and cleaners used as well as to prevent moisture buildup on walls and fixtures. Also, a sink should be nearby for easy access to wash hands before and after treatments.

• Help to keep the inside of the whirlpool clean and sterile by not touching the inside surface of the tank. All whirlpool parts as well as the treatment area should be cleaned and disinfected according to the facility's infection-control policy before each treatment.

• Select the proper water temperature, depending on the specific patient and the objectives of the treatment, and fill the whirlpool to the desired level, adding any appropriate chemical additives.

• Allow the whirlpool to agitate for 5 minutes to ensure the additives are fully blended.

Essential steps

• Explain to the patient the purpose of the whirlpool treatment and what to expect during the treatment.

• If the patient has a cardiopulmonary condition, monitor vital signs before, during, and after treatment to document the patient's tolerance to the treatment.

• Wash hands and put on applicable personal protective equipment (usually goggles, gloves, a mask, and a gown, depending on the patient and the facility's specific infection-control guidelines).

• Inspect the body part to be immersed for skin quality, including color, temperature, and edema, and test for temperature sensitivity.

• Remove and dispose of any dressings according to infection-control guidelines. If the dressing adheres to the wound, allow it to be immersed in the water with the extremity. After it's adequately loosened, remove and dispose of the dressing as above. This procedure minimizes patient discomfort and helps to prevent disruption of the underlying wound bed.

• Transfer the patient to the Hubbard tank stretcher or the lift chair, safely securing him before lowering him into the tank.

• If another type of whirlpool unit is indicated or if the patient is ambulatory, position the patient comfortably in an elevated chair or locked wheelchair as appropriate before immersing the extremity in the whirlpool.

ALERT When immersing a patient's hand or upper extremity, avoid placing the hand in a dependent position because this encourages edema.

• Pad the patient with clean towels as needed, making sure to keep them out of the water.

• Turn on the whirlpool and adjust the aeration to the desired level of agitation. Avoid positioning the agitator directly at any body part that may not tolerate the added force or may be damaged by the agitation action. If it's the patient's first treatment, begin with a low level of agitation and gradually increase if able.

• The duration of the whirlpool treatment will depend on the treatment goals. If the whirlpool modality is used strictly for its thermal effects, the standard duration of treatment is 20 minutes. When used as a precursor to debridement, a treatment of 5 to 20 minutes is adequate, depending on the quantity of necrotic tissue present. A duration of 10 to 20 minutes is typical when used for exercise.

• A treatment should be stopped immediately if any sudden change in status occurs, such as unstable vital signs and signs and symptoms of dehydration or fluid imbalance.

• Turn off the agitator at the end of the treatment, rewash your hands, and put on clean gloves (sterile gloves if doing wound care), goggles, a mask, and a gown.

• Assist the patient out of the whirlpool, using the hydraulic lift or assisting the immersed extremity out of the water.

• Dry the extremity with clean towels (or sterile towels if an open wound is present). If performing wound care or debridement, maintain a sterile field while all prescribed dressings and treatments are applied.

• Reinspect the patient's skin and monitor vital signs.

• Properly dispose of all trash and used supplies. Drain, clean, and disinfect the whirlpool according to your facility's infection-control policy.

• Document the treatment, including skin status, vital signs, and any adverse reactions to treatment.

Special considerations

• Whirlpool temperature varies according to the goals of the treatment and the condition being treated. For patients with compromised circulation, extreme temperatures may prove detrimental. Consider the following temperature guidelines.

–Water in a "tepid" whirlpool is 80° to 92° F (26.6° to 33.3° C) and is indicated when heat is contraindicated and in patients with peripheral vascular disease. This temperature range is also effective for wound cleansing and for softening necrotic tissue prior to debridement.

–Water in a "neutral" whirlpool employs temperatures in the range of 92° to 96° F (33.3° to 35.6° C). This

temperature range yields mild thermal and circulatory effects, in addition to the same tissue effects as a tepid whirlpool. Neutral whirlpools are typically used for ischemia and to promote sedation and analgesia.

–Water in "thermal" whirlpools varies from 96° to 104° F (35.6° to 40° C) and has very few indications. Its effects will vary, depending on the amount of immersed surface area and the duration of treatment. Typically, vasodilation and reflex vasodilation result. Patients with cardiopulmonary disease shouldn't be subjected to whirlpool temperatures higher than 100° F (37.8° C) to avoid the risk of decreased blood pressure when vasodilation occurs.

• A contrast bath is a hydrotherapy technique requiring two whirlpools or tubs: one thermal in the "hot" temperature range (100° to 110° F [37.8° to 43.3° C]) and one "cold" (50° to 64° F [10° to 17.8° C]). Contrast baths are believed to assist circulation by alternating vasodilation and vasoconstriction. The extremity to be treated is first immersed in the hot tub for 10 minutes, then into the cold tub for 1 minute, then back into the hot tub for 4 minutes. The process continues for 30 minutes, always finishing with the hot tub. The length of immersion in each tub may vary, but should generally follow a hot-to-cold ratio of 3 to 1 or 4 to 1, depending on the patient's condition.

• Contrast baths are indicated for use with arthritis, some cases of peripheral vascular disease, strains, sprains, and for toughening residual limbs. This therapy is contraindicated for patients with Buerger's disease, small vessel vascular disease, or for any patient who shouldn't be exposed to whirlpools in the thermal temperature range.

Massage

Massage is the systematic, mechanical stimulation of the soft tissues of the body by means of rhythmically applied pressure and stretching using the hands. It's performed to produce mechanical or reflexive effects such as improved range of motion, to increase circulation and lymphatic drainage, to induce general relaxation, and to reduce pain. The terms soft-tissue mobilization, soft-tissue manipulation, and massage are synonymous. However, a variety of soft-tissue techniques are known. Lighter, gentler techniques such as effleurage are considered massage, whereas more aggressive techniques involving movement of deeper structures in the body are considered soft-tissue mobilization.

Massage is performed by physical therapists and massage therapists. It's indicated for patients who have restricted movement limited by soft-tissue shortening or connective-tissue tightness. Nerve entrapment and circulation and lymphatic deficits stemming from soft-tissue restrictions can be successfully treated with massage.

Massage therapies are contraindicated in the presence of acute inflammation or open wounds as well as in patients with extremely fragile tissue, as in brittle diabetes. It shouldn't be performed in the lower extremity when deep vein thrombosis is present.

Equipment

Treatment table ✧ nonabsorbable massage cream ✧ sheet or towel

Preparation of equipment

• Adjust the height of the treatment table to your comfort level.
• Warm the massage cream.

Essential steps

• Explain the procedure to the patient.
• Ask the patient to remove clothing from the area to be massaged, if appropriate.
• Drape the exposed area with a sheet or towel to maintain privacy.
• Massage the affected area using your hands and the massage cream. There are many soft-tissue techniques that can be applied to assist in the patient's well-being. The chosen technique will depend on the patient's condition and the skill level of the therapist.
• Initially, apply gentle gliding strokes over the skin without moving deep muscle masses (effleurage) to allow the patient to accommodate to touch and to allow the superficial tissues to loosen.
• If appropriate, progress to more aggressive techniques, such as kneading, transverse friction, and pressure point release, to facilitate soft-tissue movement to the direction desired.

Special considerations

• Massage should always be used in conjunction with other forms of treatment such as exercise.
• Limb massage is generally done from the distal to the proximal part; if the limb is swollen, the proximal part must be massaged before the distal part.
• Circulation and lymphatic flow are greatly enhanced by soft-tissue mobilization. If there has been prolonged use of medications, soft-tissue mobilization may free toxins that have accumulated in the tissues over time. As a result, the patient may experience fatigue or nausea after treatment.
• In the presence of connective-tissue restriction, soft-tissue treatment may result in a histamine response. Tissue that responds this way is best treated

with gentle techniques. Sensitivity can be checked by drawing the thumb lightly along the patient's back and watching the autonomic response. Initially, the thumb pressure will cause decreased circulation and thus a lightening of the area. This will be followed by a reddening of the area. If the reddening is enhanced, the patient may have a heightened autonomic system, warranting gentle technique.

Mechanical compression

Compression therapy, in any form, is used to exert external pressure on the body for the purpose of improving circulation and fluid balance and to modify the appearance of soft tissue such as a scar. Compression is often performed in the form of bandaging or with specialized stockings that closely fit the extremity.

Mechanical compression pumps, also known as intermittent pneumatic compression devices, help to address circulation, fluid balance, and tissue formation. Typically, the pump is connected to a nylon sleeve that is wrapped around the body part; the sleeve fills with air and compresses the extremity. There are two types of pumps: nonsequential and sequential. A *nonsequential* pump uses a sleeve fitted with a single internal bladder that inflates intermittently to compress a limb or a residual limb. Some nonsequential pumps also use cooled water instead of air to provide a form of cold compression, if desired. In a *sequential* pump, the sleeve contains several bladders that inflate and deflate one after the other, beginning distally and moving proximally.

Patients can use mechanical compression devices independently at home after they have been instructed

in their use. In the clinical setting, a physical therapist (PT) or PT assistant should operate the device.

Mechanical compression is used to treat conditions contributing to poor lymphatic or venous drainage and to shape tissues. Common indications include postmastectomy lymphedema, venous insufficiency, amputations (new residual limbs), and rehabilitation of scars and severe burns.

Mechanical compression is contraindicated in patients with heart failure or pulmonary edema; recent or acute deep vein thrombosis, thrombophlebitis, or pulmonary embolism; obstruction of the lymph or venous system (can occur with tumors in the area or with radiation damage); significant kidney dysfunction; severe arterial insufficiency or ulcers due to arterial insufficiency; local infection; severe hypoproteinemia; and acute trauma.

Equipment

Mechanical compression pump with the appropriate size sleeve ✧ stockinette ✧ sphygmomanometer ✧ stethoscope ✧ alerting device, if appropriate ✧ and private or semiprivate treatment area

Essential steps

• Explain the procedure to the patient and tell the patient what kind of sensations will be felt during the treatment.
• Check the patient's sensory response to pressure and check skin integrity.
• Remove any clothing or jewelry from the treatment area.
• Place the patient in a comfortable position with the involved extremity elevated to approximately 30 degrees.
• Determine the patient's blood pressure, using the noninvolved arm.

• Apply a stockinette to the involved extremity. Make sure that the stockinette is lying smoothly over the extremity, covering it completely.

• Apply the compression sleeve and attach the hose to the sleeve and the device.

• Set the appropriate parameters on the device, including inflation and deflation time, inflation pressure, and total treatment time. Some sequential units will also allow you to set the pressure individually for each bladder. Inflation pressure for use with an upper-extremity sleeve shouldn't exceed 60 mm Hg and for the lower extremity shouldn't exceed 80 mm Hg. *Don't exceed the patient's diastolic blood pressure.* Usually the pressure is applied in a 3 to 1 ratio of inflation time to deflation time; however, the greater the inflation pressure, the lower the ratio. Total treatment time also varies widely, depending on the underlying clinical condition. Most treatment applications are 2 to 3 hours long, applied twice per day.

• With the unit on the continuous position (where there is no deflation time), turn the pressure up to the desired level. Then switch the compression to the set "on-off" cycle. Encourage the patient to exercise a little during the off part of the cycle.

• Give the patient an alerting device in case he needs your assistance.

• Check the patient's blood pressure in the noninvolved arm after 15 to 30 minutes, especially if the patient has a history of hypertension.

• When the treatment is complete, remove the sleeve and inspect the patient's skin. Note any areas of irritation and be sure to provide better protection, such as a thicker stockinette, for those areas during future treatments.

• Perform any necessary girth measurements or evaluation procedures and measure blood pressure again.

• To maintain reduction in the extremity, apply a pressure bandage or compression garment after the intermittent compression treatment.

Special considerations

• Use mechanical compression cautiously in patients with cancer; compression may promote metastasis due to increased circulation. Note that the method is often used after a mastectomy to control lymphedema while the patient is continuing treatment. Controversy exists regarding the use of compression with cancer patients. Consultation with the patient's primary care provider is strongly recommended.

• Use with caution on patients with impaired sensory or mental abilities, in those with uncontrolled hypertension, and in those with a recent history of stroke or transient ischemic attack.

Superficial heating agents

Superficial heating agents are used to produce a tissue temperature rise in superficial tissues. The depth of penetration is limited to the first $\frac{3}{8}''$ to $\frac{3}{4}''$ (1 to 2 cm) of tissue. These heating agents come in several forms. The agents most commonly used to produce a superficial tissue temperature rise include hot packs, paraffin, whirlpool bath (see "Hydrotherapy," page 361), and fluidotherapy.

Hot packs are canvas bags filled with hydrophilic silicate and stored on racks in hot water. *Paraffin* is a mixture of mineral oil and paraffin heated in a thermostatically controlled bath unit.

Fluidotherapy is a dry heating agent consisting of finely ground cellulose particles (ground corncobs) in a cabinet. Heat and air are forced through the particles, causing them to flow like a liquid around the area being treated. This form of superficial heat is most often applied to the distal end of extremities.

With proper instruction from a physical therapist (PT) or PT assistant, hot packs and paraffin treatments can be readily performed at home by the patient independently or with the help of a caregiver. In a clinical setting, the PT or a PT assistant should apply these modalities. Fluidotherapy is provided with a specialized piece of equipment that should only be used by a PT or a PT assistant in a clinical setting.

Superficial heating agents can be used to treat subacute or chronic traumatic and inflammatory conditions, to reduce pain, to enhance tissue extensibility, and to reduce muscle spasm.

Superficial heating agents are contraindicated in patients with acute inflammatory conditions, malignancies, significant cardiac insufficiency, active bleeding (such as from trauma), lack of sensation in the area to be treated, unreliable thermoregulation (often seen with young children and the elderly), existing fevers, significant peripheral vascular disease, or devitalized tissues caused by X-ray therapy.

 WOMEN'S HEALTH During the third trimester of pregnancy, a woman may experience ligamentous laxity due to hormonal changes. This can raise the risk of joint instability. Because superficial heat can further increase ligamentous laxity, women in the last trimester of pregnancy shouldn't receive a hot pack on a joint structure before any moderate or vigorous activities that might stretch the ligaments over that joint.

Equipment

Hot pack
Hydroculator unit (158° to 170° F [70° to 76.7° C] water temperature) ✧ hot packs in a variety of shapes and sizes ✧ commercial hot pack covers (may be substituted with terry towels, using two towels for one commercial cover) ✧ timer ✧ a call bell or other alerting device ✧ private or semiprivate treatment area

Paraffin
Paraffin and mineral oil (commercially premixed paraffin and oil compounds are available) ✧ paraffin bath unit or thermostatically controlled unit ✧ thermometer ✧ plastic bags or plastic wrap ✧ towels ✧ sink ✧ soap ✧ a bell or alerting device

Fluidotherapy
Fluidotherapy unit of appropriate size for the area to be treated ✧ bell or alerting device

Preparation of equipment
Paraffin
Melt a 6 to 1 or 7 to 1 mixture of paraffin to oil in the thermostatically controlled paraffin bath or large crock-pot. Melt the paraffin at a temperature up to 130° F (54.4° C), but keep it at 125° to 127° F (51.7° to 52.8° C) for treatment. Because of paraffin's low specific heat, it can feel cooler than other materials heated to the same temperature; therefore, it's safe to apply directly to the patient's skin. Using a thermometer, check the temperature of the bath before proceeding to make sure it's at an acceptable temperature.

Essential steps
Hot pack application
• Explain the procedure to the patient and tell the patient what kind of

sensations to expect during treatment.

• Inspect the area to be treated for possible skin irritations, and check for level of sensation to temperature in the treatment area.

• Ask the patient to remove all jewelry and clothing from the area to be treated.

• Position the patient for comfort and modesty.

• Remove the hot pack from the hydroculator unit by using the tabs on the pack. Wrap it in six to eight layers of dry toweling or three to four layers of commercial hot pack covers.

• Place the pack on top of the body part to be treated and secure it well. It's best to place the pack on top of or over the body part, but you may have to address patient comfort or positioning restraints by having the patient lie on top of the pack or resting a limb on top of it. In this case, add more toweling to compensate for the weight of the body part compressing the insulating layers.

• Provide the patient with a bell or another alerting device to use if your assistance is needed during the treatment.

• The treatment should last 15 to 30 minutes.

• Check on the patient and the treated area after the first 5 minutes. Signs of excessive redness may indicate that the pack is too hot and additional towel layers need to be added. If blistering is present, discontinue the treatment immediately and apply a cold pack to decrease the effects of burning.

• At the conclusion of the treatment, remove the pack and dry the area. Check the skin condition again. A regular response is mild hyperemia in the area. Skin mottling and severe hyperemia aren't normal responses and their cause should be investigated before continuing with hot pack or

any other superficial heating treatments.

• Return the pack to the hydroculator tank for its next use.

Paraffin application (dip-wrap method)

• Explain the procedure to the patient and tell the patient what kind of sensations to expect during treatment.

• Wash and dry the area to be treated (or, if appropriate, have the patient do this) to minimize contamination of the paraffin.

• Ask the patient to remove all jewelry from the area to be treated.

• Check the body part to be treated for temperature sensation and skin integrity. Don't proceed if the patient has an open wound.

• Immerse the body part in the bath using a dipping motion. Instruct the patient to move slowly and steadily; then lift the body part out of the bath. Warn the patient not to touch the sides or bottom of the bath, which are very hot.

• Repeat this dipping motion 6 to 12 times, allowing the wax layer to harden slightly between dips into the paraffin.

• Wrap the treated body part in a plastic bag or plastic wrap and then in a towel. The plastic wrap keeps the wax from sticking to the towel, and the towel is used as insulation to slow the cooling process.

• Rest the treated body part in an elevated position, if possible.

• Remind the patient not to move the body part because this may crack the wax coating.

• Tell the patient the paraffin "glove" may stay in place for up to 20 minutes.

• When the treatment is complete, remove the towel and plastic layer and simply peel back the glove. You may return the glove to the paraffin

bath for remelting, if this is permitted by your facility's policy.
• Check the skin condition again. Mild hyperemia should be expected; however, skin mottling and severe hyperemia aren't normal responses and their cause should be investigated before continuing with paraffin or any other superficial heating treatments.
• After the bath treatment, the patient's skin will be very oily and slippery. This may be a desired result, but if the patient is to continue the session with upper-extremity exercises, advise him to wash the body part so that he won't lose his grip on any equipment.

Fluidotherapy

• Explain the procedure to the patient and tell the patient what kind of sensations to expect during treatment.
• Ask the patient to remove all jewelry and clothing from the area to be treated.
• Cover any open wounds with a plastic barrier to prevent the cellulose particles from contaminating the wound.
• Place the body part in the appropriate portal of the unit. Most units will have portals on the sides and on the top.
• Secure the sleeve to prevent particles from escaping the cabinet.
• Set the temperature control between 110° and 118° F (43.4° and 47.8° C).
• Adjust the level of agitation based on patient comfort and desired results.
• Provide the patient with a bell or another alerting device to use if your assistance is needed during the treatment.
• The treatment should last from 20 to 30 minutes.
• At the end of the treatment, remove the body part from the portal, being careful not to spill particles from the cabinet.
• Check the skin condition for any possible adverse reactions. The patient might demonstrate mild hyperemia; however, any other response should be investigated before continuing with therapy.

Ultrasound therapy

Ultrasound is a form of deep heat application that is produced by high-frequency sound waves. These are produced by a piezoelectric crystal within the transducer of the ultrasound unit. When an alternating electric current is imposed upon the crystal, it begins to vibrate. The frequency of the resulting waves is determined by the size of the crystal and the frequency of the current across the crystal. When these waves travel through tissue, they generate molecular motion in the form of heat, which eventually increases tissue temperature.

The depth of penetration of the sound waves depends on their frequency. At 1 MHz, the sound waves aren't easily absorbed by the more superficial structures and therefore penetrate deeper, usually to a depth of $1\frac{1}{8}''$ to $2''$ (3 to 5 cm). With a higher frequency, such as 3 MHz, the sound waves are absorbed more readily in the superficial tissues because of the work required to create a faster flow of sound waves. The frequency range used for therapeutic ultrasound is from 0.75 MHz to 3 MHz, with a therapeutic intensity range of 0.5 to 2 watts/cm^2.

Ultrasound also produces therapeutically desirable nonthermal effects, such as cavitation and acoustical streaming, which don't involve increasing the tissue temperature. The pulse wave itself also has therapeutic effects that aren't related to rises in tissue temperature. Selection of thermal or nonthermal ultrasound is based on the desired clinical outcome as well as the acuity of the condition being treated. Therapeutic ultrasound should only be performed by a physical therapist (PT) or PT team member in the clinical setting.

Thermal ultrasound is used in subacute or chronic inflammatory conditions for the purpose of enhancing tissue extensibility, improving nutrition to the involved area, and reducing muscle spasm and guarding. It's also indicated for removing plantar warts.

Nonthermal ultrasound is used to increase cell membrane permeability, improve healing of open wounds, help drive topical medications deeper into tissues, increase tissue extensibility, and decrease scar formation (via separation of collagen fibers).

Ultrasound therapy shouldn't be used over areas of malignancy or any abnormal growth, tissues devitalized by X-ray therapy, the orbits of the eyes, the reproductive organs, any area where a thrombus is present, the carotid sinuses or cervical ganglia, areas of hemorrhage, the spinal cord after a laminectomy without fusion, and certain cement products commonly used in arthroplasty procedures. It also shouldn't be used directly over implanted medical devices, such as pacemakers and implantable cardioverter-defibrillators. Ultrasound therapy is also contraindicated in infection and severe arterial disease.

Ultrasound should be used cautiously over areas where sensation isn't fully intact, over epiphyseal plates of actively growing children, over recent fractures, and over breast implants.

ALERT For years, therapists have been told not to sonate over the epiphyseal plates of children because it was believed that ultrasound would alter the cells of the new bony growth. However, this warning was based on research that didn't use proven therapeutic technique and, therefore, shouldn't have been considered in the application of therapeutic ultrasound. More recent research has demonstrated beneficial effects on fracture healing by therapeutic levels of ultrasound. Ultrasonic treatments in children shouldn't be contraindicated but should be used cautiously with regard to the intensity and dosage used.

Equipment

Ultrasound unit with frequency ranges appropriate for targeted tissue ❖ conductive medium (This is usually a conductive gel or lotion specially prepared for use with an ultrasound machine. Other conductive mediums may include water and mineral oil.) ❖ towels ❖ hospital-grade electrical outlet ❖ private or semiprivate treatment area

Essential steps

• Explain the procedure to the patient and tell the patient what kind of sensations to expect during treatment. In the case of thermal ultrasound, the patient may feel a mild warming sensation, but this isn't as intense as the sensation generated by a hot pack.
• Ask the patient to remove all jewelry and clothing from the area to be treated.
• Position the patient for comfort and modesty. Also make sure that the position of the equipment doesn't impede the therapist's ability to apply the treatment safely.
• Check the patient for intact temperature sensation and skin integrity.
• Select the appropriate machine parameters: lower frequencies (1 MHz) for deeper tissues and higher frequencies (3 MHz) for more superficial tis-

DETERMINING ULTRASOUND TREATMENT TIME

Several different equations can be used to determine treatment time for ultrasound therapy. One method is to provide 5 minutes of sonication for every 25 in² of tissue to be treated. Another method is to take the size of the area to be treated and divide it by the effective radiating area (ERA) of the transducer (from the manufacturer's specifications) multiplied by a quotient based on the condition's acuity. For subacute conditions, use 1.5; for chronic conditions, use 1.0; and for maximal thermal effects, use 0.8, as shown in the equation below. Although this method is more specific, it takes time to perform the calculations and it hasn't been proven more effective than other dosage calculation methods.

For subacute conditions:

$$\frac{\text{Size of area to be treated}}{1.5 \times \text{ERA}} = \text{minutes of ultrasound treatment}$$

sues. Pulsed or continuous mode and intensity should be selected based on desired clinical results.

• Select a transducer size. Most units will come with at least two sizes. Choose one with an effective radiating area that is approximately one-half the size of the area to be treated. It's best to choose a transducer that is too small rather than one that is too large.

• Calculate your treatment time. (See *Determining ultrasound treatment time*.)

• Apply a conductive gel or lotion to both the patient and the transducer, making sure to apply enough to last throughout the treatment.

Direct method of application

• Check the unit to be sure that all dials are set to zero.

• Place the transducer on the patient and turn on the machine.

• Move the transducer within the treatment area in a circular or stroking fashion. The speed of movement should be about 4 cm/second. It's important to keep the transducer moving, particularly if you have chosen a continuous setting.

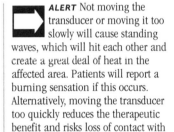 *ALERT* Not moving the transducer or moving it too slowly will cause standing waves, which will hit each other and create a great deal of heat in the affected area. Patients will report a burning sensation if this occurs. Alternatively, moving the transducer too quickly reduces the therapeutic benefit and risks loss of contact with the patient as well as exposes the transducer to the air.

• Slowly increase the intensity to the desired level while continuing to move the transducer. It's important to be able to easily operate the intensity control while continuing the transducer motion to avoid administering too little or too much energy. Good patient positioning and careful unit placement will help with this activity.

• When the treatment is completed, wipe the conductive medium from the patient and transducer with a towel or washcloth.

• Return all of the unit's controls to the zero position for its next use.

• Assess the patient's response to the treatment.

Aqueous method of application

• Place the patient's limb in the container of water.

• Check the machine to be sure that all dials are set to zero.
• Place the transducer in the water and turn on the machine
• Keeping the transducer ½" to 1" (1.3 to 2.5 cm) away from the body part, move the transducer in a circular or stroking motion over or around the area being treated. The speed of movement should be about 4 cm/second. It's important to keep the transducer moving, particularly if you have chosen a continuous setting. Also be sure to keep the transducer under the water at all times.
• Slowly turn up the intensity to the desired level while continuously moving the transducer. It's important to be able to easily operate the intensity control while continuing the transducer motion.

• When the treatment is complete, turn off the unit and dry the patient's extremity.
• Return all controls to the zero position for the machine's next use.
• Assess the patient's response to the treatment.

Special considerations

• In aqueous ultrasound application, if the targeted area is an irregular shape, it's best to use degassed water, in an appropriate size container, as your conductive medium. Tap water can be used if necessary, but you will have to continually wipe the air bubbles from your patient and the transducer.

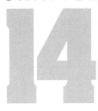

Wound care
Managing the healing process

Anatomy and physiology of the skin

The skin, considered the body's largest organ, consists of two major layers: the epidermis and dermis. A third layer of subcutaneous tissue lies beneath the dermis. Although each of these layers is composed of different types of tissues and cells and performs different functions, they're interrelated

A wound occurs whenever the skin's integrity is altered. Superficial wounds, such as minor cuts and abrasions, usually heal spontaneously in a few days. However, more extensive wounds and chronic wounds require thorough assessment and meticulous care and treatment. Understanding the rationale and measures used for wound treatment requires knowledge of the anatomy and physiology of the skin, the healing process (including methods for wound healing and the phases of wound healing), and the factors affecting wound healing. To achieve successful wound healing, the physical therapist must carefully follow every step in wound management, including assessment, planning, implementation, evaluation, and documentation.

Epidermis

The epidermis is the outermost layer of the skin. It typically renews itself every 4 to 6 weeks, serving as a physical barrier to the outside. The epidermis is thin and avascular and is composed of five sublayers, or *strata*:
- stratum corneum (outermost)
- stratum lucidum
- stratum granulosum
- stratum spinosum
- stratum germinativum (innermost).

For more information, see *Layers of the skin*.

Within the epidermis are three major cell types: keratinocytes, melanocytes, and Langerhans' cells.

Keratinocytes occur chiefly in the uppermost layer of the epidermis and produce keratin, a tough protein that provides the waterproof covering for the body. As these cells are shed or worn from the skin surface, they are continually replaced by new cells from deeper skin layers.

Melanocytes release melanin, a dark pigment that provides color tone to the skin and filters ultraviolet rays. Exposure to ultraviolet light can stimulate melanin formation.

Langerhans' cells, a part of the body's immune system, assist in the initial processing of antigens that enter the epidermis, thereby protecting the skin from allergic reactions. These cells are gradually destroyed by prolonged exposure to ultraviolet radiation, but are replaced by new cells.

Dermis

Directly beneath the epidermis lies the dermis, a thicker, inner layer secured to the epidermis by the stratum germinativum sublayer. The dermis supports and nourishes the epidermis. It's composed of two layers of elastic connective tissue containing blood vessels, lymphatic vessels, nerves, sweat glands, and hair follicles.

Fibroblasts in the dermis produce collagen, giving the skin its strength. Elastin, another protein, forms fibers that help the skin retain its elastic properties. This fibroelastic structure allows the skin to resist external injury. The dermis is secured to the subcutaneous tissue and other under-

LAYERS OF THE SKIN

The skin is composed of two major layers — the epidermis and dermis. As shown below, the epidermis consists of five strata. Subcutaneous tissue lying beneath the dermis consists of loose connective tissue that attaches the skin to underlying structures.

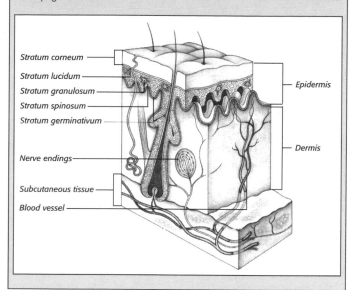

Stratum corneum
Stratum lucidum
Stratum granulosum
Stratum spinosum
Stratum germinativum

Epidermis

Nerve endings

Dermis

Subcutaneous tissue
Blood vessel

lying structures, such as fascia, muscle, and bone, by thick bundles of collagen.

Subcutaneous tissue

The subcutaneous tissue is composed of dense connective and adipose tissue and contains major blood vessels, lymphatics, and nerves. It acts as a heat insulator and provides a nutritional reserve for use during illness or starvation. This layer also acts as a mechanical shock absorber.

Physiologic functions

The skin's primary function is protection. It acts as a physical barrier to the outside environment of microorganisms and other materials to

which it's continuously exposed. Other functions include:
• regulating body temperature through vasoconstriction, vasodilation, and sweating
• providing a mechanism for sensations, such as touch, pressure, pain, and temperature
• maintaining fluid and electrolyte balance
• assisting with the excretion of waste products
• synthesizing vitamin D when exposed to sunlight, which provides the stimulus for calcium and phosphate metabolism
• shaping body image.

Aside from physiologic function, the skin also facilitates communication (for example, through facial expressions and blushing) and it also provides numerous clues to a person's age, ethnicity, gender, and other personal characteristics.

Wound healing

Regardless of their origin, wounds physically disrupt the normal structure and function of the skin and underlying tissue. When a wound occurs, healing occurs. However, certain factors can promote or delay the healing process.

Forms of wound healing

Wound healing or repair is typically classified according to how the wound closes. Wounds heal by primary intention, secondary intention, or tertiary intention.

Wounds with minimal tissue loss and well-approximated edges (close together) may heal by primary intention, (for example, by surgically suturing the edges). Such wounds have a lower risk of infection and heal with minimal scarring, usually in 4 to 14 days.

Wounds with substantial tissue loss that can't be closed surgically (such as pressure ulcers) heal by secondary intention. In these wounds, closure is achieved through the formation of connective tissue or scars (contractions). The connective tissue must completely fill the wound before skin cells can advance from the wound margins to cover the entire wound surface. Healing in this manner is associated with a higher risk of infection and a longer healing time.

Finally, surgical wounds left open for 3 to 5 days to allow resolution of edema or infection or drainage of exudate before being closed surgically with sutures, staples, or skin closures, heal by tertiary intention.

Phases of wound healing

The healing process begins at the moment of injury, proceeding through a cascade of physiologic events. These events are divided into three distinct phases: the inflammatory phase, the proliferative phase, and the maturation phase.

Inflammatory phase

During the inflammatory phase, tissue trauma stimulates an acute inflammatory response characterized by local erythema, heat, edema, and tenderness of the affected tissues, accompanied by pain and a serous exudate. The inflammatory changes serve to initiate hemostasis; fight bacterial invasion primarily through the action of granulocytic leukocytes, particularly polymorphonuclear leukocytes and neutrophils; remove wound debris through the action of macrophages; and encourage epithelial cells to grow. This phase lasts approximately 4 to 6 days.

Proliferative phase

During the proliferative phase, the wound is filled with new connective tissue and capillary networks (granulation). Granulation tissue, appearing as red, beefy, shiny, granular tissue, consists of macrophages, fibroblasts, immature collagen, blood vessels, and ground substance. The fibroblasts stimulate collagen production as the granulation tissue proliferates. This collagen provides strength and structure to the tissues. The wound's surface gradually decreases as granulation tissue fills in the wound and brings its edges closer together.

During the final stages of this phase, epithelial cells migrate across the moist wound surface to cover the wound. However, for epithelialization to occur, the underlying tissue must be viable and contain an adequate vascular supply.

Maturation phase

In the maturation phase, also called the differentiation or remodeling phase, the closed wound matures as the collagen scar undergoes repeated degradation and resynthesis by macrophages and other tissue-repairing cells providing strength to the area. If the concurrent processes of collagen synthesis and breakdown aren't balanced, scar tissue may be either weakened or overdeveloped. This balance is adversely affected by factors, such as reduced capillary oxygen levels and nutritional deficiencies, especially those involving vitamins and amino acids.

Factors affecting wound healing

Optimum conditions must be met for a wound to heal properly. Various factors, whether local or systemic, can affect these conditions.

Local factors

Local factors occurring directly within the wound include:
• *pressure,* which, if sustained or too great, disrupts the blood supply and delays healing
• *dryness,* which causes the cells to dehydrate resulting in the formation of a scab or crust and delays healing (Moisture enhances epithelialization.)
• *trauma, edema, or infection,* which interferes with oxygen and nutrient transport to the wound, delaying healing
• *necrosis,* which must be removed for repair and healing to occur

AGE-RELATED SKIN CHANGES

Dramatic changes occur in all skin layers as a person ages. In the younger adult, skin cells turn over approximately every 3 weeks; in the normal older adult, this turnover slows to once every 2 months. Skin elasticity declines due to progressive degeneration of collagen and elastin. Photosensitivity increases as the number of melanocytes declines. Loss of melanocytes also results in fraying of the hair and fading normal skin color, coupled with reduced capillary blood supply.

Diminished adhesion between the dermis and epidermis causes increased wrinkling and slackness, especially in the extremities, neck, and face. Wrinkling is exacerbated by prolonged sun exposure.

A diminishing blood supply reduces the skin's thermoregulatory function, causing older adults to feel colder in the extremities. The blood vessels themselves become more fragile, leading to easy bruising and formation of senile purpura.

Loss of fat from the subcutaneous tissue predisposes older adults to pressure ulcer formation, especially at the scapulae, trochanters, knees, and other bony prominences.

Ultimately, these changes can impact and possibly impede wound healing.

• *incontinence,* which alters the skin's integrity and delays healing.

Systemic factors

Systemic factors, which involve the entire body, can also affect wound healing. Possible systemic factors impeding wound healing may include:
• age of the skin (See *Age-related skin changes.*)
• obesity or emaciation

• chronic diseases, such as heart disease, diabetes, cancer, and peripheral vascular disease
• impaired nutritional status
• vascular insufficiencies
• immunosuppression and radiation therapy.

Wound assessment

Any effective treatment plan begins with a thorough assessment. However, this assessment takes on an even greater significance for a patient with a wound. It must provide an accurate baseline depiction of the wound for comparison with future assessments to determine the progress of healing. The key to the assessment is identifying populations at risk for wounds such as pressure ulcers. This information, coupled with information about the characteristics of the wound, the patient's nutritional status, and laboratory and diagnostic test results, provides a complete picture for determining the most effective strategy for managing the wound.

Risk assessment

Pressure ulcers are one of the most common types of wounds, primarily resulting from pressure to an area applied with great force for a short period of time or less force over a longer period of time. Most pressure ulcers develop over bony prominences where friction and shearing forces combine with pressure to break down skin and underlying tissue. As a result, circulation is impaired, tissues become hypoxic, and cells die. Certain factors are commonly associated with increasing a patient's risk for pressure ulcers. These may include

prolonged bed rest or immobility, dehydration, impaired circulation, malnutrition, immunosuppression, incontinence, decreased pain awareness, paralysis, significant obesity or emaciation, corticosteroid therapy, and a history of previous pressure ulcers.

Various tools have been developed to identify factors most commonly contributing to pressure ulcer development and to provide a quantitative, objective measure of the patient's risk of pressure ulcers. Two examples are the Norton Scale and the Braden Scale. (See *Using the Norton Scale,* opposite, and *Using the Braden Scale*, pages 380 and 381.)

Wound characteristics

Accurate assessment of wound characteristics is essential in selecting the most appropriate form of wound care management. Wound characteristics include etiology, classification, location, size, appearance, and drainage. For all of these parameters, be sure to use correct terminology and consistent units of measurement.

Etiology

Determining the cause of the wound is essential for correct classification and management. Wounds caused by vascular insufficiency are typically classified by depth, and those caused by pressure are commonly classified by stages. Other essential data include the patient's underlying medical condition (such as diabetes or malnutrition), which may adversely impact wound development or healing, and a wound history, including onset, duration, and previous treatments and outcomes.

USING THE NORTON SCALE

You use the Norton scale to assess the following five conditions and assign appropriate scores. A total score of 14 or less indicates the risk of pressure ulcer development. A score under 12 indicates high risk.

Name _Sally Peters_   Date _3/11/00_

Physical condition		Mental condition		Activity		Mobility		Continence	
Good	4	Alert	4	Walks	4	Full	4	Good	4
Fair	3	Apathetic	3	Walks with help	3	Slightly limited	3	Occasional incontinence	3
Poor	2	Confused	2	Sits in chair	2	Very limited	2	Frequent incontinence	2
Very poor	1	Stuporous	1	Remains in bed	1	Immobile	1	Urine and fecal incontinence	1

TOTAL _3_   TOTAL _3_   TOTAL _2_   TOTAL _3_   TOTAL _3_

Total score   _14_

Adapted with permission from Norton, D., et al. *An Investigation of Geriatric Nursing Problems in the Hospital.* London: National Corporation for the Care of Old People (now the Centre for Policy on Ageing), 1962.

Classification

Although numerous classification systems exist, wounds are generally classified by stage, depth, or color.

By stage

When a classification by stage is used, the wound is identified by the tissue layer involved. This type of classification provides only an anatomic description of the wound's depth. It doesn't describe the wound in its entirety. Pressure ulcers are typically classified by stages. (See *Pressure ulcer staging,* pages 382 and 383.)

By depth

When wounds result from a cause other than pressure, they are typically classified as partial- or full-thickness wounds. Partial-thickness wounds extend through the epidermis and into, but not through, the dermis. These wounds heal primarily by reepithe-lialization. Full-thickness wounds extend through both layers, the epidermis and dermis, and possibly into the subcutaneous tissue, muscle, and bone. These types of wounds heal by granulation, contraction, and reepithelialization. Classifying a wound by depth doesn't account for the tissue layer exposed, the color of the wound, or the status of the surrounding skin.

By color

When color is used to classify a wound, three colors are typically described: red, yellow, and black. Red denotes a wound that is healthy and clean with a layer of pink granulation tissue that eventually changes to beefy red. Yellow denotes a need for cleaning because of exudate or slough. Black indicates the presence of eschar, necrotic tissue that provides a medium for microorganism growth and also slows healing. When a

(Text continues on page 383.)

USING THE BRADEN SCALE

To use the Braden scale, assess the patient for each category, assign a score of 1 to 4, and then calculate the total score. If the patient's score is 16 or less, consider him at high risk for pressure ulcer development.

Sensory perception Ability to respond appropriately to pressure-related discomfort	1. Completely limited Patient is unresponsive to painful stimuli (doesn't moan, flinch, or grasp) or has limited ability to feel pain over most of body surface due to diminished level of consciousness or sedation.	2. Very limited Patient responds only to painful stimuli, can't communicate discomfort except by moaning or restlessness, or has a sensory impairment that limits the ability to feel pain or discomfort over half of body.
Moisture Degree to which skin is exposed to moisture	1. Constantly moist Skin is moistened almost constantly by perspiration, urine, and so on. Dampness is detected every time patient is moved or turned.	2. Moist Skin is usually but not always moist. A linen change is required at least once each shift.
Activity Degree of physical activity	1. Bedbound Patient is confined to bed.	2. Chairbound Patient's ability to walk is severely limited or nonexistent. Patient can't bear his own weight or must be assisted into a chair or wheelchair.
Mobility Ability to change and control body position	1. Completely immobile Patient doesn't make even slight changes in body or extremity position without assistance.	2. Very limited Patient makes occasional slight changes in body or extremity position but is unable to make frequent or significant changes independently.
Nutrition Usual food intake pattern	1. Very poor Patient never eats a complete meal and rarely eats more than one-third of any food offered. Patient eats two servings or less of protein (meat or dairy products) per day, takes fluids poorly, doesn't take a liquid dietary supplement, or is NPO or maintained on clear liquids or I.V. fluids for more than 5 days.	2. Probably inadequate Patient rarely eats a complete meal and generally eats only about one-half of any food offered. Patient eats three servings of protein (meat or dairy products) per day, occasionally will take a dietary supplement, or receives less than an optimum amount of liquid diet or tube feeding.
Friction and shear	1. Problem Patient requires moderate to maximum assistance in moving. Complete lifting without sliding against sheets is impossible and he frequently slides down in the bed or chair, requiring repositioning with maximum assistance. Spasticity, contractures, or agitation lead to almost constant friction.	2. Potential problem Patient moves feebly or requires minimum assistance. During a move, skin slides to some extent against sheets, the chair, restraints, or other devices. Patient maintains relatively good position in a chair or bed most of the time but occasionally slides down.

		DATE OF ASSESSMENT	1/3/00			
3. Slightly limited Patient responds to verbal commands but can't always communicate discomfort or need to be turned or has some sensory impairment that limits his ability to feel pain or discomfort in one or two extremities.	4. No impairment Patient responds to verbal commands and has no sensory deficit that would limit his ability to feel or voice pain or discomfort.		3			
3. Occasionally moist Skin is occasionally moist, and an extra linen change is required approximately once per day.	4. Rarely moist Skin is usually dry and linen requires changing only at routine intervals.		3			
3. Walks occasionally Patient walks occasionally during the day but only for very short distances, with or without assistance. Patient spends most of each shift in a bed or chair.	4. Walks frequently Patient walks outside the room at least twice per day and inside the room at least once every 2 hours during waking hours.		4			
3. Slightly limited Patient independently makes frequent though slight changes in body or extremity position.	4. No limitations Patient makes major and frequent changes in position without assistance.		4			
3. Adequate Patient eats over one-half of most meals and eats a total of four servings of protein (meat or dairy products) each day. Occasionally, patient will refuse a meal but will usually take a supplement if offered or is on a tube feeding or total parenteral nutrition regimen.	4. Excellent Patient eats most of every meal and never refuses a meal. Patient usually eats a total of four or more servings of protein (meat or dairy products) daily. Patient occasionally eats between meals and doesn't require supplementation.		3			
3. No apparent problem Patient moves in a bed or chair independently and has sufficient muscle strength to lift up completely during the move. Patient maintains good position in a bed or chair at all times.			3			
		TOTAL SCORE	20			

PRESSURE ULCER STAGING

The staging system described below is based on the recommendations of the National Pressure Ulcer Advisory Panel (NPUAP) [Consensus Conference, 1991] and the Agency for Health Care Policy and Research (Clinical Practice Guidelines for Treatment of Pressure Ulcers, 1992). The stage 1 definition was updated by the NPUAP in 1997.

Stage 1
A stage 1 pressure ulcer is an observable pressure-related alteration of intact skin whose indicators, as compared to the adjacent or opposite area on the body, may include changes in one or more of the following: skin temperature (warmth or coolness), tissue consistency (firm or boggy feel), and sensation (pain or itching). The ulcer appears as a defined area of persistent redness in lightly pigmented skin; in darker skin tones, the ulcer may appear with persistent red, blue, or purple hues.

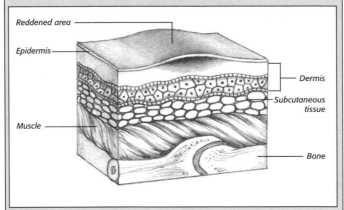

Stage 2
A stage 2 pressure ulcer is characterized by partial-thickness skin loss involving the epidermis or dermis. The ulcer is superficial and presents clinically as an abrasion, blister, or shallow crater.

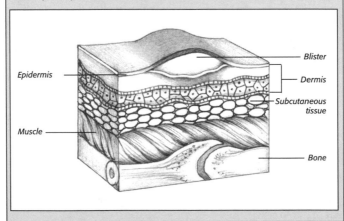

PRESSURE ULCER STAGING (continued)

Stage 3

A stage 3 pressure ulcer is characterized by full-thickness skin loss involving damage or necrosis of subcutaneous tissue, which may extend down to, but not through, underlying fasciae. The ulcer presents clinically as a deep crater with or without the undermining of adjacent tissue.

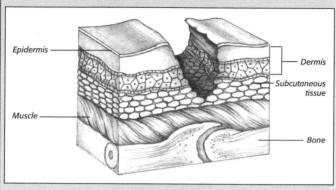

Stage 4

Full-thickness skin loss with extensive destruction, tissue necrosis, or damage to muscle, bone, or support structures (for example, tendon or joint capsule) characterizes a stage 4 pressure ulcer. Tunneling and sinus tracts may be associated with stage 4 pressure ulcers.

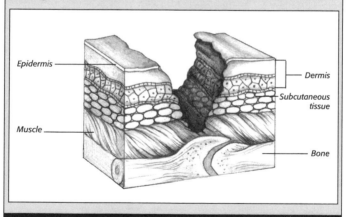

wound shows more than one color, it's classified by the predominant color. This three-color concept was adapted by Marion Laboratories and is used in wound assessment to help direct treatment.

Location

The wound assessment must document the wound's exact location. Be sure to include a complete description of the area involved along with any major landmarks. Often, a standard form using anatomic diagrams is most useful for noting the exact area of the body affected. If multiple wounds are present, each of the areas can be identified by circling the body area on the diagram or marking each area with a different letter.

Size

Typically, wounds are measured for length, width, and depth in centimeters, or by measuring volume. Tunneling, if present, is measured for depth and direction.

Accurate and consistent measurements establish landmarks so that the size of the wound can be measured using the longest and widest measurements in centimeters. Measurements can be taken according to a "clock" orientation, with 12 o'clock aligning to the patient's head.

To measure depth, insert a sterile flexible applicator into the wound and mark the location of the wound's margins with a pen. Then note the depth from the tip of the applicator to the pen mark. Also note depth and location of any tunneling and undermining. After inserting a sterile flexible applicator into the wound and tunnel area, identify the direction of the tunnel as if the applicator was a hand on a clock. Then measure the depth as you would for any wound.

A quick size measurement can be made by multiplying the wound's length by its width. Comparing the surface area measurement on a weekly basis will provide a percent of healing outcome measurement. In addition, the outline of the wound can be traced on transparent paper with a permanent marker; done weekly, this can be used to monitor the healing wound's decreasing size.

If the wound is a pressure ulcer, the stage of the ulcer aids in assessing its size. For example, only length and width measurements are used for a stage 1 pressure ulcer because the

epidermis is intact and there is no measurable depth. Because a stage 2 pressure ulcer extends through the epidermis, length, width, and depth are measured. For stage 3 and 4 pressure ulcers, length, width, depth, and tunneling are assessed.

To obtain the most accurate ongoing assessment of wound size, position the patient in the same manner each time you measure the wound. Be sure to avoid pulling or stretching the tissue while measuring. If appropriate, tracings, photographs, and digital (video) images may also be taken initially and at subsequent intervals to provide a permanent medical record of the wound. If photographs are used, label them with the patient's name and date. Also include a measuring device, such as a small ruler, in the photograph to demonstrate the true size of the wound.

Appearance

Wound appearance includes the color of the wound bed and margins, the status of the surrounding skin, including its color and temperature, and any evidence of exposed bone or foreign objects, such as sutures, staples, or metal. When documenting wound appearance, be as specific as possible and use precise descriptions.

Drainage

Drainage from a wound may be normal or abnormal depending on its color, consistency, amount, and odor. Drainage color and consistency are described as serous (clear, watery plasma), serosanguineous (plasma containing red blood cells), sanguineous (bloody plasma), and purulent (thick, white blood cells and living or dead organisms).

When describing the amount of drainage, try to quantify it using common measures, such as "the size of a dime or quarter" and "a 2-inch circular area on the dressing." If this isn't possible, use descriptive terms, such as "scant," "light," "moderate," "heavy," "large," and "copious."

Other characteristics

When assessing a patient's wound, investigate the possibility of underlying local or systemic factors that may affect healing. Also note any verbal or nonverbal indicators of pain or complaints of tenderness because these may indicate infection, underlying tissue destruction not yet visible, or vascular insufficiency. Conversely, don't overlook the patient's apparent *lack* of pain — this may indicate neuropathy or nerve damage.

Nutritional status

A balanced diet with adequate nutrient intake is vital for the growth and maintenance of all tissues. For patients with wounds or those at risk for wounds, this takes on even greater importance because adequate nutrition is necessary for the healing process. Although each nutrient is involved in specific aspects of wound healing, these nutrients work together to ensure use, absorption, and transport of other nutrients. (See *Nutrient roles in wound healing*, page 386.)

One of the goals of wound treatment is to provide sufficient calories to maintain the patient's weight and prevent weight loss. Generally, protein intake is increased to ensure a positive nitrogen balance and replace any protein lost through the wound. Vitamins and minerals should meet or exceed the recommended daily allowances. Supplements, such as vitamin C and zinc, may be needed to promote wound healing.

Laboratory and diagnostic tests

Laboratory and diagnostic tests provide valuable information about the patient's general health and condition of all the body systems. Blood tests, such as white blood cell count, red blood cell count, hemoglobin, and hematocrit, are routinely performed to evaluate the patient's overall health status. Additionally, total serum protein, albumin, transferrin, and total lymphocyte counts are performed to evaluate the patient's nutritional status. Coagulation studies, such as activated partial thromboplastin time and prothrombin time, may be obtained to evaluate the patient's ability to achieve hemostasis.

Because the transport of oxygen and nutrients is necessary for cellular growth and function, additional tests may be performed to evaluate the patient's vascular status and determine the adequacy of blood flow. These may include:

• *Ankle-brachial index (ABI):* ABI compares systolic blood pressure in the ankle arteries with systolic blood pressure in the brachial artery. A normal ABI is 1 to 1.2; an ABI of 0.8 or less indicates an obstruction.

• *Doppler ultrasonography:* Doppler ultrasonography evaluates blood flow using sound waves to produce a tone that correlates directly with blood flow velocity.

• *Duplex ultrasonography:* Duplex ultrasonography evaluates arterial or venous blood flow using ultrasonic imaging and Doppler ultrasound techniques.

• *Impedance plethysmography:* Impedance plethysmography measures changes in blood volume in the calf secondary to temporary venous occlusion.

• *Arteriography* and *venography:* Arteriography and venography use radiopaque contrast medium to visual-

NUTRIENT ROLES IN WOUND HEALING

Nutrient	Roles in wound healing
Calcium	Aids action of tissue collagenases Helps promote normal hemostasis during the inflammatory phase
Carbohydrates	Provide glucose for wound repair Form ground substance during proliferative phase
Copper	Strengthens scar tissue Provides cross-linkages associated with collagen formation
Fats	Supply cellular energy Produce prostaglandins, which mediate activity of the inflammatory phase
Iron	Forms collagen during the proliferative phase
Magnesium	Aids in protein synthesis and energy release Maintains muscle and nerve tissue function
Manganese	Synthesizes collagen during the proliferative phase
Protein	Supports cellular proliferation Synthesizes collagen
Vitamin A	Allows epithelialization Promotes collagen synthesis
Vitamin B	Provides cofactors for enzyme systems
Vitamin C	Promotes collagen synthesis Aids neutrophil formation Required for normal fibroblastic activity
Zinc	Promotes protein synthesis Enhances collagen synthesis

ize arteries or veins and blood flow through them.

If a wound infection is suspected, aerobic and anaerobic wound cultures are taken to identify the causative organism. A bacterial count of greater than 100,000 per gram of tissue indicates an infection.

Outcome measures

Wound assessment is an ongoing activity. Continuous monitoring and accurate documentation of any changes in the wound are crucial. To ensure accurate, consistent monitoring and continuity of care and to promote communication among health care team members, numerous tools exist to monitor wound healing. The Pressure Sore Status Tool shown on the following pages is one example. (See *Gauging pressure sore status,* pages 387 to 390.)

Wound management

All wounds need to be cleaned and, if necessary, debrided. Both of these
(Text continues on page 390.)

GAUGING PRESSURE SORE STATUS

The Pressure Sore Status Tool provides a means for monitoring pressure ulcers based on 15 items. Of these, 13 items are given a numeric score, which can be plotted on the Pressure Sore Status Continuum. Thus, a quick glance at the continuum can provide information about the progress of the wound and the need for a possible change in the treatment plan.

PRESSURE SORE STATUS TOOL

Name: _David Stevens_

Complete the rating sheet to assess pressure sore status. Evaluate each item by picking the response that best describes the wound and entering the score in the item score column for the appropriate date.

Location: anatomic site. Circle, identify right (R) or left (L), and use an "X" to mark the site on body diagrams.

✓ (Sacrum and coccyx) ___ Lateral ankle
___ Trochanter   ___ Medial ankle
___ Ischial tuberosity ___ Heel
___ Other site

Shape: overall wound pattern. Assess this by observing perimeter and depth. Circle and date the appropriate description.

___ Irregular   ___ Linear or elongated
3/9 (Round or oval)   ___ Bowl or boat
___ Square or rectangle ___ Butterfly
___ Other shape

Item	Assessment	Date	Date	Date
		3/9 Score	Score	Score
1. Size	1 = Length × width less than 4 cm² 2 = Length × width 4 to 16 cm² 3 = Length × width 16.1 to 36 cm² 4 = Length × width 36.1 to 80 cm² 5 = Length × width greater than 80 cm²	1		
2. Depth	1 = Nonblanchable erythema on intact skin 2 = Partial-thickness skin loss involving epidermis or dermis 3 = Full-thickness skin loss involving damage or necrosis of subcutaneous tissue; may extend down to but not through underlying fasciae; or mixed partial- and full-thickness wounds; or tissue layers obscured by granulation tissue 4 = Obscured by necrosis 5 = Full-thickness skin loss with extensive destruction, tissue necrosis, or damage to muscle, bone, or supporting structures	2		

(continued)

GAUGING PRESSURE SORE STATUS (continued)		Date	Date	Date
Item	Assessment	3/9 Score	Score	Score
3. Edges	1 = Indistinct, diffuse, none clearly visible 2 = Distinct, outline clearly visible, attached, even with wound base 3 = Well-defined, not attached to wound base 4 = Well-defined, not attached to base, rolled-under, thickened 5 = Well-defined, fibrotic, scarred or hyperkeratotic	2		
4. Undermining	1 = Undermining less than 2 cm in any area 2 = Undermining 2 to 4 cm involving less than 50% of wound margins 3 = Undermining 2 to 4 cm involving greater than 50% of wound margins 4 = Undermining greater than 4 cm in any area 5 = Tunneling or sinus tract formation	1		
5. Necrotic tissue type	1 = None visible 2 = White-gray nonviable tissue or nonadherent, yellow slough 3 = Loosely adherent, yellow slough 4 = Adherent, soft, back eschar 5 = Firmly adherent, hard, black eschar	1		
6. Necrotic tissue amount	1 = None visible 2 = Less than 25% of wound bed covered 3 = 25% to 50% of wound bed covered 4 = Greater than 50% and less than 75% of wound bed covered 5 = 75% to 100% of wound bed covered	1		
7. Exudate type	1 = None or bloody 2 = Serosanguineous (thin, watery, pale red or pink) 3 = Serous (thin, watery, clear) 4 = Purulent (thin or thick, opaque, tan or yellow) 5 = Foul-smelling, purulent (thick, opaque, yellow or green with odor)	2		
8. Exudate amount	1 = None 2 = Scant 3 = Small 4 = Moderate 5 = Large	2		

GAUGING PRESSURE SORE STATUS (continued)

Item	Assessment	Date 3/9 Score	Date Score	Date Score
9. Skin color surrounding wound	1 = Pink or normal for ethnic group 2 = Bright red or blanches to touch 3 = White or gray pallor or hypopigmented 4 = Dark red or purple or nonblanchable 5 = Black or hypopigmented	2		
10. Peripheral tissue edema	1 = Minimal swelling around wound 2 = Nonpitting edema extends less than 4 cm around wound 3 = Nonpitting edema extends 4 cm or more around wound 4 = Pitting edema extends less than 4 cm around wound 5 = Crepitus or pitting edema extends 4 cm or more around wound	1		
11. Peripheral tissue induration	1 = Minimal firmness around wound 2 = Induration less than 2 cm around wound 3 = Induration 2 to 4 cm, extending less than 50% around wound 4 = Induration 2 to 4 cm, extending 50% or more around wound 5 = Induration greater than 4 cm in any area	1		
12. Granulation tissue	1 = Skin intact or partial-thickness wound 2 = Bright, beefy red; 75% to 100% of wound filled or tissue overgrowth 3 = Bright, beefy red; less than 75% and greater than 25% of wound filled 4 = Pink or dull, dusky red and fills 25% or less of wound 5 = No granulation tissue present	1		
13. Epithelialization	1 = 100% wound covered and surface intact 2 = 75% to less than 100% of wound covered or epithelial tissue extends greater than 0.5 cm into wound bed 3 = 50% to less than 75% of wound covered or epithelial tissue extends to less than 0.5 cm into wound bed 4 = 25% to less than 50% of wound covered 5 = Less than 25% of wound covered	1		
Total score		18		
Signature	*Pat Sloan*			

(continued)

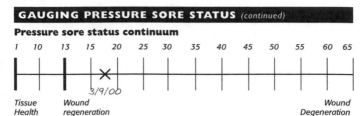

Pressure sore status continuum

| 1 | 10 | 13 | 15 | 20 | 25 | 30 | 35 | 40 | 45 | 50 | 55 | 60 | 65 |

X
3/9/00

Tissue   *Wound*   *Wound*
Health   *regeneration*   *Degeneration*

Plot the total score on the Pressure Sore Status Continuum by putting an "X" on the line and the date beneath the line. Plot multiple scores with their dates to see regeneration or degeneration of the wound at a glance.

Adapted with permission from Sussman, C., and Bates-Jensen, B., eds. *Wound Care: A Collaborative Practice Manual for Physical Therapists and Nurses.* Gaithersburg, Md.: Aspen Publishers, 1998.

measures permit wound assessment and healthy tissue regeneration and minimize the risk of infection. Diabetic, arterial and venous ulcers may all require different forms of management. (See *Grading diabetic ulcers,* opposite; *Treatment algorithm for diabetic ulcers,* page 392; *Treatment guidelines for arterial ulcers,* page 393; and *Treatment algorithm for venous ulcers,* page 394.)

Cleansing

Cleansing the wound removes bacteria and debris, preserves the surrounding skin surface to minimize the extent of chemical and mechanical trauma, and protects healthy granulation tissue. Wounds are usually cleaned with normal saline solution because it's cost effective and readily available. Saline solution supplies moisture to encourage healing and minimizes fluid shifting in healthy cells because it's isotonic. Acetic acid, hydrogen peroxide, sodium hypochlorite (Dakin's solution), and povidone-iodine are also used for cleaning certain types of wounds, but they are also more likely to cause tissue damage and delay healing.

The choice of which solution to use depends on the characteristics of the wound, the presence of infection, and the risks and benefits to the patient. For example, povidone-iodine kills gram-negative and gram-positive bacteria, fungi, viruses, protozoa, and yeasts. Acetic acid suppresses the growth of *Pseudomonas aeruginosa.* Sodium hypochlorite solution is helpful in dissolving necrotic tissue and also in managing suppurative wounds.

When cleaning any wound, always follow standard precautions, wiping from the cleanest area toward less clean areas and using a new pad or swab for each stroke. If a wound needs to be irrigated, use a bulb or piston syringe or a gravity drip to generate low pressure.

Debridement

Debridement is the selective removal of necrotic, nonviable tissue from a wound to prevent or control infection and promote healing. Usually performed on serious burns, debridement removes hard black eschar, yellowish, stringy slough and, if necessary, underlying muscle and fat tissue. Debridement is performed to

GRADING DIABETIC ULCERS

When you've evaluated the diabetic patient's ulcer and determined its grade using the Wagner ulcer grade classification, follow the treatment guidelines listed below.

Wagner grade and characteristics	Interventions
Grade 0 • Preulcer lesion • Healed ulcer • Presence of bony deformity	• Maintain skin integrity. • Observe for changes.
Grade 1 • Superficial ulcer without subcutaneous tissue involvement	• Use padding and accommodative devices. • Debride callus. • Instruct patient on foot care, footwear selection, and when to seek medical attention.
Grade 2 • Penetration through the subcutaneous tissue, possibly exposing bone, tendon, ligament, or joint capsule	• Follow grade 1 protocol. • Apply topical silver sulfadiazine. • Use antiseptic soaks. • Apply occlusive or nonocclusive dressing. • Use gauze dressing on plantar surface. • Evaluate weekly until healing occurs.
Grade 3 • Osteitis, abscess, or osteomyelitis	• Follow grade 1 protocol. • Rule out osteomyelitis (X-ray, bone scan, bone biopsy). • Provide non-weight-bearing surface. • Apply topical antimicrobial cream, ointment, or amorphous hydrogel. • Use gauze dressing on plantar surface. • Use occlusive dressing on dorsal surface. • Seek surgical consultation.
Grade 4 • Gangrene of a digit	• Follow grade 1 protocol. • Rule out osteomyelitis (X-ray, bone scan, bone biopsy). • Use antiseptic soaks. • Apply topical antimicrobial cream, ointment, or amorphous hydrogel. • Use gauze dressing on plantar surface. • Use occlusive dressing on dorsal surface. • Seek surgical consultation.
Grade 5 • Gangrene requiring foot amputation	• Refer for surgical intervention.

Adapted with permission from Glugla, M., and Mulder, G.D. "The Diabetic Foot: Medical Management of Food Ulcers," in *Chronic Wound Care*, edited by Krasner, D. King of Prussia, Pa.: Health Management Publications, Inc., 1990.

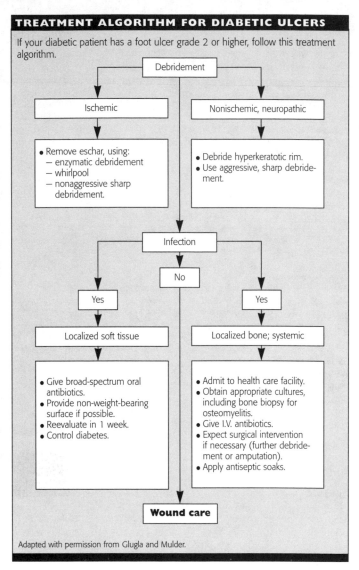

TREATMENT ALGORITHM FOR DIABETIC ULCERS

If your diabetic patient has a foot ulcer grade 2 or higher, follow this treatment algorithm.

Adapted with permission from Glugla and Mulder.

enhance the wound healing process and to prevent infection. Four basic methods of debridement include mechanical (using dressings or water), surgical (or sharp), enzymatic, and autolytic. (See *Guide to wound debridement,* page 395.)

Mechanical debridement

Mechanical debridement requires the use of an outside force to remove dead tissue. This can be accomplished using wet-to-dry dressings, hydrotherapy, or pulsatile lavage (wound irrigation using pressure ranging from 4 to 15 psi). Mechanical debridement is used primarily for moist necrotic wounds.

Surgical debridement

In surgical, or sharp, debridement, dead or devitalized tissue is removed with a sharp instrument or laser. This type of debridement, performed once or in a sequential fashion, can be done at the patient's bedside or in the operating room. Surgical debridement is indicated for extensively devitalized tissue, callus formation, and thick adherent eschar as well as in situations where the patient exhibits signs of advancing infection.

Enzymatic debridement

In enzymatic debridement, specific enzyme-containing ointments or solutions are used to break down necrotic tissue. An example of an enzymatic debriding agent is collagenase ointment. Such agents require a moist environment. If dry eschar is present, it must be incised (crosshatched) first for the agent to be effective. Enzymatic debridement works best on moist necrotic wounds.

Autolytic debridement

In autolytic debridement, necrotic tissue is broken down by the body's own white blood cells and enzymes. This is usually accomplished by applying a moisture-retaining dressing to the wound. The wound surface remains moist, promoting rehydration of the dead tissue. The wound fluid contains white blood cells and enzymes, which break down the necrotic tissue. (For more information, see "Dressings," page 394.)

TREATMENT GUIDELINES FOR ARTERIAL ULCERS

Because arterial ulcers result from inadequate blood supply, treatment depends on the extent of vascular insufficiency. Most patients with these ulcers benefit from a revascularization procedure such as femoral-popliteal bypass. However, when surgery isn't an option — as with a frail elderly patient — patient comfort and prevention of wound deterioration become the goals of therapy.

To prevent deterioration, use the following topical treatments:
- enzymatic debridement
- wet-to-damp dressings
- alginates
- amorphous hydrogels
- nonadherent, nonocclusive dressings.

Don't surgically debride these wounds; further trauma will increase wound size because of inadequate blood supply. Also, don't use occlusive dressings; the wounds can deteriorate rapidly under dressings that prevent close observation.

Adapted with permission from Hess, C.T. *Nurse's Clinical Guide to Wound Care*, 3rd ed. Springhouse, Pa.: Springhouse Corp., 2000.

Adjunctive wound care

In addition to cleansing and debriding wounds, other methods of wound care may be used. These adjunctive measures include dressings, support surfaces, compression, ultrasound, electrical stimulation, hyperbaric oxygen, and tissue growth factors. It's important to plan carefully to obtain the best treatment outcome. A decision tree can be very helpful. (See *Topical treatment algorithm for wound care,* pages 396 and 397.)

TREATMENT ALGORITHM FOR VENOUS ULCERS

Use this algorithm to plan your care for a patient with a venous ulcer. However, if your patient also has arterial complications, obtain a vascular consultation before beginning therapy.

Debridement

Yes → **Necrotic tissue**

- Remove eschar, using:
  - wet-to-dry debridement
  - whirlpool
  - sharp debridement.

Yes → **Fibrotic tissue**

- Leave small amounts intact.
- Remove moderate to large amounts using:
  - wet-to-dry debridement
  - whirlpool
  - sharp debridement
  - enzymatic debridement.

Infection

Yes → **Localized**

- Give oral antibiotics.
- Verify no occlusion.

No

Compression

Yes → **Systemic**

- Admit to health care facility.
- Give I.V. antibiotics.
- Verify no occlusion.

Yes

- Therapy may include:
  - antiembolism stockings
  - elastic bandages
  - sequential compression therapy.

No

- Contraindicated in:
  - infection
  - weeping dermatitis
  - arterial disease
  - heart failure.

Adapted with permission from Hess.

Dressings

Selection of the type of wound dressing — dry or moist — depends on the color, depth, and amount of wound exudate; the condition of the tissue and surrounding skin; presence of infection; and any underlying medical conditions that may impact the wound or wound healing.

(Text continues on page 398.)

GUIDE TO WOUND DEBRIDEMENT

The table below lists the major advantages and disadvantages of the four basic methods of wound debridement.

Method	Advantages	Disadvantages
Mechanical debridement: wet-to-dry dressings	• Readily available • Easily performed • Familiar to most health care providers	• Nonselective • May cause pain on removal • Rarely applied correctly • May remove healthy along with necrotic tissue
Mechanical debridement: hydrotherapy	• Softens necrotic tissue • Increases circulation • Loosens debris • Removes topical agents	• Nonselective • Possible maceration or damage to tissue • May increase edema • Procedure is painful and frightening • Washes away exogenous enzymes
Mechanical debridement: pulsatile lavage	• Cleans debris, exudate, and residual agents out of wound • Softens necrotic tissue • Increases circulation • Easily performed • Reduces bacterial growth	• Nonselective • Painful to patient • May disrupt newly granulated and healthy tissue • May dehydrate wound • May increase edema • Wound is chilled by lavage solutions
Surgical or sharp debridement	• Quickly restores wound from necrotic to healthy state • Highly selective • Often combined with other methods to speed removal of necrotic tissue	• Requires high skill level • Not recommended for ischemic ulcers unless collateral circulation is present • Patient premedication necessary • Increased risk for bleeding
Enzymatic debridement	• Useful with other types of debridement • Requires less skill to perform than sharp debridement • Product choices provide selective debridement	• Nonselective • Expensive • Requires secondary dressing • May require up to 30 days for debridement to occur • Uncomfortable to patient • May cause maceration of surrounding tissue
Autolytic debridement	• Noninvasive, very safe • Relatively painless for patient • Requires minimal professional expertise • Easily performed • Doesn't disrupt healthy tissue • Useful with other forms of debridement • Inexpensive • Possibly very selective • Wide variety of semipermeable to nonpermeable dressings available	• Longest duration of all methods • May cause maceration of surrounding tissue • May promote bacterial growth • Contraindicated for infected wounds

TOPICAL TREATMENT ALGORITHM FOR WOUND CARE

Use this chart to help you effectively assess, plan, intervene, and evaluate wounds. You'll need to exclude patients with diabetic or neurotrophic ulcers and those with stage 3 or 4 osteomyelitis, systemic infection, or venous stasis ulcers.

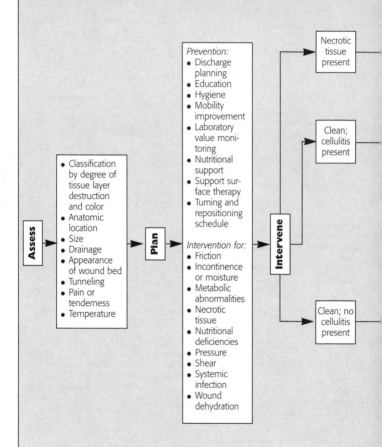

Adapted with permission from Hess.

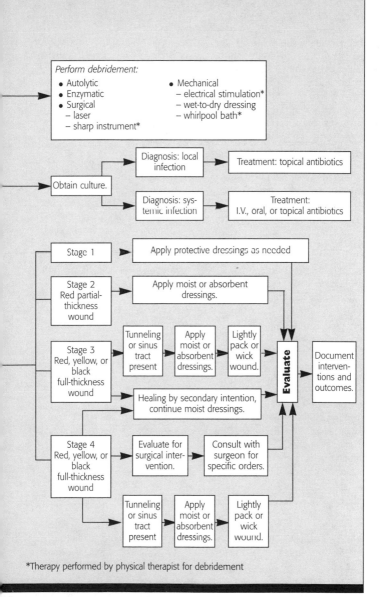

Perform debridement:
- Autolytic
- Enzymatic
- Surgical
  - laser
  - sharp instrument*
- Mechanical
  - electrical stimulation*
  - wet-to-dry dressing
  - whirlpool bath*

Obtain culture. → Diagnosis: local infection → Treatment: topical antibiotics

Obtain culture. → Diagnosis: systemic infection → Treatment: I.V., oral, or topical antibiotics

Stage 1 → Apply protective dressings as needed

Stage 2 Red partial-thickness wound → Apply moist or absorbent dressings.

Stage 3 Red, yellow, or black full-thickness wound → Tunneling or sinus tract present → Apply moist or absorbent dressings. → Lightly pack or wick wound.

Healing by secondary intention, continue moist dressings.

Stage 4 Red, yellow, or black full-thickness wound → Evaluate for surgical intervention. → Consult with surgeon for specific orders.

Tunneling or sinus tract present → Apply moist or absorbent dressings. → Lightly pack or wick wound.

Evaluate → Document interventions and outcomes.

*Therapy performed by physical therapist for debridement

Although most familiar, dry gauze dressings have several drawbacks. They are fibrous and permeable to microorganisms, possibly increasing the risk of infection. They tend to shed fibers easily, possibly exposing the wound to further contamination. Because they are highly absorptive, gauze dressings dry out the wound surface quickly and adhere to it as well, often causing injury to the wound when removed.

Moist wound coverings include films, foams, hydrogels, biosynthetics, collagens, composites, contact layers, hydrocolloids, alginates, and hydroactive dressings. (See *Guide to moist wound dressings,* pages 400 and 401.)

Support surfaces

A variety of support surfaces are available to control pressure, friction, and shear (parallel forces resulting from the interplay of gravity and friction causing stretching and twisting of the tissues and blood vessels). When used properly, they can also decrease or control moisture and inhibit bacterial growth. These surfaces aid in managing tissue load, creating an environment that enhances soft tissue viability and promotes wound healing. The Agency for Health Care Policy and Research (AHCPR) has identified support surfaces as an important adjunct to pressure ulcer prevention and treatment. Research has so far failed to show that one support surface performs better than another.

There are two types of support surfaces. *Static* support surfaces maintain constant inflation by using materials that conform to the body surface. *Dynamic* support surfaces use alternating inflation and deflation to spread the pressure load over a large surface.

Support surfaces are further categorized as pressure-reducing or pressure-relieving support surfaces. The major difference between the two is the consistency of the device in lowering pressure.

Support surfaces are available for beds, chairs, and all clinical stretchers and tables. Proper positioning and turning are essential to achieve the best outcome and wound healing.

Pressure-reducing support surfaces

Pressure-reducing support surfaces, as the name implies, reduce pressure; however, they don't reduce this pressure consistently in all positions or on all body surfaces. Typically, this type of support surface is indicated for patients at risk for pressure ulcers who can be turned and who have existing skin breakdown that is limited to only one sleep surface.

Pressure-reducing support surfaces include mattress overlays or replacement mattresses. Foam, air, or gel mattress overlays and water-filled mattresses are examples of static pressure-reducing support surfaces. Alternating-pressure air mattresses are an example of a dynamic pressure-reducing support surface.

When using a mattress overlay, the patient may experience "bottoming out." This occurs when the patient's body sinks down and the support surface is compressed and unable to function properly. As a result, the patient's body is lying directly on the hospital bed mattress; thus pressure isn't reduced in that area. To prevent this, monitor your patient by placing a flat, outstretched hand between the overlay and the patient's body part. If you feel less than 1″ (2.5 cm) of the support surface, bottoming out has occurred. Perform this check when the patient is in different positions. Always check for bottoming out in the areas at high risk for breakdown when the patient is in different positions. For example, when the patient is supine, check for bottoming out in the sacral area and at the heels.

Pressure-relieving support surfaces

Pressure-relieving support surfaces differ from pressure-reducing support surfaces because they consistently reduce the pressure in any body part and in most body areas. Pressure-relieving support surfaces are indicated for patients who are at high risk for pressure ulcers, who can't turn independently, and who have skin breakdown in more than one body surface area.

The major types of pressure-reducing support surfaces available include low air loss, fluidized air, and kinetic therapies. Low air loss therapy consists of a bed frame containing a series of air pillows that are connected and covered by a low-friction material. Each air pillow contains a controlled amount of air that can be calibrated for the individual patient. This type of therapy relieves pressure when the patient is placed in any position.

Fluidized air therapy provides air and fluid support. It consists of a bed frame containing silicone-coated glass beads that act as a fluid when infiltrated by a stream of air. The beads are alkaline and can trap microorganisms. However, the warm, dry air may also increase fluid loss through evaporation, placing the patient at risk for dehydration.

Kinetic therapy provides continuous passive motion. This is achieved in one of two ways: the bed frame moves or air cushions inflate and deflate, moving the patient from side to side or causing a pulsating motion.

Selection of support surfaces

The choice of support surface for your patient is highly individualized. However, general guidelines have been developed by the AHCPR to aid in this selection process. The AHCPR recommends:

• placing any patient at risk for developing pressure ulcers on a dynamic (pressure-reducing) support surface
• using a static support surface if the patient can assume different positions without weight bearing on an existing pressure ulcer and without bottoming out
• using a dynamic support surface if the patient can't assume different positions without weight bearing on an existing pressure ulcer, if the patient fully compresses the static support surface, or if the pressure ulcer shows no evidence of healing.

The AHCPR also recommends low air loss or fluidized air therapy for patients with large stage 3 and 4 pressure ulcers in multiple areas. In addition to these recommendations, other factors need to be considered, including:

• tissue history
• patient's body build
• location of the highest pressure
• number of hours spent on the surface per day
• effects of shear and friction
• environmental factors, such as temperature, humidity, and moisture (including moisture from incontinence)
• deficits increasing or decreasing the risk of pressure ulcer development
• cost
• availability for reimbursement.

Regardless of the support surface chosen and used, proper positioning, meticulous skin care, and adequate nutritional intake are the keys to maximizing the effectiveness of the

(Text continues on page 402.)

GUIDE TO MOIST WOUND DRESSINGS

The chart below highlights some of the most common types of moist wound dressings. These dressings produce a moist wound environment that is conducive to wound healing.

Type	Indications
Films (transparent polyurethane or similar synthetic film, coated on one side with a water-resistant, hypoallergenic adhesive)	• Minor burns and scalds • Abrasions and lacerations • Incisional sites • I.V. catheter insertion sites • Superficial pressure areas
Foams (spongelike polymer dressing composed of different layers, which are hydrophilic on wound side and hydrophobic on outside)	• Superficial and cavity-type wounds • Leg ulcers • Pressure ulcers • Sutured incisions • Skin grafts • Minor burns • Secondary dressing over amorphous hydrogels
Hydrogels (water- or glycerin-based amorphous gels or sheets)	• Dry and sloughy wounds • Simple partial-thickness burns • Leg ulcers • Pressure ulcers • Extravasation injuries • Necrotic wounds
Hydrocolloids (occlusive, adhesive hydroactive wafers, pastes, powders or granules that form a gel and may contain pectin or gelatin, which can leave a residue in the wound)	• Superficial leg ulcers • Burns • Donor sites after hemostasis • Small cavity wounds in combination with hydrocolloids
Alginates (hydrophilic, nonwoven fiber derived from seaweed that converts to a firm gel or fiber mat when activated by wound exudate; has alginic acid as the main factor converted to a mixed calcium and sodium salt)	• Exuding wounds • Leg ulcers • Cavity wounds • Pressure ulcers • Infected wounds
Hydroactive (similar to hydrocolloids without gel formation; a multilayer absorbent polymer gel with adhesive backing)	• Exuding wounds • Leg ulcers • Pressure ulcers • Minor burns

Advantages	Disadvantages	Examples
• Conforms well to body area • Allows visual monitoring • Permeable to oxygen • Fair moisture-vapor transmission • No dissolution into wound	• Unable to absorb large amounts of exudate • Unable to maintain body temperature in the wound • Easily detached by mechanical forces • Possible wound tissue trauma from adhesive	• OpSite • BIOCLUSIVE • Tegaderm
• Good exudate absorption • Maintains body temperature in wound site • Little or no irritation of healing tissue upon removal • Good biocompatibility to periwound tissue	• Tape or covering required • Doesn't allow visual monitoring of the wound	• Allevyn • HYDRA-SORB • Lyofoam
• Good moisture vapor transmission • Cools wound temperature • Fills in dead space • Allows visual monitoring of wound • Enhances autolytic debridement • Doesn't adhere to healthy tissue	• Requires covering and adhesive to keep in place • More expensive • Tends to dry out • Unable to absorb large amounts of exudate • Unable to keep bacteria out of the wound alone	• Carrasyn Gel • DuoDERM Gel
• Easily molded • Self-adhesive • Provides some absorption • Impermeable to bacteria and contaminants • Remains in place for 3 to 5 days, decreasing trauma • Promotes debridement	• Not recommended for infected wounds or wounds with tunneling or heavy exudate • Not transparent • Occlusive (limits gas exchange)	• Comfeel • Tegasorb • DuoDERM
• Highly absorbent (up to 20 times its weight), excellent for medium or heavy exudate • Doesn't irritate upon removal • Easy to conform	• More expensive than other dressings • Easily disturbed by mechanical forces • Very permeable; requires secondary dressing	• AlgiDERM • CURASORB • Sorbsan
• Highly effective over joint areas • Expands and contracts without constrictive effects • Highly absorbable • Waterproof • Semipermeable to water vapor	• Not for use with infected or nonexuding wounds • Care necessary when applied to fine or easily damaged skin	• TIELLE • Cutinova (thin, hydro, or foam)

COMPARING TYPES OF COMPRESSION THERAPY

The chart below highlights some of the major similarities and differences among different types of compression therapy.

Type of therapy	Indications	Advantages
Elastic wraps	• Dependent edema • Nonambulatory patients with edema	• Easy to apply and remove • Inexpensive • Increased patient independence with self-application
Paste bandages	• Inability to comply with other compression methods • Inability to wrap legs every day • Temporary assistance while awaiting custom-fit devices	• Doesn't require daily changing • Application only every 4 to 7 days
Compression stockings	• Venous disease • Lymphedema	• Graduated compression • Stockings last 4 to 7 months • Variety of stockings available • Cosmetically acceptable appearance
Intermittent sequential compression devices	• Edema without ulcers • Unsuccessful treatment with customized pressure stockings or elastic bandages • Lower-extremity ulcers	• Gradual compression provided by pump • Intermittent use only • Easy to use

support surface to promote optimal wound healing.

Compression therapy

Compression therapy helps promote the movement of excess fluid in the tissues (edema) back to the vascular space. Compression therapy is indicated for patients with vascular or lymphatic disease and those who are experiencing increased interstitial fluid volume secondary to cirrhosis, renal failure, protein-calorie malnutrition, or hormonal drug therapy. Compression therapy can be used in conjunction with leg elevation and exercise to decrease edema. It can also be used alone when leg elevation

and exercise have failed to reduce edema.

A variety of compression therapy devices are available, including elastic wraps, paste bandages such Unna's boot, graduated compression stockings, and intermittent sequential compression devices. The level of support provided by each of these devices varies. For example, elastic wraps and paste bandages provide low compression while intermittent sequential compression devices provide moderate to high compression. (See *Comparing types of compression therapy*.)

Keep in mind that compression therapy is contraindicated in patients with an ankle-brachial index less

Disadvantages

• Requires removal at night
• Patient teaching and practice necessary for correct application

• No showering while in place
• Odor possible on removal
• Increased risk for new wounds if applied incorrectly

• Difficulty in application for patients with musculoskeletal hand problems such as arthritis
• Not always covered by insurance
• Consistent wearing required for positive effect
• Contraindicated in patients with extensive leg ulcers or circumferential wounds

• Restriction to bed or chair while using device
• Additional compression therapy needed when device isn't in use

than 0.5 because this value suggests compromised arterial blood flow.

Ultrasound

Ultrasound provides mechanical vibration through the use of sound waves. It affects the inflammatory and proliferative phases of wound healing. Applied in the inflammatory phase, ultrasound causes mast cells to degranulate and release histamines and other chemical mediators. These are thought to attract neutrophils and monocytes to the injured area, thus accelerating the acute inflammatory phase and promoting healing. Applied in the proliferative phase, ultrasound stimulates fibro-

blasts to secrete collagen, accelerating wound contraction and strengthening healing tissue.

The lowest intensity of ultrasound is used to produce the desired result. Typically, the wound bed and margins are covered with a hydrogel dressing. If the wound has a cavity, this is usually filled with an aqueous gel and then covered with the dressing. Next, the therapist applies conductive gel to the dressing and begins treating the wound by moving the transducer over the area. Usually, acute wounds are treated once or twice per day until inflammation subsides, then two to three times weekly. If appropriate, the area surrounding the wound may also be treated with ultrasound to provide mild heating, which stimulates circulation. In either case, if the patient complains of pain, the intensity should be reduced or the treatment discontinued to prevent complications.

Electrical stimulation

Electrical stimulation uses an electric current to transfer energy to a wound. This current is transferred through a surface electrode applied to the area. The electrode is in wet contact with the external skin surface or wound bed. When electrical stimulation is used, two electrodes are necessary to complete the circuit. Electrodes are usually applied over a wet conductive substance (such as saline-soaked gauze) in the wound bed and on the skin at a distance away from the wound.

The theory behind electrical stimulation is the belief that the body has its own bioelectric system, which influences wound healing. It does this by attracting the cells involved in healing, changing cell membrane permeability, and enhancing cellular secretion. When a break in the skin occurs, a current called the *current of injury*, is generated between the skin and inner tissues and continues until the break is repaired. Healing is stopped or incomplete if the current no long flows while the wound is open. A moist wound environment is also needed for this bioelectric system to function properly. Thus, applying electrical stimulation is believed to mimic the natural current of injury, initiating or accelerating the wound healing process.

Keeping a wound moist with normal saline solution is preferred because it's similar to the electrolyte composition of the wound fluid and, therefore, maintains the optimal bioelectric charge. Dressings, such as moist saline gauze, amorphous hydrogels, and occlusive dressings, help promote the body's current of injury by maintaining wound moisture.

Electrical stimulation also affects each of the phases of wound healing. In the inflammatory phase, it increases blood flow, promotes phagocytosis, enhances tissue oxygenation, and attracts and stimulates fibroblasts and epithelial cells. In the proliferation phase, electrical stimulation continues its effect on fibroblasts and epithelial cells. It also stimulates protein synthesis, improves membrane transport, produces a stronger collagen matrix, and stimulates wound contraction. In the maturation phase, it stimulates epidermal cell reproduction and migration and produces a thinner, smoother scar.

Electrical stimulation is indicated for all stages of pressure ulcers; ulcers secondary to diabetes; venous, ischemic, or vasculitic ulcers; traumatic, surgical, or burn wounds; and wound flaps.

Hyperbaric oxygen therapy

Hyperbaric oxygen therapy (HBOT) significantly increases the oxygen supply to the tissues in a hypoperfused, infected wound. This increased oxygenation enhances collagen deposition and bacterial clearance, thus improving wound healing.

HBOT is used as an adjunct to treatment for bone infections, such as osteomyelitis; complications of radiation therapy, such as soft-tissue damage and osteoradionecrosis; and certain chronic, nonhealing wounds, such as diabetic ulcers, selected vascular ulcers, and some pressure ulcers. It's also used for treatment of gas gangrene, compromised skin grafts and flaps, compartment syndrome, crush injuries, and necrotizing soft-tissue infections.

HBOT may be administered in a multipatient, air-filled chamber. When it's performed this way, patients inhale 100% oxygen at greater than 1 atmosphere of pressure by way of a mask or hood. Alternatively, a smaller chamber attached to an oxygen device may be used to provide HBOT to a localized area. In this method, the highly concentrated oxygen is absorbed directly into the tissues.

Tissue growth factors

Tissue growth factors involve the use of a small amount of the patient's blood that is isolated, concentrated, and then applied topically to the wound or a genetically engineered product that is similarly applied. Growth factors help speed wound healing by attracting macrophages to the wound to fight infection and by stimulating production of new connective tissue and new blood vessels.

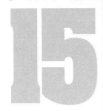

Medications
Augmenting physical therapies

Antianxiety medications

Alprazolam

Apo-Alpraz, Novo-Alprazol, Nu-Alpraz, Xanax

Indications
- Anxiety
- Panic disorders

Adverse reactions
CNS: drowsiness, light-headedness, headache, confusion, tremor, dizziness, syncope, depression, insomnia, nervousness
CV: hypotension, tachycardia
EENT: blurred vision, nasal congestion
GI: dry mouth, nausea, vomiting, diarrhea, constipation
Skin: dermatitis
Other: muscle rigidity, weight gain or loss

Special considerations
- Schedule therapy sessions when the drug reaches peak blood levels for the potential benefit of gaining the patient's full cooperation.
- Use cautiously in patients with hepatic, renal, or pulmonary disease.
- The drug shouldn't be prescribed for daily stress or for long-term use (more than 4 months).
- The drug shouldn't be withdrawn abruptly after long-term use; withdrawal symptoms may occur. Abuse or addiction is possible.
- The patient should avoid hazardous activities that require alertness and good psychomotor coordination until the central nervous system effects of the drug are known.
- The patient should avoid alcohol while taking the drug.

Buspirone hydrochloride

BuSpar

Indications
- Anxiety disorders
- Short-term relief of anxiety

Adverse reactions
CNS: dizziness, drowsiness, nervousness, insomnia, headache, light-headedness, fatigue, numbness
GI: dry mouth, nausea, diarrhea, abdominal distress
Other: blurred vision

Special considerations
- Use cautiously in patients with hepatic or renal failure.
- Be aware that the drug has shown no potential for abuse and hasn't been classified as a controlled substance. However, it isn't recommended for the relief of daily stress.
- The patient should avoid hazardous activities that require alertness and good psychomotor coordination until the central nervous system effects of the drug are known.
- The patient should avoid alcohol use while taking the drug.
- Schedule therapy sessions when the drug reaches peak blood levels for the potential benefit of gaining the patient's full cooperation.

Clonazepam

Klonopin, Rivotril

Indications
- Lennox-Gastaut syndrome
- Atypical absence seizures
- Akinetic and myoclonic seizures
- Panic disorder

Adverse reactions
CNS: drowsiness, ataxia, behavioral disturbances (especially in children),

slurred speech, tremor, confusion, psychosis, agitation
CV: palpitations
EENT: nystagmus, abnormal eye movements, sore gums
GI: constipation, gastritis, change in appetite, nausea, anorexia, diarrhea
GU: dysuria, enuresis, nocturia, urine retention
Hematologic: leukopenia, thrombocytopenia, eosinophilia
Respiratory: respiratory depression, chest congestion, shortness of breath
Skin: rash

Special considerations

• Use cautiously in children and in patients with chronic respiratory disease or open-angle glaucoma.
• Patients being treated for seizures unrelated to epilepsy should be identified as potentially at risk for a seizure during the therapy session.
• If ataxic adverse effects persist, coordination exercises may help resolve this problem.
• In the presence of skin conditions (dermatitis or rashes), discontinue therapeutic modalities that might exacerbate these conditions.
• Patients may benefit from a quiet setting if seizures are exacerbated by environmental stimuli.
• Assess an elderly patient's response closely. Elderly patients are more sensitive to the drug's central nervous system (CNS) effects.
• Monitor the patient for oversedation.
• The patient should avoid driving and other potentially hazardous activities that require mental alertness until the drug's CNS effects are known.
• Parents should monitor a child's school performance because clonazepam may interfere with attentiveness in school.
• Patients should never abruptly stop taking the drug because seizures may occur.

Diazepam

Apo-Diazepam, Atenex, Diazemuls, Diazepam Intensol, Novo-Dipam, PMS-Diazepam, Valium, Valrelease, Vivol, Zetran

Indications

• Anxiety
• Acute alcohol withdrawal
• Before endoscopic procedures
• Muscle spasm
• Preoperative sedation
• Cardioversion
• Adjunct in seizure disorders
• Status epilepticus and severe recurrent seizures

Adverse reactions

CNS: drowsiness, slurred speech, tremor, transient amnesia, fatigue, ataxia, headache, insomnia, paradoxical anxiety, hallucinations
CV: hypotension, cardiovascular collapse, bradycardia
EENT: diplopia, blurred vision, nystagmus
GI: nausea, constipation
GU: incontinence, urine retention, altered libido
Respiratory: respiratory depression
Skin: rash
Other: physical or psychological dependence, acute withdrawal syndrome after sudden discontinuation in physically dependent persons, pain, phlebitis at injection site, dysarthria, jaundice, neutropenia

Special considerations

• The drug should be avoided during pregnancy, especially during the first trimester.
• Patients should avoid activities that require alertness and good psychomotor coordination until the central nervous system effects of the drug are known.
• Patients should avoid alcohol while taking the drug.

• Schedule therapy sessions when the drug reaches peak blood levels for the potential benefit of gaining the patient's full cooperation.

Hydroxyzine hydrochloride

Atarax

Indications
• Anxiety
• Pruritus due to allergies
• Psychiatric and emotional emergencies, including acute alcoholism
• Nausea and vomiting (excluding nausea and vomiting of pregnancy)
• Antepartum and postpartum adjunctive therapy

Adverse reactions
CNS: drowsiness, involuntary motor activity
GI: dry mouth
Other: marked discomfort at I.M. injection site, hypersensitivity reactions (such as wheezing, dyspnea, and chest tightness)

Special considerations
• If the patient is taking other central nervous system (CNS) drugs, observe for oversedation.
• Patients should avoid hazardous activities that require alertness and good psychomotor coordination until the CNS effects of the drug are known.
• Patients should avoid alcohol while taking the drug.
• Patients may use hard candy or sugarless gum to help relieve dry mouth.

Lorazepam

Apo-Lorazepam, Ativan, Lorazepam Intensol, Novo-Lorazem, Nu-Loraz

Indications
• Anxiety
• Insomnia due to anxiety

• Preoperative sedation

Adverse reactions
CNS: drowsiness, amnesia, insomnia, agitation, sedation, dizziness, weakness, unsteadiness, disorientation, depression, headache
EENT: visual disturbances
GI: abdominal discomfort, nausea, change in appetite
Other: acute withdrawal syndrome (following sudden discontinuation in physically dependent persons)

Special considerations
• The drug should be avoided during pregnancy, especially during the first trimester.
• Use cautiously in elderly, acutely ill, or debilitated patients.
• The possibility of abuse and addiction exists. Don't withdraw the drug abruptly after long-term use; withdrawal symptoms may occur.
• Patients should avoid hazardous activities that require alertness or good psychomotor coordination until the drug's central nervous system effects are known.
• Patients should avoid alcohol while taking the drug.

Cardiac medications

Amlodipine besylate

Norvasc

Indications
• Chronic stable angina
• Hypertension
• Vasospastic angina (Prinzmetal's [variant] angina)

Adverse reactions
CNS: headache, somnolence, fatigue, dizziness, light-headedness, paresthesia
CV: edema, flushing, palpitations

GI: nausea, abdominal pain
Other: dyspnea, muscle pain, rash, pruritus

Special considerations

• Monitor the patient carefully. Some patients, especially those with severe obstructive coronary artery disease, have developed increased frequency, duration, or severity of angina — even acute myocardial infarction — after the initiation of calcium channel blocker therapy or at the time of dosage increase.

• Monitor blood pressure frequently during initiation of therapy. Because drug-induced vasodilation has a gradual onset, acute hypotension is rare.

• Notify the primary care provider if signs of heart failure, such as swelling of hands and feet and shortness of breath, occur.

• Make sure patients have the drug nearby during therapy sessions. Because such activities as exercise and functional training increase myocardial oxygen demand, anginal attacks may occur during therapy.

• Be aware of the cardiac limitations of patients with angina. Use caution so as not to overtax the heart to the extent that renders antianginal drugs ineffective.

• Blunted exercise response must be considered for cardiac conditioning activities. Exercise workloads need to be adjusted accordingly.

• Hypotension is possible when applying systemic heat and when large muscle groups are exercised.

• Patients need to continue taking the drug, even when feeling better.

• Patients may take sublingual nitroglycerin as needed when anginal symptoms are acute. If the patient continues nitrate therapy during the titration of the amlodipine dosage, urge continued compliance.

Atenolol

Apo-Atenol, Nu-Atenol, Tenormin

Indications

• Hypertension
• Angina pectoris
• To reduce cardiovascular mortality and the risk of reinfarction in patients with acute myocardial infarction

Adverse reactions

CNS: fatigue, lethargy, vertigo, drowsiness, dizziness
CV: bradycardia, hypotension, heart failure, intermittent claudication
GI: nausea, diarrhea
Respiratory: dyspnea, bronchospasm
Skin: rash
Other: fever, leg pain

Special considerations

• There is a potential for increased arrhythmias or changes in the nature of arrhythmias.

• Monitor electrocardiogram or pulses for rate and regularity.

• Faintness or dizziness may signal the presence of cardiotoxic drug effects and increased arrhythmias.

• Sudden posture changes may produce dizziness.

• Patients need to take the drug exactly as prescribed — at the same time every day.

• Patients shouldn't stop taking the drug suddenly and should call the primary care provider if unpleasant adverse reactions occur.

• Patients should learn how to take a pulse and should withhold the drug and call the primary care provider if their pulse rate is below 60 beats/ minute.

• Female patients should notify the primary care provider if pregnancy occurs because the drug will need to be discontinued.

Bepridil hydrochloride

Vascor

Indications
• Chronic stable angina in patients who can't tolerate or who fail to respond to other agents

Adverse reactions
CNS: dizziness, drowsiness, nervousness, headache, insomnia, paresthesia, asthenia, tremor
CV: edema, flushing, palpitations, tachycardia, ventricular arrhythmias (including torsades de pointes), ventricular tachycardia, ventricular fibrillation
EENT: tinnitus
GI: nausea, diarrhea, constipation, abdominal discomfort, dry mouth, anorexia
Respiratory: dyspnea, shortness of breath
Skin: rash
Other: flu syndrome, significant muscle fatigue and weakness caused by long-term use

Special considerations
• Monitor the patient for adverse reactions. Bepridil has been associated with severe ventricular arrhythmias, including torsades de pointes.
• The dosage shouldn't be adjusted more frequently than every 10 to 14 days because of bepridil's long half life and the time it takes to reach steady-state blood levels.
• Be aware of the cardiac limitations of patients with angina. Use caution so as not to overtax the heart to the extent that renders antianginal drugs ineffective.
• Blunted exercise response must be considered for cardiac conditioning activities. Exercise workloads need to be adjusted accordingly.

• Hypotension is possible when applying systemic heat and when large muscle groups are exercised.
• Patients should take the drug exactly as directed.

Carvedilol

Coreg

Indications
• Hypertension
• Heart failure

Adverse reactions
CNS: dizziness, fatigue, headache, hypoesthesia, insomnia, pain, paresthesia, somnolence, vertigo
CV: aggravated angina pectoris, atrioventricular block, bradycardia, chest pain, fluid overload, hypertension, hypotension, postural hypotension, syncope
EENT: abnormal vision
GI: abdominal pain, diarrhea, melena, nausea, periodontitis, vomiting
GU: abnormal renal function, albuminuria, hematuria, impotence, urinary tract infection
Hematologic: purpura, thrombocytopenia
Metabolic: dehydration, glycosuria, gout, hypercholesterolemia, hyperglycemia, hypertriglyceridemia, hypervolemia, hypovolemia, hyperuricemia, hypoglycemia, hyponatremia, weight gain
Respiratory: bronchitis, dyspnea, pharyngitis, rhinitis, sinusitis, upper respiratory tract infection
Other: allergy, arthralgia, back pain, edema, fever, malaise, myalgia, peripheral edema, sudden death, viral infection

Special considerations
• Use cautiously in hypertensive patients with left-sided heart failure, in perioperative patients who receive anesthetics that depress myocardial function (such as ether, cyclopro-

pane, and trichloroethylene), and in diabetic patients receiving insulin or oral antidiabetic agents and in those subject to spontaneous hypoglycemia. Also use with caution in patients with thyroid disease (may mask hyperthyroidism; withdrawal may precipitate thyroid storm or exacerbation of hyperthyroidism), pheochromocytoma, Prinzmetal's (variant) angina, bronchospastic disease, or peripheral vascular disease (may precipitate or aggravate symptoms of arterial insufficiency). Also use cautiously in breast-feeding women.

• Patients on beta-adrenergic blocker therapy with a history of severe anaphylactic reaction to several allergens may be more reactive to repeated challenge (accidental, diagnostic, or therapeutic). They may be unresponsive to dosages of epinephrine typically used to treat allergic reactions.

• Monitor patients with heart failure for worsened condition, renal dysfunction, or fluid retention; diuretics may need to be increased.

• Monitor diabetic patients closely; carvedilol may mask the signs of hypoglycemia or hyperglycemia may be worsened.

• Sudden posture changes may produce orthostatic hypotension.

• Use cautiously in conjunction with systemically applied heat (whirlpool or Hubbard tank).

• Exercise may cause vasodilation in skeletal muscle.

• Exercise tolerance may be impaired.

• Patients shouldn't interrupt or discontinue the drug without medical approval.

• Heart failure patients should call the primary care provider if weight gain or shortness of breath occurs.

• Patients may experience low blood pressure when standing. If dizziness or fainting (rare) occur, the patient should sit or lie down.

• Patients shouldn't perform hazardous tasks during initiation of ther-

apy. If dizziness or fatigue occur, the patient should call for an adjustment in dosage.

• Diabetic patients should report changes in blood glucose levels promptly.

• Patients who wear contact lenses may experience decreased lacrimation.

Digoxin

Digoxin, Lanoxicaps, Lanoxin, Novodigoxin

Indications
• Heart failure
• Paroxysmal supraventricular tachycardia
• Atrial fibrillation
• Atrial flutter

Adverse reactions
CNS: fatigue, generalized muscle weakness, agitation, hallucinations, headache, malaise, dizziness, vertigo, stupor, paresthesia
CV: arrhythmias (most commonly, conduction disturbances with or without atrioventricular block, premature ventricular contractions, and supraventricular arrhythmias). (Arrhythmias may lead to increased severity of heart failure and hypotension.)
EENT: yellow-green halos around visual images, blurred vision, light flashes, photophobia, diplopia
GI: anorexia, nausea, vomiting, diarrhea

Special considerations
• Toxic effects on the heart may be life threatening and require immediate attention.

• Excessive slowing of the pulse rate (60 beats/minute or less) may be a sign of digitalis toxicity. Patients should stop taking the drug and notify the primary care provider.

• Acute heart failure may occur in patients with myocardial disease due to a

lack of therapeutic drug effects or the toxic effects of some cardiac drugs.
• Be alert for signs of heart failure, such as increased dyspnea, rales, cough, and frothy sputum.
• Be alert for signs of digitalis toxicity, such as dizziness, confusion, nausea, and arrhythmias.
• Patients on diuretics may exhibit excessive fatigue and weakness as early signs of fluid and electrolyte depletion.
• Patients and responsible family members should be aware of drug action, dosage regimen, how to take pulse, reportable signs, and follow-up care.
• Patients should eat potassium-rich foods.
• Patients shouldn't substitute one brand of digoxin for another.

Diltiazem hydrochloride

Apo-Diltiaz, Cardizem, Cardizem CD, Cardizem SR, Dilacor-XR

Indications
• Vasospastic angina (Prinzmetal's [variant] angina)
• Classic chronic stable angina pectoris
• Atrial fibrillation or flutter
• Paroxysmal supraventricular tachycardia
• Hypertension

Adverse reactions
CNS: headache, dizziness, asthenia, somnolence
CV: edema, arrhythmias, flushing, bradycardia, hypotension, conduction abnormalities, heart failure, atrioventricular block, abnormal electrocardiogram (ECG)
GI: nausea, constipation, abdominal discomfort
Hepatic: acute hepatic injury
Skin: rash

Special considerations
• Monitor blood pressure and heart rate during the initiation of therapy and dosage adjustments.
• If systolic blood pressure is below 90 mm Hg or heart rate is below 60 beats/minute, withhold dose and notify the primary care provider.
• Be aware that because activities, such as exercise and functional training, increase myocardial oxygen demand, anginal attacks may occur during therapy.
• Be aware of the cardiac limitations of patients with angina. Use caution so as not to overtax the heart to the extent that renders antianginal drugs ineffective.
• Blunted exercise response must be considered for cardiac conditioning activities. Exercise workloads need to be adjusted accordingly.
• Hypotension is possible when applying systemic heat and when large muscle groups are exercised.
• Be aware of the potential for increased arrhythmias or changes in the nature of arrhythmias.
• Monitor ECG or pulses for rate and regularity.
• Faintness or dizziness may signal the presence of cardiotoxic drug effects and increased arrhythmias.
• Sudden posture changes may produce dizziness.
• Patients should avoid hazardous activities during the initiation of therapy.
• Patients should maintain compliance with medical regimen.
• Patients may take sublingual nitroglycerin concomitantly as needed when anginal symptoms are acute.
• Patients should swallow Dilacor-XR whole; they shouldn't open, crush, or chew it.

Enalapril maleate

Vasotec

Indications
• Hypertension
• Heart failure

Adverse reactions
CNS: headache, dizziness, fatigue, vertigo, asthenia, syncope
CV: hypotension, chest pain
GI: diarrhea, nausea, abdominal pain, vomiting
GU: decreased renal function (in patients with bilateral renal artery stenosis or heart failure)
Hematologic: neutropenia, thrombocytopenia, agranulocytosis.
Respiratory: dry, persistent, tickling, nonproductive cough; dyspnea
Skin: rash
Other: angioedema

Special considerations
• Whirlpool may produce profound hypotension. Use it cautiously.
• Monitor blood pressure response to the drug closely.
• Use caution when patients sit up or stand up suddenly. Use of a vasodilator may cause postural hypotension.
• Light-headedness can occur, especially during the first few days of therapy.
• Patients need to use caution in hot weather and during exercise. Inadequate fluid intake, vomiting, diarrhea, and excessive perspiration can lead to light-headedness and syncope.
• Patients should report breathing difficulty or swelling of face, eyes, lips, or tongue. Angioedema (including laryngeal edema) may occur, especially after the first dose.
• Patients should report signs of infection, such as fever and sore throat.
• When administered along with a diuretic, be alert for signs of fluid and electrolyte depletion, such as excessive fatigue and weakness.

Isosorbide dinitrate

Apo-ISDN, Cedocard-SR, Coradur, Coronex, Dilatrate SR, Isonate, Isorbid, Isordil, Isordil Tembids, Isordil Titradose, Isotrate, Novosorbide, Sorbitrate

Isosorbide mononitrate

Imdur, ISMO, Monoket

Indications
• Acute anginal attacks (sublingual and chewable tablets of isosorbide dinitrate only)
• Prophylaxis in situations likely to cause anginal attacks

Adverse reactions
CNS: headache (sometimes with throbbing), dizziness, weakness
CV: orthostatic hypotension, tachycardia, palpitations, ankle edema, fainting
GI: nausea, vomiting
Skin: cutaneous vasodilation, flushing, rash
Other: hypersensitivity reactions, sublingual burning

Special considerations
• Monitor blood pressure and intensity and the duration of the drug response.
• May cause headaches, especially at the beginning of therapy. Dosage may be reduced temporarily, but tolerance usually develops. Treat headache with aspirin or acetaminophen.
• Make sure patients have isosorbide dinitrate nearby during therapy sessions. Because such activities as exercise and functional training increase myocardial oxygen demand, anginal attacks may occurs during therapy.
• Be aware of the cardiac limitations of patients with angina. Use cautions so as not to overtax the heart to the

extent that renders antianginal drugs ineffective.

• Blunted exercise response must be considered for cardiac conditioning activities. Exercise workload should be adjusted accordingly.

• Hypotension is possible when applying systemic heat and when large muscle groups are exercised.

• Patients need to take medication regularly, as prescribed. and to keep it accessible at all times.

• Patients should be warned not to abruptly discontinue the drug because of coronary vasospasm with increased anginal symptoms and the potential risk of myocardial infarction.

• Patients should take the tablet sublingually at the first sign of an attack. The tablet should be wet with saliva and placed under the tongue until absorbed, and the patient should sit down and rest. The dose may be repeated every 10 to 15 minutes for a maximum of three doses. If the drug doesn't provide relief, medical help should be obtained immediately.

• Patients who experience a tingling sensation with sublingual isosorbide dinitrate should try holding the tablet in the buccal pouch.

• Patients should be aware of the difference between oral and sublingual forms.

• Patients should take oral form of isosorbide dinitrate on an empty stomach, either 30 minutes before or 1 to 2 hours after meals. They should also swallow oral tablets whole and chew chewable tablets thoroughly before swallowing.

• Patients can minimize orthostatic hypotension by changing to upright position slowly, going up and down stairs carefully, and lying down at the first sign of dizziness.

• Store the drug in a cool place, in a tightly closed container, away from light.

Metoprolol succinate

Toprol-XL

Metoprolol tartrate

Apo-Metoprolol, Apo-Metoprolol (Type L), Betaloc, Durules, Lopresor, Lopresor SR, Lopressor, Novometoprol, Nu-Metop

Indications
• Hypertension
• Early intervention in acute myocardial infarction (metoprolol tartrate)
• Angina pectoris

Adverse reactions
CNS: fatigue, dizziness, depression
CV: bradycardia, hypotension, heart failure, atrioventricular block
GI: nausea, diarrhea
Respiratory: dyspnea, bronchospasm
Skin: rash

Special considerations
• Monitor blood glucose levels closely in diabetic patients because the drug masks common signs of hypoglycemia.

• Monitor blood pressure frequently. Know that metoprolol masks common signs of shock.

• Store the drug at room temperature and protect it from the light. Discard the solution if it's discolored or contains particles.

• There's potential for increased arrhythmias or changes in the nature of arrhythmias.

• Monitor electrocardiogram or pulses for rate and regularity.

• Faintness or dizziness may signal the presence of cardiotoxic drug effects and increased arrhythmias.

• Sudden posture changes may produce dizziness.

• Patients should take the drug exactly as prescribed and take it with meals.

• Patients shouldn't stop taking the drug suddenly and should notify the primary care provider about unpleasant adverse reactions. The drug must be withdrawn gradually over 1 to 2 weeks.

Nifedipine

Adalat, Adalat CC, Adalat FT, Adalat P.A., Apo-Nifed, Novo-Nifedin, Nu-Nifed, Procardia, Procardia XL

Indications

• Vasospastic angina (Prinzmetal's [variant] angina)
• Classic chronic stable angina pectoris
• Hypertension

Adverse reactions

CNS: dizziness, light-headedness, flushing, headache, weakness, syncope, nervousness
CV: peripheral edema, hypotension, palpitations, heart failure, myocardial infarction, pulmonary edema
EENT: nasal congestion.
GI: nausea, diarrhea, constipation, abdominal discomfort
Respiratory: dyspnea, cough
Skin: rash, pruritus
Other: muscle cramps, hypokalemia

Special considerations

• Monitor blood pressure regularly, especially in patients who are taking beta-adrenergic blockers or antihypertensives.

• Make sure patients have the drug nearby during therapy sessions. Because such activities as exercise and functional training increase myocardial oxygen demand, anginal attacks may occur during therapy.

• Be aware of the cardiac limitations of patients with angina. Use caution so as not to overtax the heart to the extent that renders antianginal drugs ineffective.

• Blunted exercise response must be considered for cardiac conditioning activities. Exercise workloads need to be adjusted accordingly.

• Hypotension is possible when applying systemic heat and when large muscle groups are exercised.

• Patients should maintain drug therapy compliance. Patients may take sublingual nitroglycerin as needed when anginal symptoms are acute.

• Patients may briefly develop anginal exacerbation when beginning drug therapy or when dosage is increased.

• Patients should swallow extended-release tablets without breaking, crushing, or chewing.

• Patients shouldn't switch brands. Procardia XL and Adalat CC aren't therapeutically equivalent because of major differences in their pharmacokinetics.

Nitroglycerin (glyceryl trinitrate)

Deponit, Minitran, Nitro-Bid, Nitro-Bid I.V., Nitrocine, Nitrodisc, Nitro-Dur, Nitrogard, Nitroglyn, Nitrol, Nitrolingual, Nitrong, Nitrostat, Nitro-Time, NTS, Transderm-Nitro, Tridil

Indications

• Prophylaxis against chronic anginal attacks
• Acute angina pectoris
• Prophylaxis to prevent or minimize anginal attacks before stressful events
• Hypertension associated with surgery
• Heart failure associated with myocardial infarction
• Angina pectoris in acute situations
• To produce controlled hypotension during surgery (by I.V. infusion)

Adverse reactions

CNS: headache (sometimes throbbing), dizziness, weakness
CV: orthostatic hypotension, tachycardia, flushing, palpitations, fainting.
GI: nausea, vomiting
Skin: cutaneous vasodilation, contact dermatitis (patch), rash
Other: hypersensitivity reactions, sublingual burning

Special considerations

• Remove the transdermal patch before defibrillation. Because of its aluminum backing, the electric current may cause arcing that can result in damage to paddles and burns to the patient.
• The drug may cause headaches, especially at the beginning of therapy. The dosage may be reduced temporarily, but tolerance usually develops. Treat headaches with aspirin or acetaminophen.
• Make sure patients have the drug nearby during therapy sessions. Because such activities as exercise and functional training increase myocardial oxygen demand, anginal attacks may occur during therapy.
• Be aware of the cardiac limitations of patients with angina. Use caution so as not to overtax the heart to the extent that renders antianginal drugs ineffective.
• Blunted exercise response must be considered for cardiac conditioning activities. Exercise workloads should be adjusted accordingly.
• Hypotension is possible when applying systemic heat and when large muscle groups are exercised.
• Patients should take nitroglycerin regularly, as prescribed, and have it accessible at all times.
• Abrupt discontinuation of the drug causes coronary vasospasms.
• Patients should know how to administer the prescribed form of nitroglycerin.
• Patients should take sublingual tablet at the first sign of an attack. The tablet should be wet with saliva and placed under the tongue until absorbed, and the patient should sit down and rest. The dose may be repeated every 5 minutes for a maximum of three doses. If the drug doesn't provide relief, medical help should be obtained immediately.
• Patients who complain of a tingling sensation with the sublingual drug should try holding tablet in the buccal pouch.
• To minimize orthostatic hypotension, patients should change to upright position slowly, go up and down stairs carefully, and lie down at the first sign of dizziness.

Propranolol hydrochloride

Apo-Propranolol, Inderal, Inderal LA, Novopranol, pms Propranolol

Indications

• Angina pectoris
• Mortality reduction after myocardial infarction (MI)
• Supraventricular, ventricular, and atrial arrhythmias
• Tachyarrhythmias caused by excessive catecholamine action during anesthesia
• Hyperthyroidism
• Pheochromocytoma
• Hypertension
• Prevention of frequent, severe, uncontrollable, or disabling migraine or vascular headache
• Essential tremor
• Hypertrophic subaortic stenosis
• Adjunct therapy in pheochromocytoma

Adverse reactions

CNS: fatigue, lethargy, vivid dreams, hallucinations, mental depression, light-headedness, insomnia

CV: bradycardia, hypotension, heart failure, intermittent claudication, intensification of atrioventricular block
GI: nausea, vomiting, diarrhea, abdominal cramping
Respiratory: bronchospasm
Skin: rash
Other: fever, agranulocytosis

Special considerations

• Use cautiously in patients with renal impairment, nonallergic bronchospastic diseases, or hepatic disease and in those taking other antihypertensives. Because propranolol blocks some symptoms of hypoglycemia, use cautiously in patients with diabetes mellitus. Also use cautiously in patients with thyrotoxicosis because the drug may mask some signs of that disorder. Elderly patients may experience enhanced adverse reactions and may need dosage adjustments.
• The drug masks common signs of shock and hypoglycemia.
• Be aware of the potential for increased arrhythmias or a change in the nature of arrhythmias.
• Monitor electrocardiogram or pulses for rate and regularity.
• Faintness or dizziness may signal the presence of cardiotoxic drug effects and increased arrhythmias.
• Sudden posture changes may produce dizziness.
• Patients should continue taking this drug as prescribed even when feeling well.
• Patients should take propranolol with food.
• Patients shouldn't discontinue the drug suddenly because this can exacerbate angina and precipitate MI.

Sotalol

Betapace, Sotacor

Indications

• Documented, life-threatening ventricular arrhythmias

• Hypertension
• Angina

Adverse reactions

CNS: asthenia, headache, dizziness, weakness, fatigue, sleep problems, light-headedness
CV: bradycardia, arrhythmias, heart failure, atrioventricular block, proarrhythmic events (polymorphic ventricular tachycardia, premature ventricular contractions, ventricular fibrillation), edema, palpitations, chest pain, electrocardiogram (ECG) abnormalities, hypotension
GI: nausea, vomiting, diarrhea, dyspepsia
Respiratory: dyspnea, bronchospasm

Special considerations

• Monitor serum electrolytes regularly, especially if the patient is receiving diuretics. Electrolyte imbalances, such as hypokalemia or hypomagnesemia, may enhance QT-interval prolongation and increase the risk of serious arrhythmias, such as torsades de pointes.
• Be aware of the potential for increased arrhythmias or changes in the nature of arrhythmias.
• Monitor the ECG or pulses for rate and regularity.
• Faintness or dizziness may signal the presence of cardiotoxic drug effects and increased arrhythmias.
• Sudden posture changes may produce dizziness.
• Patients should be aware of the importance of taking the drug as prescribed, even when feeling well. The drug shouldn't be discontinued suddenly.

Terazosin hydrochloride

Hytrin

Indications

• Hypertension

• Symptomatic benign prostatic hypertrophy

Adverse reactions
CNS: asthenia, dizziness, headache, nervousness, paresthesia, somnolence
CV: palpitations, postural hypotension, tachycardia, peripheral edema
EENT: nasal congestion, sinusitis, blurred vision
GI: nausea
GU: impotence
Respiratory: dyspnea
Other: back pain, muscle pain

Special considerations
• Sudden posture changes may produce orthostatic hypotension.
• Give cautiously with the use of systemically applied heat (whirlpool or Hubbard tank).
• Exercise may cause vasodilation in skeletal muscle.
• Exercise tolerance may be impaired.
• Patients shouldn't discontinue the drug suddenly, but should call the primary care provider if adverse reactions occur.
• Patients should avoid hazardous activities that require mental alertness, such as driving or operating heavy machinery, for 12 hours after the first dose.

Verapamil

Apo-Verap, Calan, Isoptin, Novo-Veramil, Nu-Verap

Verapamil hydrochloride

Calan, Calan SR, Isoptin, Isoptin SR, Novo-Veramil, Verelan

Indications
• Vasospastic angina (also called Prinzmetal's [variant] angina)

• Classic chronic, stable angina pectoris
• Chronic atrial fibrillation
• Supraventricular arrhythmias
• Hypertension

Adverse reactions
CNS: dizziness, headache, asthenia
CV: transient hypotension, heart failure, pulmonary edema, bradycardia, atrioventricular block, ventricular asystole, ventricular fibrillation, peripheral edema
GI: constipation, nausea
Hepatic: elevated liver enzymes
Skin: rash

Special considerations
• Use cautiously in elderly patients, in patients with increased intracranial pressure, and in patients with hepatic or renal disease.
• All patients receiving I.V. verapamil should be on a cardiac monitor. Monitor the R-R interval.
• Monitor blood pressure at the start of therapy and during dosage adjustments.
• Assist the patient with ambulation because dizziness may occur.
• Sublingual nitroglycerin may be taken as needed when anginal symptoms are acute.
• Be aware of the potential for increased arrhythmias or changes in the nature of arrhythmias.
• Monitor electrocardiogram or pulses for rate and regularity.
• Faintness or dizziness may signal the presence of cardiotoxic drug effects and increased arrhythmias.
• Sudden posture changes may produce dizziness.
• Make sure patients have the drug nearby during therapy sessions. Because such activities as exercise and functional training increase myocardial oxygen demand, anginal attacks may occur during therapy.
• Be aware of the cardiac limitations of patients with angina. Use caution

so as not to overtax the heart to the extent that renders antianginal drugs ineffective.

• Blunted exercise response must be considered for cardiac conditioning activities. Exercise workloads need to be adjusted accordingly.

• Hypotension is possible when applying systemic heat and when large muscle groups are exercised.

Nervous system medications

Amitriptyline hydrochloride

Apo-Amitriptyline, Elavil, Endep, Levate, Novotriptyn

Indications
• Depression

Adverse reactions
CNS: coma, seizures, hallucinations, delusions, disorientation, ataxia, tremor, peripheral neuropathy, anxiety, insomnia, restlessness, drowsiness, dizziness, weakness, fatigue, headache, extrapyramidal reactions
CV: myocardial infarction, stroke, arrhythmias, heart block, orthostatic hypotension, tachycardia, electrocardiogram changes, hypertension
EENT: blurred vision, tinnitus, mydriasis, increased intraocular pressure.
GI: dry mouth, nausea, vomiting, anorexia, epigastric distress, diarrhea, constipation, paralytic ileus
GU: urine retention
Hematologic: agranulocytosis, thrombocytopenia, leukopenia, eosinophilia
Skin: rash, urticaria, photosensitivity
Other: diaphoresis, hypersensitivity reaction, edema. *After abrupt withdrawal of long-term therapy:* nausea, headache, malaise (doesn't indicate addiction)

Special considerations
• Amitriptyline has strong anticholinergic effects and is one of the most sedating tricyclic antidepressants. Be aware that anticholinergic effects have a rapid onset even though the therapeutic effect is delayed for weeks.
• If signs of psychosis occur or increase, expect the primary care provider to reduce the dosage. Record mood changes. Monitor the patient for suicidal tendencies and allow only a minimum supply of the drug.
• A full dose of the drug should be taken at bedtime, but patients should be aware of possible morning orthostatic hypotension.
• Patients should avoid alcohol use while taking this drug.
• Patients need to consult with their primary care provider before taking other medications.
• Patients should avoid activities that require alertness and good psychomotor coordination until the drug's central nervous system effects are known. Drowsiness and dizziness usually subside after a few weeks.
• Dry mouth may be relieved with sugarless hard candy or gum. Saliva substitutes may be needed.
• To prevent photosensitivity reactions, patients should avoid prolonged exposure to the sun.

Bupropion hydrochloride

Wellbutrin

Indications
• Depression

Adverse reactions
CNS: headache, seizures, anxiety, confusion, delusions, euphoria, hostility, impaired sleep quality, insomnia, sedation, tremor, akinesia, akathisia, agitation, dizziness, fatigue

CV: arrhythmias, hypertension, hypotension, palpitations, syncope, tachycardia
EENT: auditory disturbances, blurred vision
GI: dry mouth, taste disturbance, increased appetite, constipation, dyspepsia, nausea, vomiting, weight loss, anorexia, weight gain, diarrhea
GU: impotence, menstrual complaints, urinary frequency, decreased libido, urine retention
Skin: pruritus, rash, cutaneous temperature disturbance, excessive diaphoresis
Other: arthritis, fever, chills

Special considerations
• Know that many patients experience a period of increased restlessness, especially at the initiation of therapy. This may include agitation, insomnia, and anxiety
• Patients who experience seizures often have predisposing factors, including a history of head trauma, prior seizures, or central nervous system (CNS) tumors, or may be taking a drug that lowers the seizure threshold.
• Monitor the patient with a history of bipolar disorders closely. Antidepressants can cause manic episodes during the depressed phase of bipolar disorder.
• Patients should avoid alcohol while taking the drug because it may contribute to the development of seizures.
• Patients should avoid hazardous activities that require alertness and good psychomotor coordination until the drug's CNS effects are known.

Carbidopa-levodopa
Sinemet, Sinemet CR
Indications
• Idiopathic Parkinson's disease
• Postencephalitic parkinsonism
• Symptomatic parkinsonism resulting from carbon monoxide or manganese intoxication

Adverse reactions
CNS: choreiform, dystonic, dyskinetic movements; involuntary grimacing, head movements, myoclonic body jerks, ataxia, tremor, and muscle twitching; bradykinetic episodes; psychiatric disturbances, such as anxiety, disturbing dreams, and euphoria; malaise; fatigue; severe depression; suicidal tendencies; dementia; delirium; hallucinations (may necessitate reduction or withdrawal of the drug); confusion; insomnia; agitation
CV: orthostatic hypotension, cardiac irregularities
EENT: blepharospasm, blurred vision, diplopia, mydriasis or miosis, oculogyric crises, excessive salivation
GI: dry mouth, bitter taste, nausea, vomiting, anorexia, weight loss (may occur at start of therapy), constipation, flatulence, diarrhea, abdominal pain
GU: urinary frequency, urine retention, urinary incontinence, darkened urine, priapism
Hematologic: hemolytic anemia, thrombocytopenia, leukopenia, agranulocytosis
Hepatic: hepatotoxicity
Other: dark perspiration, hyperventilation, hiccups, phlebitis

Special considerations
• Be aware that therapeutic and adverse reactions occur more rapidly with carbidopa-levodopa than with levodopa alone. Observe and monitor vital signs, especially while adjusting dosage. Report significant changes.
• Muscle twitching and blepharospasm may be early signs of drug overdose; report immediately.
• Schedule therapy sessions with the peak effects of drug therapy (usually approximately 1 hour after medication is taken). Optimal effects can be achieved if the therapy session is scheduled after the breakfast dose (maximum drug efficacy and low fatigue levels in patients).

• For patients who have stopped taking the drug temporarily: Maintain joint range of motion and cardiovascular fitness. This helps the patient resume activity when medications are reinstated.

• Monitor blood pressure as orthostatic hypotension may occur and may predispose the patient to falls.

• The drug should be taken with food to minimize GI upset.

• Patients and caregivers shouldn't increase dosage without the primary care provider's orders.

• Patients should be aware of possible dizziness and orthostatic hypotension, especially at the start of therapy. They should change position slowly and dangle legs before getting out of bed. Elastic stockings may control this adverse reaction in some patients.

• Patients should report adverse reactions as well as therapeutic effects.

• Patients should be aware that pyridoxine (vitamin B$_6$) doesn't reverse the beneficial effects of carbidopa-levodopa. Multivitamins can be taken without losing control of symptoms.

Cyclobenzaprine hydrochloride

Flexeril

Indications
• Short-term treatment of muscle spasm

Adverse reactions
CNS: drowsiness, headache, insomnia, fatigue, asthenia, nervousness, confusion, paresthesia, dizziness, depression, seizures

CV: tachycardia, syncope, arrhythmias, palpitations, hypotension, vasodilation

EENT: blurred vision, visual disturbances

GI: dyspepsia, abnormal taste, constipation, dry mouth, nausea

GU: urine retention, urinary frequency

Skin: rash, urticaria, pruritus

Other: with high doses, adverse reactions similar to those of other tricyclic antidepressants

Special considerations
• Use cautiously in patients with a history of urine retention, acute angle-closure glaucoma, and increased intraocular pressure as well as elderly and debilitated patients.

• Be alert for nausea, headache, and malaise, which may occur if the drug is stopped abruptly after long-term use.

• Watch for symptoms of overdose, including cardiac toxicity. Notify the primary care provider immediately and have physostigmine available.

• The safety and efficacy of the drug in children under 15 years haven't been established.

• Therapy sessions may have to be scheduled when the sedative effects of the drug are minimal.

• It's important to facilitate the substitution of normal physiologic motor control for previously used spastic tone in those individuals who obtained support from their hypertonic muscles.

• Patients should report urinary hesitancy or urine retention. If constipation is a problem, increasing fluid intake and taking a stool softener may be helpful.

• Patients should avoid activities that require alertness until the drug's central nervous system (CNS) effects are known.

• Patients shouldn't combine the drug with alcohol or other CNS depressants.

Fluoxetine hydrochloride

Prozac

Indications
• Depression
• Obsessive-compulsive disorder

• Treatment of binge-eating and vomiting behavior in patients with moderate to severe bulimia nervosa

Adverse reactions

CNS: nervousness, anxiety, insomnia, headache, drowsiness, fatigue, tremor, dizziness, asthenia
CV: palpitations, hot flashes
EENT: nasal congestion, pharyngitis, cough, sinusitis
GI: nausea, diarrhea, dry mouth, anorexia, dyspepsia, constipation, abdominal pain, vomiting, flatulence, increased appetite
GU: sexual dysfunction
Respiratory: upper respiratory infection, respiratory distress
Skin: rash, pruritus, diaphoresis
Other: flulike syndrome, muscle pain, weight loss, fever

Special considerations

• Use cautiously in patients at high risk for suicide and those with a history of hepatic, renal, or cardiovascular disease; diabetes mellitus; or seizures.
• Use antihistamines or topical corticosteroids as ordered to treat rashes or pruritus.
• Avoid taking the drug in the afternoon because fluoxetine commonly causes nervousness and insomnia.
• The drug may cause dizziness or drowsiness in some patients. Patients should avoid driving and other hazardous activities that require alertness and good psychomotor coordination until the drug's central nervous system effects are known.
• Patients should consult the primary care provider before taking other prescription or over-the-counter drugs.
• Warn patients to avoid foods containing tryptophan.

Haloperidol

Apo-Haloperidol, Haldol, Novo-Peridol, Peridol

Haloperidol decanoate

Haldol decanoate, Haldol LA

Haloperidol lactate

Haldol, Haldol Concentrate, Haloperidol Injection, Haloperidol Intensol

Indications

• Psychotic disorders
• Nonpsychotic behavior disorders
• Tourette's syndrome

Adverse reactions

CNS: severe extrapyramidal reactions, tardive dyskinesia, sedation, drowsiness, lethargy, headache, insomnia, confusion, vertigo, seizures
CV: tachycardia, hypotension, hypertension, electrocardiogram changes
EENT: blurred vision
GI: dry mouth, anorexia, constipation, diarrhea, nausea, vomiting, dyspepsia
GU: urine retention, menstrual irregularities, gynecomastia, priapism
Hematologic: leukopenia, leukocytosis
Skin: rash, other skin reactions, diaphoresis
Other: neuroleptic malignant syndrome (rare), altered liver function tests, jaundice

Special considerations

• Use cautiously in elderly and debilitated patients; in patients with a history of seizures or EEG abnormalities, severe cardiovascular disorders, allergies, glaucoma, or urine retention; and in patients taking anticonvulsants, anticoagulants, antiparkinsonian drugs, or lithium.
• Monitor the patient for tardive dyskinesia, which may occur after pro-

longed use. This complication may not appear until months or years later and may disappear spontaneously or persist for life, despite discontinuation of the drug.

• Watch the patient for neuroleptic malignant syndrome (extrapyramidal effects, hyperthermia, autonomic disturbance), which is rare but often fatal. This syndrome isn't necessarily related to the length of drug use or the type of neuroleptic. Over 60% of affected patients are men.

• Be alert for early signs of motor involvement (posture, balance, or involuntary movements). If this occurs, bring it to the attention of the medical staff immediately.

• Haloperidol is the least sedating of the antipsychotics; however, patients should still avoid activities that require alertness and good psychomotor coordination until the drug's central nervous system effects are known. Drowsiness and dizziness usually subside after a few weeks.

• Patients should avoid alcohol while taking this drug.

• Patients can relieve dry mouth with sugarless gum or hard candy.

Imipramine hydrochloride

Apo-Imipramine, Impril, Norfranil, Novopramine, Tipramine, Tofranil

Imipramine pamoate

Tofranil-PM

Indications
• Depression
• Childhood enuresis

Adverse reactions
CNS: drowsiness, dizziness, excitation, tremor, confusion, hallucinations, anxiety, ataxia, paresthesia, nervousness, EEG changes, seizures, extrapyramidal reactions
CV: orthostatic hypotension, tachycardia, electrocardiogram changes, hypertension, myocardial infarction, stroke, arrhythmias, heart block, precipitation of heart failure
EENT: blurred vision, tinnitus, mydriasis
GI: dry mouth, constipation, nausea, vomiting, anorexia, paralytic ileus, abdominal cramps
GU: urine retention
Skin: rash, urticaria, photosensitivity, pruritus
Other: diaphoresis, hypersensitivity reaction. *After abrupt withdrawal of long-term therapy:* nausea, headache, malaise (doesn't indicate addiction)

Special considerations
• If signs of psychosis occur or increase, expect the primary care provider to reduce the dosage. Record mood changes. Monitor the patient for suicidal tendencies, and allow only a minimum supply of the drug.
• Patients can relieve dry mouth with sugarless hard candy or gum. Saliva substitutes may also be necessary.
• Patients should take a full dose at bed time and should be aware of possible morning orthostatic hypotension.
• Patients should avoid alcohol while taking this drug.
• Patients should avoid hazardous activities that require alertness and good psychomotor coordination until the drug's central nervous system effects are known. Drowsiness and dizziness usually subside after a few weeks.
• Patients shouldn't stop taking the drug suddenly.
• To prevent photosensitivity reactions, patients should use sunblock, wear protective clothing, and avoid prolonged exposure to strong sunlight.

Paroxetine hydrochloride

Paxil

Indications
• Depression
• Panic disorder

Adverse reactions
CNS: somnolence, dizziness, insomnia, tremor, nervousness, anxiety, paresthesia, confusion, headache, agitation
CV: palpitations, vasodilation, orthostatic hypotension
EENT: lump or tightness in throat, dysgeusia
GI: dry mouth, nausea, constipation, diarrhea, flatulence, vomiting, dyspepsia, increased appetite, abdominal pain
GU: ejaculatory disturbances, male genital disorders (including anorgasmy, erectile difficulties, delayed ejaculation or orgasm, impotence, and sexual dysfunction), urinary frequency and other urinary disorders, female genital disorders (including anorgasmy and difficulty with orgasm)
Skin: rash, pruritus
Other: asthenia, diaphoresis, myopathy, myalgia, myasthenia, decreased libido, yawning

Special considerations
• Use cautiously in patients with a history of seizure disorders or mania and in those with severe, concomitant systemic illness.
• Use cautiously in patients at risk for volume depletion, and monitor appropriately.
• If signs of psychosis occur or increase, expect the primary care provider to reduce the dosage. Record mood changes. Monitor the patient for suicidal tendencies and allow him only a minimum supply of the drug.
• Patients should avoid activities that require alertness and good psychomo-

tor coordination until the drug's central nervous system effects are known.
• Patients should avoid alcohol and consult the primary care provider before taking other prescription or over-the-counter drugs.

Phenobarbital (phenobarbitone)

Ancalixir, Barbita, Solfoton

Phenobarbital sodium (phenobarbitone sodium)

Luminal

Indications
• All forms of epilepsy
• Febrile seizures
• Status epilepticus
• Sedation
• Insomnia
• Preoperative sedation

Adverse reactions
CNS: drowsiness, lethargy, hangover, paradoxical excitement in elderly patients, somnolence
CV: bradycardia, hypotension
GI: nausea, vomiting
Hematologic: exacerbation of porphyria
Respiratory: respiratory depression, apnea
Skin: rash, erythema multiforme, Stevens-Johnson syndrome, urticaria, pain, swelling, thrombophlebitis, necrosis, nerve injury at injection site.
Other: angioedema, physical and psychological dependence.

Special considerations
• Elderly patients are more sensitive to the drug's effects.
• Watch for signs of barbiturate toxicity, such as coma, asthmatic breath-

ing, cyanosis, clammy skin, and hypotension. Overdose can be fatal.

• Patients shouldn't stop taking the drug abruptly because seizures may worsen. Call the primary care provider immediately if adverse reactions develop.

• Patients being treated for conditions unrelated to epilepsy should be identified as potentially at risk for a seizure during a therapy session.

• If ataxic adverse effects persist, coordination exercises may help resolve this problem.

• In the presence of skin conditions (dermatitis or rashes), discontinue therapeutic modalities that might exacerbate these conditions.

• Some patients may benefit from a quiet setting (no noise or lights) if seizures are exacerbated by environmental stimuli.

• Patients should be aware that phenobarbital is available in many sizes and strengths and they'll need to check prescriptions and refills closely.

• Full therapeutic effects aren't seen for 2 to 3 weeks, except when loading dose is used.

• Patients should avoid driving and other potentially hazardous activities that require mental alertness until the drug's central nervous system effects are known.

• Female patients who use oral contraceptives should consider another birth-control method;this drug may enhance contraceptive hormone metabolism and decrease its effect.

Phenytoin (diphenylhydantoin)

Dilantin-125, Dilantin Infatab

Phenytoin sodium

Dilantin, Phenytex

Phenytoin sodium (extended)

Dilantin Kapseals

Indications
• Control of generalized tonic-clonic and complex partial (temporal lobe) seizures
• Prevention and treatment of seizures occurring during neurosurgery
• Status epilepticus

Adverse reactions
CNS: ataxia, slurred speech, dizziness, insomnia, nervousness, twitching, headache, mental confusion, decreased coordination
CV: periarteritis nodosa
EENT: nystagmus, diplopia, blurred vision, gingival hyperplasia (especially in children)
GI: nausea, vomiting, constipation
Hematologic: thrombocytopenia, leukopenia, agranulocytosis, pancytopenia, macrocythemia, megaloblastic anemia
Hepatic: toxic hepatitis
Skin: scarlatiniform or morbilliform rash; bullous, exfoliative, or purpuric dermatitis; lupus erythematosus; Stevens-Johnson syndrome; hirsutism; toxic epidermal necrolysis; photosensitivity; pain, necrosis, and inflammation at injection site; discoloration of skin ("purple-glove syndrome") if given by I.V. push in back of hand
Other: lymphadenopathy, hyperglycemia, osteomalacia, hypertrichosis

Special considerations
• Be aware that elderly patients tend to metabolize phenytoin slowly and may require lower dosages.
• Phenytoin requirements usually increase during pregnancy.
• Be aware that the drug should be discontinued if a rash appears. If the rash is scarlatiniform or morbilliform, the drug may be resumed after the rash clears. If the rash reappears,

therapy should be discontinued. If the rash is exfoliative, purpuric, or bullous, the drug shouldn't be resumed.

• Mononucleosis may decrease phenytoin levels. Monitor for increased seizure activity.

• Patients being treated for conditions unrelated to epilepsy should be identified as potentially at risk for a seizure during therapy sessions.

• If ataxic adverse effects persist, coordination exercises may help resolve this problem.

• In the presence of skin conditions (dermatitis or rashes), discontinue therapeutic modalities that might exacerbate these conditions.

• Some patients may benefit from a quiet setting (no noise and light) if seizures are exacerbated by environmental stimuli.

• Patients should avoid driving and other potentially hazardous activities that require mental alertness until the drug's central nervous system effects are known.

• The patient shouldn't stop taking the drug abruptly.

• Good oral hygiene and regular dental examinations are important while taking this drug. Gingivectomy may be necessary periodically if dental hygiene is poor.

• The drug may color urine pink, red, or reddish brown.

Risperidone

Risperdal

Indications

• Psychosis

Adverse reactions

CNS: somnolence, extrapyramidal symptoms, headache, insomnia, agitation, anxiety, tardive dyskinesia, aggressiveness

CV: tachycardia, chest pain, orthostatic hypotension, prolonged QT interval

EENT: rhinitis, coughing, upper respiratory infection, sinusitis, pharyngitis, abnormal vision

GI: constipation, nausea, vomiting, dyspepsia

Skin: rash, dry skin, photosensitivity

Other: arthralgia, back pain, fever, neuroleptic malignant syndrome (rare)

Special considerations

• Obtain baseline measures of blood pressure before starting therapy and monitor regularly. Watch for orthostatic hypotension, especially during initial dosage titration.

• Monitor the patient for tardive dyskinesia, which may occur after prolonged use. It may not appear until months or years later and may disappear spontaneously or persist for life, despite discontinuation of the drug.

• Assess for neuroleptic malignant syndrome (extrapyramidal effects, hyperthermia, autonomic disturbance). It's rare, but frequently fatal. It isn't necessarily related to length of drug use or type of neuroleptic, but over 60% of patients are men.

• Patients should avoid activities that require alertness until the drug's central nervous system effects are known.

• Patients should rise slowly, avoid hot showers, and use extra caution during the first few days of therapy to avoid fainting.

• Patients should avoid alcohol.

• Patients should use sunblock and wear protective clothing outdoors.

• Female patients should notify the primary care provider if they are or plan to become pregnant during the therapy.

Sertraline hydrochloride

Zoloft

Indications

• Depression

- Obsessive-compulsive disorder
- Panic disorder

Adverse reactions

CNS: headache, tremor, dizziness, insomnia, somnolence, paresthesia, hypoesthesia, fatigue, nervousness, anxiety, agitation, hypertonia, twitching, confusion
CV: palpitations, chest pain, hot flashes
GI: dry mouth, nausea, diarrhea, loose stools, dyspepsia, vomiting, constipation, thirst, flatulence, anorexia, abdominal pain, increased appetite
GU: male sexual dysfunction
Skin: rash, pruritus
Other: diaphoresis, myalgia

Special considerations

• Record mood changes. Monitor the patient for suicidal tendencies and allow only a minimum supply of the drug.
• Patients should use caution when performing hazardous tasks that require alertness.
• Patients should avoid alcohol and notify the primary care provider before taking over-the-counter drugs.

Trazodone hydrochloride

Desyrel, Trazon, Trialodine

Indications

• Depression

Adverse reactions

CNS: drowsiness, dizziness, nervousness, fatigue, confusion, tremor, weakness, hostility, anger, nightmares, vivid dreams, headache, insomnia
CV: orthostatic hypotension, tachycardia, hypertension, syncope, shortness of breath
EENT: blurred vision, tinnitus, nasal congestion
GI: dry mouth, dysgeusia, constipation, nausea, vomiting, anorexia

GU: urine retention, priapism (possibly leading to impotence), decreased libido, hematuria
Hematologic: anemia
Skin: rash, urticaria
Other: diaphoresis

Special considerations

• Record mood changes. Monitor the patient for suicidal tendencies and allow only a minimum supply of the drug.
• Patients should avoid activities that require alertness and good psychomotor coordination until the drug's central nervous system effects are known. Drowsiness and dizziness usually subside after the first few weeks.
• Caregivers should know how to recognize the signs of suicidal tendency or suicidal ideation.

Valproate sodium

Depakene, Depacon

Valproic acid

Depakene

Divalproex sodium

Depakote, Depakote Sprinkle, Epival

Indications

• Simple and complex absence seizures
• Mixed seizure types (including absence seizures)
• Mania
• Prophylaxis for migraine headache (Depakote only)
• Complex partial seizures

Adverse reactions

Note: Because the drug usually is used in combination with other anticonvulsants, the adverse reactions reported may not be caused by valproic acid alone.

CNS: sedation, emotional upset, depression, psychosis, aggressiveness, hyperactivity, behavioral deterioration, muscle weakness, tremor, ataxia, headache, dizziness, incoordination

EENT: nystagmus, diplopia

GI: nausea, vomiting, indigestion, diarrhea, abdominal cramps, constipation, increased appetite and weight gain, anorexia, pancreatitis. (*Note:* A lower incidence of GI effects occurs with divalproex sodium.)

Hematologic: thrombocytopenia, increased bleeding time, petechiae, bruising, eosinophilia, hemorrhage, leukopenia, bone marrow suppression

Hepatic: elevated liver enzymes, toxic hepatitis

Skin: rash, alopecia, pruritus, photosensitivity, erythema multiforme

Special considerations

• Never withdraw the drug suddenly because this may worsen seizures. Call the primary care provider immediately if adverse reactions develop.

• Be aware that serious or fatal hepatotoxicity may follow nonspecific symptoms, such as malaise, fever, and lethargy. Notify the primary care provider immediately because the drug will need to be discontinued in the presence of suspected or apparent substantial hepatic dysfunction.

• Patients at high risk for hepatotoxicity include those with congenital metabolic disorders, mental retardation, or organic brain disease; those taking multiple anticonvulsants; and children under age 2.

• Patients being treated for conditions unrelated to epilepsy should be identified as potentially at risk for a seizure during the therapy session.

• If ataxic adverse effects persist, coordination exercises may also help resolve this problem.

• In the presence of skin conditions (dermatitis or rashes), discontinue therapeutic modalities that might exacerbate these conditions.

• Some patients may benefit from a quiet setting (no noise or lights) if seizures are exacerbated by environmental stimuli.

• Avoid driving and other potentially hazardous activities that require mental alertness until the drug's central nervous system effects are known.

Zolpidem tartrate

Ambien

Indications

• Short-term management of insomnia

Adverse reactions

CNS: daytime drowsiness, light-headedness, abnormal dreams, amnesia, dizziness, headache, hangover, sleep disorder, lethargy, depression

CV: palpitations

EENT: sinusitis, pharyngitis, dry mouth

GI: nausea, vomiting, diarrhea, dyspepsia, constipation, abdominal pain.

Skin: rash

Other: back or chest pain, flulike symptoms, hypersensitivity reactions, myalgia, arthralgia

Special considerations

• Be aware that hypnotics should be used only for short-term management of insomnia (usually 7 to 10 days).

• The smallest effective dose should be used in all patients.

• Take precautions to prevent hoarding or self-overdosing by patients who are drug-dependent, depressed, or suicidal or who have a history of drug abuse.

• Patient should avoid alcohol.

• Patients should avoid performing activities that require mental alertness or physical coordination.

Pain medications

Codeine phosphate

Paveral

Codeine sulfate

Indications
- Mild to moderate pain
- Nonproductive cough

Adverse reactions
CNS: sedation, clouded sensorium, euphoria, dizziness, light-headedness
CV: hypotension, bradycardia
GI: nausea, vomiting, constipation, dry mouth, ileus
GU: urine retention
Respiratory: respiratory depression
Skin: pruritus, flushing, diaphoresis
Other: physical dependence

Special considerations
- Codeine and aspirin or acetaminophen are often prescribed together to provide enhanced pain relief.
- Monitor respiratory and circulatory status. Be aware that respiratory response to exercise may be blunted.
- In patients being weaned off opioid drugs, muscles aches and pains may occur. To ease symptoms, try physical agents (such as heat or electrotherapy) and manual techniques (such as massage and relaxation techniques).
- To minimize GI distress caused by oral administration, patients should take this drug with milk or meals.
- Patients should ask for or take the drug before pain is intense.
- Ambulatory patients should use caution when getting out of bed or walking. Outpatients should avoid driving and other potentially hazardous activities that require mental alertness until the drug's central nervous system effects are known.
- Patients should avoid alcohol while taking the drug.

Ibuprofen

Advil, Apo-Ibuprofen, Bayer Select Pain Relief Formula, Children's Advil, Children's Motrin, Excedrin IB Caplets and Tablets, Genpril Caplets and Tablets, Haltran, Ibuprin, Ibuprohm Caplets and Tablets, Ibu-Tab, Medipren, Medipren Caplets, Menadol, Midol IB, Motrin, Motrin-IB Caplets and Tablets, Novo-Profen, Nuprin Caplets and Tablets, Pamprin-IB, Pedia Profen, Rufen, Saleto-200, Saleto-400, Saleto-600, Saleto-800, Trendar

Indications
- Rheumatoid arthritis
- Osteoarthritis
- Arthritis
- Mild to moderate pain
- Dysmenorrhea
- Fever
- Juvenile arthritis

Adverse reactions
CNS: headache, dizziness, nervousness, aseptic meningitis
CV: peripheral edema, fluid retention, edema
EENT: tinnitus
GI: epigastric distress, nausea, occult blood loss, peptic ulceration, diarrhea, constipation, dyspepsia, flatulence, heartburn, decreased appetite
GU: acute renal failure, azotemia, cystitis, hematuria
Hematologic: prolonged bleeding time, anemia, neutropenia, pancytopenia, thrombocytopenia, aplastic anemia, leukopenia, agranulocytosis
Hepatic: elevated enzymes
Respiratory: bronchospasm
Skin: pruritus, rash, urticaria, Stevens-Johnson syndrome

Special considerations

• Be aware that because of their anti-inflammatory and antipyretic actions, nonsteroidal anti-inflammatory drugs (NSAIDs) may mask the signs and symptoms of infection.

• Know that blurred or diminished vision and changes in color vision have occurred.

• To reduce adverse GI reactions, patients should take the drug with meals or milk.

• The drug is available over the counter in several brands (200 mg). Patients shouldn't exceed 1.2 g daily or self-medicate for extended periods without consulting the primary care provider. The drug also shouldn't be given to patients under age 12.

• The full therapeutic effect for arthritis may be delayed 2 to 4 weeks. Although the analgesic effect occurs at low dosage levels, the anti inflammatory effect doesn't occur at dosages below 400 mg four times per day.

• Concomitant use with aspirin, alcohol, or corticosteroids may increase the risk of GI adverse reactions.

• Serious GI toxicity, including peptic ulceration and bleeding, can occur in patients taking NSAIDs even if they have no GI symptoms. Patients should be aware of signs and symptoms of GI bleeding and the need to notify the primary care provider immediately if these signs and symptoms occur.

• Patients should avoid hazardous activities that require mental alertness until the drug's central nervous system effects are known.

• The drug may cause a photosensitivity reaction; patients should wear sunscreen.

Indomethacin

Apo-Indomethacin, Indochron E-R, Indocid SR, Indocin, Indocin SR, Novo-Methacin

Indomethacin sodium trihydrate

Apo-indomethacin, Indocid PDA, Indocin I.V., Novo-Methacin

Indications

• Moderate to severe rheumatoid arthritis or osteoarthritis
• Ankylosing spondylitis
• Acute gouty arthritis
• Acute painful shoulders (bursitis or tendinitis)
• To close a hemodynamically significant patent ductus arteriosus in premature infants (I.V. form only)

Adverse reactions
Oral and rectal forms

CNS: headache, dizziness, depression, drowsiness, confusion, somnolence, fatigue, peripheral neuropathy, seizures, psychic disturbances, syncope, vertigo
CV: hypertension, edema, heart failure
EENT: blurred vision, corneal and retinal damage, hearing loss, tinnitus
GI: nausea, anorexia, diarrhea, peptic ulceration, GI bleeding, constipation, dyspepsia, pancreatitis
GU: hematuria, acute renal failure
Hematologic: hemolytic anemia, aplastic anemia, agranulocytosis, leukopenia, thrombocytopenic purpura, iron deficiency anemia
Skin: pruritus, urticaria, Stevens-Johnson syndrome
Other: hypersensitivity (rash, respiratory distress, anaphylaxis, angioedema), hyperkalemia
I.V. form
GU: renal failure, hematuria, proteinuria, interstitial nephritis

Special considerations

• The drug causes sodium retention; monitor for weight gain (especially in elderly patients) and increased blood pressure in patients with hypertension.

• Because of their anti-inflammatory and antipyretic actions, nonsteroidal anti-inflammatory drugs (NSAIDs) may mask the signs and symptoms of infection.

• Concomitant use of an oral form with aspirin, alcohol, or corticosteroids may increase the risk of adverse GI reactions.

• Serious GI toxicity, including peptic ulceration and bleeding, can occur in patients taking oral NSAIDs despite the absence of GI symptoms. Patients should be aware of the signs and symptoms of GI bleeding and should notify the primary care provider immediately if these signs and symptoms occur.

• Patients should avoid hazardous activities that require mental alertness until the drug's central nervous system effects are known.

• Patients need to notify the primary care provider immediately if visual or hearing changes occur. Patients on long-term oral therapy should have regular eye examinations, hearing tests, complete blood counts, and renal function tests to monitor for toxicity.

Morphine hydrochloride

Morphitec, M.O.S., M.O.S.-S.R.

Morphine sulfate

Astramorph PF, Duramorph, Epimorph, Infumorph 200, Infumorph 500, Morphine H.P, MS Contin, MSIR, MS/L, OMS Concentrate, Oramorph SR, RMS Uniserts, Roxanol, Roxanol 100, Roxanol Rescudose, Roxanol SR, Roxanol UD, Statex

Indications
• Severe pain

Adverse reactions
CNS: sedation, somnolence, clouded sensorium, euphoria, seizures (with large doses), dizziness, nightmares (with long-acting oral forms), lightheadedness, hallucinations, nervousness, depression, syncope
CV: hypotension, bradycardia, shock, cardiac arrest, tachycardia, hypertension
GI: nausea, vomiting, constipation, ileus, dry mouth, biliary tract spasms, anorexia
GU: urine retention, decreased libido
Hematologic: thrombocytopenia
Respiratory: respiratory depression, apnea, respiratory arrest
Skin: pruritus and skin flushing (with epidural administration), diaphoresis, edema
Other: physical dependence

Special considerations
• Keep narcotic antagonists (naloxone) and resuscitation equipment available.
• When the drug is used postoperatively, the patient should turn, cough, and deep breathe and use an incentive spirometer to prevent atelectasis.
• Ambulatory patients should be cautious when getting out of bed or walking. Outpatients should avoid driving and other potentially hazardous activities that require mental alertness until the drug's central nervous system effects are known.
• Patients should avoid alcohol while taking the drug.
For postanesthesia patients:
• Muscle weakness may occur for a variable amount of time.
• Early mobilization of patients is important to prevent the pooling of mucus, which may lead to respiratory infections and atelectasis.
• Breathing exercises and postural drainage should be implemented as needed.

For acute pain relief and chronic analgesia:

• Schedule therapy when the drugs reach their peak effects.

• These drugs may produce respiratory depression or respiratory blunting to exercise.

• Muscle aches and pains may be caused by these drugs in patients who are being weaned off opioid drugs. To ease symptoms, try physical agents (such as heat and electrotherapy) and manual techniques (such as massage and relaxation techniques).

For patient-controlled analgesia (PCA):

• Monitor signs and symptoms.

• Use the Visual Analog Scale to routinely assess pain in patients receiving PCA.

• An unexplained increase in pain may be due to a PCA system that is underdelivering the analgesic drug.

• Respiratory depression or excessive sedation may be due to a PCA system that is overdosing the patient.

Naproxen

Apo-Naproxen, Naprosyn, Naprosyn-E, EC-Naprosyn, Naprosyn-SR, Naxen, Novo-Naprox, Nu-Naprox

Naproxen sodium

Aleve, Anaprox, Anaprox DS, Apo-Napro-Na, Naprelan, Novo-Naprox Sodium, Synflex

Indications
• Rheumatoid arthritis
• Osteoarthritis
• Ankylosing spondylitis
• Pain
• Dysmenorrhea
• Tendinitis
• Bursitis
• Juvenile arthritis
• Acute gout
• Mild to moderate pain
• Primary dysmenorrhea

Adverse reactions
CNS: headache, drowsiness, dizziness, vertigo
CV: edema, palpitations
EENT: visual disturbances, tinnitus, auditory disturbances
GI: epigastric distress, occult blood loss, nausea, peptic ulceration, constipation, dyspepsia, heartburn, diarrhea, stomatitis, thirst
GU: acute renal failure
Hematologic: thrombocytopenia, eosinophilia, agranulocytosis, neutropenia
Hepatic: elevated liver enzyme levels
Respiratory: dyspnea
Skin: pruritus, rash, urticaria, ecchymosis, diaphoresis, purpura
blood urea nitrogen, and serum

Special considerations
• Because nonsteroidal anti-inflammatory drugs (NSAIDs) impair the synthesis of renal prostaglandins, they can decrease renal blood flow and lead to reversible renal impairment, especially in patients with preexisting renal failure, liver dysfunction, or heart failure; in elderly patients; and in those taking diuretics. Monitor these patients closely during therapy.

• Be aware that because of their antipyretic and anti-inflammatory actions, NSAIDs may mask the signs and symptoms of infection.

• The drug is available over the counter (naproxen sodium, 200 mg). Patients shouldn't exceed 600 mg in 24 hours. Dosage in patients over age 65 shouldn't exceed 400 mg/day.

• Patients should take the drug with food or milk to minimize GI upset. A full glass of water or other liquid should also be taken with each dose.

• Serious GI toxicity, including peptic ulceration and bleeding, can occur in patients taking NSAIDs even if GI symptoms are absent. Patients should know the signs and symptoms of GI bleeding and notify the primary care provider immediately if they occur..

• Concomitant use with aspirin, alcohol, or corticosteroids may increase the risk of adverse GI reactions.

• Patients taking prescription doses of naproxen for arthritis should be aware that the full therapeutic effect may be delayed 2 to 4 weeks.

• Patients shouldn't take both naproxen and naproxen sodium at the same time because both circulate in the blood as the naproxen anion.

• Patients should avoid hazardous activities that require mental alertness until the drug's central nervous system effects are known.

Oxycodone hydrochloride

OxyContin, Oxy IR, Roxicodone, Roxicodone Intensol, Supeudol

Indications
• Moderate to severe pain

Adverse reactions
CNS: sedation, somnolence, clouded sensorium, euphoria, dizziness, light-headedness
CV: hypotension, bradycardia
GI: nausea, vomiting, constipation, ileus
GU: urine retention
Respiratory: respiratory depression.
Skin: diaphoresis, pruritus
Other: physical dependence

Special considerations
• Monitor the patient's circulatory and respiratory statuses. Withhold dose and notify the primary care provider if respirations are shallow or if the respiratory rate falls below 12 breaths/minute.

• Schedule therapy when the drugs reach their peak effects.

• The patient's respiratory response to exercise may be blunted.

• Patients should ask for the drug before pain is intense.

• Patients should take the drug with milk or after eating.

• Ambulatory patients should use caution when getting out of bed or walking. Outpatients should avoid driving and other potentially hazardous activities that require mental alertness until the drug's central nervous system effects are known.

• Patients should avoid alcohol while taking the drug.

Propoxyphene hydrochloride

Darvon, Dolene, Novopropoxyn

Propoxyphene napsylate

Darvon-N

Indications
• Mild to moderate pain

Adverse reactions
CNS: dizziness, headache, sedation, euphoria, light-headedness, weakness, hallucinations
GI: nausea, vomiting, constipation, abdominal pain
Respiratory: respiratory depression
Other: psychological and physical dependence, abnormal liver function

Special considerations
• The drug is considered a mild narcotic analgesic, but pain relief is equivalent to that provided by aspirin. Tolerance and physical dependence may occur. It may be used with aspirin or acetaminophen to maximize analgesia.

• Smokers may need an increased dosage because smoking may reduce levels of the liver enzymes responsible for metabolizing the drug.

• Respiratory response to exercise may be blunted.

• In patients being weaned off opioid drugs, muscle aches and pains may occur. To ease symptoms, try physical agents (such as heat and electrotherapy) and manual techniques (such as massage and relaxation techniques).

• To reduce GI upset, patients should take the drug with food or milk.

• Patients shouldn't exceed the recommended dosage or use with alcohol or other central nervous system (CNS) depressants. Respiratory depression, hypotension, profound sedation, and coma may result.

• Ambulatory patients should use caution when rising or walking. Outpatients should avoid driving and other hazardous activities that require mental alertness until the drug's CNS effects are known.

Tramadol hydrochloride

Ultram

Indications

• Moderate to moderately severe pain

Adverse reactions

CNS: dizziness, vertigo, headache, somnolence, central nervous system (CNS) stimulation, asthenia, anxiety, confusion, coordination disturbance, euphoria, nervousness, sleep disorder, seizures

CV: vasodilation

EENT: visual disturbances

GI: nausea, constipation, vomiting, dyspepsia, dry mouth, diarrhea, abdominal pain, anorexia, flatulence

GU: urine retention, urinary frequency, menopausal symptoms

Respiratory: respiratory depression

Skin: pruritus, diaphoresis, rash

Other: malaise, hypertonia

Special considerations

• Monitor the patient's cardiovascular and respiratory status. Withhold the dose and notify the primary care provider if respirations decrease or the rate is below 12 breaths/minute.

• Monitor bowel and bladder function. Anticipate the need for a laxative.

• For better analgesic effect, give the drug before the onset of intense pain.

• Monitor the patient at risk for seizures. The drug may reduce the seizure threshold.

• Monitor the patient for drug dependence. This drug can produce dependence similar to that of codeine or dextropropoxyphene.

• The patient's respiratory response to exercise may be blunted.

• In patients being weaned off opioid drugs, muscle aches and pains may occur. To ease symptoms, try physical agents (such as heat and electrotherapy) and manual techniques (such as massage and relaxation techniques).

• Patients should take the drug as prescribed and not increase the dosage or dosage interval unless ordered by the primary care provider.

• Ambulatory patients should use caution when rising and walking. Outpatients should avoid driving and other potentially hazardous activities that require mental alertness until the drug's CNS effects are known.

• Patients need to check with the primary care provider before taking over-the-counter medications; drug interactions can occur.

Respiratory medications

Cetirizine hydrochloride

Zyrtec

Indications

• Seasonal allergic rhinitis

- Perennial allergic rhinitis
- Chronic urticaria

Adverse reactions
CNS: somnolence, fatigue, dizziness
EENT: pharyngitis
GI: dry mouth

Special considerations
- The safety of the drug hasn't been established in children under age 12.
- Patients shouldn't drive or perform hazardous activities if experiencing somnolence, a common reaction.
- Patients shouldn't use alcohol or other central nervous system (CNS) depressants while taking the drug.
- Patients should avoid driving and other activities that require alertness until the drug's CNS effects are known.
- Coffee or tea may reduce drowsiness.
- Sugarless gum; sugarless, sour hard candy; or ice chips may help relieve dry mouth.

Diphenhydramine hydrochloride

Benadryl, Benadryl Allergy, Benylin, Compoz, Diphen AF, Diphen Cough, Diphenadryl, Hydramine, Insomnal, Nervine Nighttime Sleep-Aid, Nytol with DPH, Sleep-Eze 3, Sominex, Tusstat, Twilite

Indications
- Rhinitis
- Allergy symptoms
- Motion sickness
- Parkinson's disease
- Sedation
- Nighttime sleep aid
- Nonproductive cough

Adverse reactions
CNS: drowsiness, confusion, insomnia, headache, vertigo sedation, sleepiness, dizziness, incoordination, fatigue, restlessness, tremor, nervousness, seizures
CV: Palpitation, hypotension, tachycardia
EENT: diplopia, blurred vision, nasal congestion, tinnitus
GI: nausea, vomiting, diarrhea, dry mouth, constipation, epigastric distress, anorexia
GU: dysuria, urine retention, urinary frequency
Hematologic: hemolytic anemia, thrombocytopenia, agranulocytosis
Respiratory: thickening of bronchial secretions
Skin: urticaria, photosensitivity, rash
Other: anaphylactic shock

Special considerations
- Use with extreme caution in patients with angle-closure glaucoma, prostatic hyperplasia, pyloroduodenal and bladder-neck obstruction, asthma or chronic obstructive pulmonary disease, increased intraocular pressure, hyperthyroidism, cardiovascular disease, hypertension, and stenosing peptic ulcer.
- Schedule therapy when the peak effects of the drug occur (preferably after the breakfast dose) for maximum efficacy and low fatigue levels.
- Monitor blood pressure. Orthostatic hypotension may precipitate falls.
- Patients should take the drug 30 minutes before travel to prevent motion sickness.
- Patients should take the drug with food or milk to reduce GI distress.
- Patients should avoid alcohol and driving or other activities that require alertness until the drug's central nervous system effects are known.
- Coffee or tea may reduce drowsiness but patients should use them cautiously if palpitations develop.
- Sugarless gum; sugarless, sour hard candy; or ice chips help to relieve dry mouth.
- Patients should use sunblock because of the possibility of photosensitivity reactions.

Appendix A:
Guide to skeletal muscles

This chart names the muscles of each part of the body, along with their points of origin and insertion.

Muscle and innervation	Origin	Insertion
Muscles of the head and neck		
Muscles of the face		
Buccinator • Buccal branches of the facial nerves	• Mandible (alveolar process) • Maxillary bone	• Orbicularis oris • Skin at mouth angle
Corrugator supercilii • Temporal and zygomatic branches of the facial nerve	• Frontal bone	• Skin of eyebrow
Depressor anguli oris • Mandibular and buccal branches of the facial nerve	• Mandible (below mental foramen)	• Skin and muscles at mouth angle
Depressor labii inferioris • Mandibular and buccal branches of the facial nerve	• Mandible (between symphysis and mental foramen)	• Skin and muscles of lower lip
Epicranius frontalis • Cranial nerve VII	• Aponeurotic structure of scalp	• Skin and muscles of forehead
Epicranius occipitalis • Cranial nerve VII	• Occiptal bone	• Aponeurotic structure of scalp
Levator labii superioris • Buccal branches of the facial nerve	• Eye orbit (lower margin)	• Skin and muscles of upper lip • Wing of nose
Mentalis • Mandibular and buccal branches of the facial nerve	• Mandible (near symphysis)	• Skin of chin
Orbicularis oculi • Temporal and zygomatic branches of the facial nerve	• Frontal and maxillary bones • Medial palpebral ligament	• Skin around eye and eyelids
Orbicularis oris • Mandibular and buccal branches of the facial nerve	• Muscles surrounding mouth	• Skin surrounding mouth
Platysma • Cervical branch of the facial nerve	• Fascia over pectoralis major and deltoid muscles	• Mandible (lower border) • Skin of cheek and neck

Muscle and innervation	Origin	Insertion
Muscles of the head and neck (continued)		

Muscles of the face (continued)

Procerus • Buccal branches of the facial nerve	• Nasal bone (lower portion) • Lateral nasal cartilage (upper part)	• Skin between eyebrows
Risorius • Mandibular and buccal branches of the facial nerve	• Fascia of masseter muscle	• Skin at mouth angle
Zygomaticus major • Buccal branches of the facial nerve	• Zygomatic bone	• Skin and muscles above mouth angle
Zygomaticus minor • Buccal branches of the facial nerve	• Zygomatic bone	• Skin and muscles above mouth angle

Muscles of mastication

Lateral pterygoid • Lateral pterygoid nerve of the mandibular division of the trigeminal nerve	• Lateral pterygoid plate (lateral surface) • Sphenoid bone (great wing)	• Mandible (just below condyle)
Masseter • Masseteric branch of the mandibular division of the trigeminal nerve	• Zygomatic arch	• Mandible (angle and ramus)
Medial pterygoid • Medial pterygoid branch of the mandibular division of the trigeminal nerve	• Sphenoid bone (lateral pterygoid plate)	• Mandible (inner surface)
Temporalis • Anterior and posterior deep temporal nerves of the mandibular division of the trigeminal nerve	• Temporal fossa	• Mandible (coronoid process and ramus)

Extrinsic muscles of the tongue

Genioglossus • Hyoglossal nerve	• Mandible (internal surface)	• Near symphysis
Hyoglossus • Hyoglossal nerve	• Hyoid bone (body and greater projection)	• Tongue (sides)
Styloglossus • Hyoglossal nerve	• Temporal bone (styloid process)	• Tongue (sides)

Muscle and innervation	Origin	Insertion
Muscles of the head and neck (continued)		

Muscles of the neck

Muscle and innervation	Origin	Insertion
Digastric • Trigeminal nerve	• Mandible (lower border) • Temporal bone (mastoid notch)	• Intermediate tendon on hyoid bone
Geniohyoid • Branch of the first cervical nerve via the hyoglossal nerve	• Mandibular symphysis (inner surface)	• Hyoid bone
Mylohyoid • Mylohyoid nerve of the mandibular division of the trigeminal nerve	• Mandible (inner surface, from symphysis to angle)	• Hyoid bone
Omohyoid • Ansa cervicalis containing fibers from C1 to C3	• Scapula (superior border)	• Hyoid bone
Sternocleidomastoid • Spinal part of the accesory nerve	• Sternum (manubrium) • Clavicle (medial portion)	• Temporal bone (mastoid process)
Sternohyoid • Branches of ansa cervicalis hyoglossi, including fibers from C1 to C3	• Clavicle (manubrium and medial end)	• Hyoid bone
Sternothyoid • Branches of ansa cervicalis hyoglossi, inculding fibers from C1 to C3	• Manubrium	• Larynx (thyroid cartilage)
Stylohyoid • Facial nerve	• Temporal bone (styloid process)	• Hyoid bone
Thyrohyoid • Fibers from C1	• Larynx (thyroid cartilage)	• Hyoid bone

Muscles of the vertebral column

Muscle and innervation	Origin	Insertion
Interspinales • Dorsal primary divisions of the spinal nerves	• Vertebrae (superior surfaces of all spinous processes)	• Next superior vertebra (inferior surface of spinous process)
Intertransversarii • Anterior, lateral, and posterior branches of the ventral primary divisions of the spinal nerves	• Vertebrae (transverse processes)	• Next superior vertebra (transverse process)

Muscle and innervation	Origin	Insertion
Muscles of the head and neck (continued)		

Muscles of the vertebral column (continued)

Muscle and innervation	Origin	Insertion
Multifidi • Dorsal primary divisions of the spinal nerves	• Ilium and sacrum (posterior surface) • Vertebrae (transverse processes of lumbar, thoracic, and lower cervical)	• Vertebrae (spinous processes of lumbar, thoracic, and cervical)
Rotatores • Dorsal primary divisions of the spinal nerves	• Vertebrae (transverse processes)	• Next superior vertebra (base of spinous process)
Scalenus anterior Scalenus medius Scalenus posterior • C5 to C8	• Cervical vertebrae (transverse processes)	• Ribs (first and second)
Semispinalis capitis Semispinalis cervicis Semispinalis thoracis • Dorsal primary divisions of spinal nerves	• Vertebrae (transverse processes of all thoracic and seventh cervical)	• Vertebrae (spinous processes of second cervical through fourth thoracic) • Occipital bone
Splenius capitis Splenius cervicis • Dorsal primary divisions of the middle cervical roots • Dorsal primary divisions of the lower cervical roots	• Vertebrae spinous processes of upper thoracic and seventh cervical, from ligamentum nuchae	• Occipital bone • Temporal bone (mastoid process) • Vertebrae (transverse processes of upper three cervical)

Erector spine group

Muscle and innervation	Origin	Insertion
Iliocostalis cervicis Iliocostalis lumborum Iliocostalis thoracis • Dorsal primary divisions of the spinal nerves	• Sacrum (crest) • Vertebrae (spinous processes of lumbar and lower thoracic) • Iliac crests • Rib angles	• Rib angles • Vertebrae (transverse processes of cervical)
Longissimus capitis Longissimus cervicis Longissimus thoracis • Dorsal primary divisions of the spinal nerves	• Vertebrae (transverse processes of lumbar, thoracic, and lower thoracic)	• Next superior vertebra (transverse process) • Temporal bone (mastoid process)

Muscle and innervation	Origin	Insertion
Muscles of the head and neck (continued)		

Erector spine group (continued)

Muscle and innervation	Origin	Insertion
Spinalis cervicis Spinalis thoracis • Dorsal primary divisions of the spinal nerves	• Vertebrae (spinous process of upper lumbar, lower thoracic, and seventh cervical)	• Vertebrae (spinous processes of upper thoracic and cervical)

Muscles of respiration

Muscle and innervation	Origin	Insertion
Diaphragm • Phrenic nerve C3 to C5	• Rib cage (inferior border) • Xiphoid process • Costal cartilages • Vertebrae (lumbar)	• Central tendon of diaphragm
Intercostales externi • Intercostal nerves	• Ribs (inferior border) • Costal cartilages	• Next inferior rib (superior border)
Intercostales interni • Intercostal nerves	• Ribs (inner surface) • Costal cartilages	• Next inferior rib (superior border)
Subcostales • Intercostal nerves	• Ribs (inner surface, near angles)	• Second or third inferior rib (inner surface)
Transversus thoracis • Intercostal nerves	• Sternum (inner surface)	• Costal cartilages (inner surface)

Muscles of the shoulder

Muscle and innervation	Origin	Insertion
Levator scapulae • C3 to C4 and frequently the dorsal scapular nerve, C5	• Vertebrae (transverse processes of upper four cervical)	• Scapula (vertebral border, above spine)
Pectoralis minor • Medial pectoral nerve, C8 to T1	• Ribs (anterior surface of third through fifth)	• Scapula (coracoid process)
Rhomboideus major • Dorsal scapular nerve, C5	• Vertebrae (spinous processes of second through fifth thoracic)	• Scapula (vertebral border, below spine)
Rhomboideus minor • Dorsal scapular nerve, C5	• Vertebrae (spinous processes of seventh cervical and first thoracic)	• Scapula (vertebral border, at base of spine)
Serratus anterior • Long thoracic nerve, C5 to C7	• Ribs (outer surface of first nine)	• Scapula (ventral surface of vertebral border)

Muscle and innervation	Origin	Insertion
Muscles of the head and neck (continued)		
Muscles of the shoulder (continued)		
Subclavius • Nerve to subclavius, C5 to C6	• Ribs (outer surface of first)	• Clavicle (inferior surface of lateral portion)
Trapezius • Spinal part of accessory nerve	• Occipital bone • Ligamentum nuchae • Vertebrae (spinous processes of seventh cervical and all thoracic)	• Clavicle (lateral third) • Acromion process • Scapula (spine)

Muscles of the abdominopelvic cavity

Muscles that move the abdominal wall

External abdominal oblique • Intercostal nerves, T7 to T12	• Ribs (external surface of lower eight)	• Iliac crest (anterior half)
Internal abdominal oblique • Branches of the intercostal nerves from T8 to T12 and the iliohypogastric and ilioinguinal branches of L1	• Inguinal ligament • Iliac crest • Lumbodorsal fascia	• Linea alba • Pubic crest • Ribs (lower four)
Quadratus lumborum • T12 to L3 (or L4)	• Iliac crest • Iliolumbar ligament	• Rib (lower border of twelfth) • Vertebrae (transverse processes of upper lumbar)
Rectus abdominis • T7 to T12 and ilioinguinal (L1) and iliohypogastric nerves (T12 to L1)	• Pubic crest	• Xiphoid process • Ribs (costal cartilages of fifth through seventh)
Transversus abdominis • Branches of the iliohypogastric and ilioinguinal nerves, T7 to T12	• Inguinal ligament • Iliac crest • Lumbodorsal fascia • Ribs (costal cartilages of last six)	• Linea alba • Pubic crest

Muscles of the pelvic floor

Coccygeus • Pudendal plexus, including S4 to S5	• Ischium (spine) • Sacrospinous ligament	• Coccyx • Sacrum
Levator ani • Pudendal plexus, including S3 to S5	• Pubic bone (inner surface of superior ramus) • Lateral pelvic wall • Ischium (spine)	• Coccyx (inner surface)

Muscle and innervation	**Origin**	**Insertion**
Muscles of the upper extremities		

Muscles that move the arm

Muscle and innervation	Origin	Insertion
Coracobrachialis • Musculocutaneous nerve, C6 to C7	• Scapula (coracoid process)	• Humerus (medial surface of medial third)
Deltoid • Axillary nerve, C5 to C6	• Clavicle (lateral third) • Acromion process • Scapula (spine)	• Humerus (deltoid tuberosity)
Infraspinatus • Suprascapular nerve, C5 to C6	• Scapula (infraspinatus fossa)	• Humerus (greater tuberosity)
Latissimus dorsi • Thoracodorsal nerve, C6 to C8	• Verterbrae (spinous processes of lower six thoracic and all lumbar) • Sacrum • Ilium (posterior crest)	• Humerus (medial margin of intertubercular groove)
Pectoralis major • Medial and lateral nerves, C5 to T1	• Clavicle (medial half) • Sternum • Ribs (costal cartilages of upper six) • External oblique (aponeurosis)	• Humerus (greater tuberosity)
Subscapularis • Upper and lower subscapular nerves, C5 to C6	• Scapula (subscapular fossa)	• Humerus (lesser tuberosity)
Supraspinatus • Suprascapular nerve, C5	• Scapula (supraspinatus fossa)	• Humerus (greater tuberosity)
Teres major • Lower subscapular nerve, C5 to C6	• Scapula (dorsal surface of inferior angle)	• Humerus (lesser tuberosity)
Teres minor • Axillary nerve, C5	• Scapula (axillary border)	• Humerus (greater tuberosity)

Muscles that move the forearm

Muscle and innervation	Origin	Insertion
Anconeus • Radial nerve, C7 to C8	• Humerus (lateral epicondyle)	• Ulna (lateral surface, olecranon process)
Biceps brachii • Musculocutaneous nerve, C5 to C6, and radial nerve	• Long head: scapula (supraglenoid tuberosity) • Short head: scapula (coracoid process)	• Radius (tuberosity)

Muscle and innervation	Origin	Insertion
Muscles of the upper extremities (continued)		
Muscles that move the forearm (continued)		
Brachialis • Musculocutaneous nerve, C5 to C6, and radial nerve	• Humerus (anterior surface of distal half)	• Ulna (coronoid process)
Brachioradialis • Radial nerve, C7 to C8	• Humerus (lateral supracondylar ridge)	• Radius (styloid process)
Triceps brachii • Radial nerve, C7 to C8	• Long head: scapula (infraglenoid tuberosity) • Lateral head: humerus (posterior surface, above radial groove) • Medial head: humerus (posterior surface, below radial groove)	• Ulna (olecranon process)
Muscles that move the wrist, hand, and fingers		
Anterior superficial muscles		
Flexor carpi radialis • Median nerve, C6 to C7	• Humerus (medial epicondyle)	• Second and third metacarpals (ventral surface)
Flexor carpi ulnaris • Ulnar nerve, C8 to T1	• Humerus (medial epicondyle) • Olecranon process • Ulna (posterior surface of proximal two-thirds)	• Third through fifth metacarpals
Flexor digitorum superficialis • Median nerve, C7 to C8	• Humerus (medial epicondyle) • Ulna (coronoid process) • Radius (anterior surface)	• Second through fifth fingers (ventral surface of middle phalanges)
Palmaris longus • Median nerve, C6 to C7	• Humerus (medial epicondyle)	• Palmar aponeurosis
Pronator teres • Median nerve, C6 to C7	• Humerus (medial epicondyle) • Ulna (coronoid process)	• Radius (shaft, middle of lateral surface)

Muscle and innervation	Origin	Insertion
Muscles that move the wrist, hand, and fingers (continued)		

Anterior deep muscles

Muscle and innervation	Origin	Insertion
Flexor digitorum profundus • Median and ulnar nerves, C8 to T1	• Humerus (medial epicondyle and coronoid process) • Interosseus membrane • Ulna (ventral surface)	• Second through fifth fingers (distal phalanges, ventral surface of base)
Flexor pollicis longus • Median nerve, C8 to T1	• Radius (ventral surface) • Interosseous membrane	• Thumb (distal phalange, ventral surface of base)
Pronator quadratus • Median nerve, C8 to T1	• Ulna (distal ventral surface)	• Radius (distal ventral surface)

Posterior superficial muscles

Muscle and innervation	Origin	Insertion
Extensor carpi radialis brevis • Radial nerve, C6 to C7	• Humerus (lateral epicondyle)	• Third metacarpal (dorsal surface of base)
Extensor carpi radialis longus • Radial nerve, C6 to C8	• Humerus (lateral supracondylar ridge)	• Second metacarpal (dorsal surface of base)
Extensor carpi ulnaris • Radial nerve, C6 to C8	• Humerus (lateral epicondyle)	• Fifth metacarpal (base)
Extensor digiti minimi • Radial nerve, C6 to C8	• Tendon of extensor digitorum	• Fifth finger (tendon of extensor digitorum, on dorsum)
Extensor digitorum • Radial nerve, C6 to C8	• Humerus (lateral epicondyle)	• Second through fifth fingers (dorsal surface of phalanges)

Posterior deep muscles

Muscle and innervation	Origin	Insertion
Abductor pollicis longus • Radial nerve, C7	• Radius and ulna (posterior surface of middle portions) • Interosseous membrane	• First metacarpal (base)
Extensor indicis • Radial nerve, C6 to C8	• Ulna (posterior surface of distal end) • Interosseous membrane	• Second finger (tendon of extensor digitorum)

Muscle and innervation	Origin	Insertion
Muscles that move the wrist, hand, and fingers (continued)		

Posterior deep muscles (continued)

Muscle and innervation	Origin	Insertion
Extensor pollicis brevis • Radial nerve, C6 to C7	• Radius (posterior surface of middle portion)	• Thumb (base of first phalanx) • Interosseous membrane
Extensor pollicis longus • Radial nerve, C6 to C8	• Ulna (posterior surface of middle end) • Interosseous membrane	• Thumb (base of last phalanx)
Supinator • Radial nerve, C6	• Humerus (lateral epicondyle)	• Radius (proximal end, lateral surface of shaft)

Intrinsic muscles of the hand

Muscle and innervation	Origin	Insertion
Abductor digiti minimi manus • Ulnar nerve, C8 to T1	• Pisiform • Flexor carpi ulnaris (tendon)	• Fifth finger (base of proximal phalanx)
Abductor pollicis brevis • Median nerve, C8 to T1	• Flexor retinaculum • Scaphoid • Trapezium	• Thumb (proximal phalanx)
Adductor pollicis • Ulnar nerve, C8 to T1	• Capitate • Second and third metacarpals	• Fifth finger (base of proximal phalanx)
Flexor digiti minimi brevis manus • Ulnar nerve, C8 to T1	• Flexor retinaculum	• Fifth finger (base of proximal phalanx)
Flexor pollicis brevis • Superficial head: median nerve, C8 to T1; deep head: ulnar nerve, C8 to T1	• Flexor retinaculum • Trapezium • First metacarpal	• Thumb (base of proximal phalanx)
Interossei dorsales manus • Ulnar nerve, C8 to T1	• Metacarpals (adjacent sides)	• Second through fourth fingers (proximal phalanx)
Interossei palmares • Ulnar nerve, C8 to T1	• Second metacarpal (medial side) • Fourth and fifth metacarpals (lateral side)	• Same finger (proximal phalanx)

Muscle and innervation	Origin	Insertion
Muscles that move the wrist, hand, and fingers (continued)		

Intrinsic muscles of the hand (continued)

Muscle and innervation	Origin	Insertion
Lumbricales manus • First and second lumbricals by the median nerve, C8 to T1, and third and fourth lumbricals by the ulnar nerve, C8 to T1	• Tendons of flexor digitorum profundus	• Tendons of extensor digitorum
Opponens digiti minimi • Ulnar nerve, T1	• Flexor retinaculum • Hamate	• Fifth finger (metacarpal)
Opponens pollicis • Median nerve (sometimes by branch of ulnar nerve), C8 to T1	• Flexor retinaculum • Trapezium	• Thumb (metacarpal, lower border)
Palmaris brevis • Ulnar nerve, C8 to T1	• Flexor retinaculum	• Hand (skin on ulnar border)

Muscles of the lower extremities		

Muscles that move the femur (thigh)

Muscle and innervation	Origin	Insertion
Adductor brevis • Obturator nerve, L2 to L4	• Pubis (inferior ramus)	• Femur (linea aspera)
Adductor longus • Obturator nerve, L2 to L4	• Pubis (crest and symphysis)	• Femur (linea aspera)
Adductor magnus • Obturator nerve, L2 to L4, and tibial portion of the sciatic nerve, L2 to L4	• Pubis and ischium (inferior rami) • Ischial tuberosity	Femur (linea aspera, adductor tuberosity)
Gemellus inferior • Nerve to quadratus femoris, L4 to S1	• Ischial tuberosity	• Femur (greater trochanter)
Gemellus superior • Nerve to obturatorius internus, L5 to S2	• Ischial spine	• Femur (greater trochanter)
Gluteus maximus • Inferior gluteal nerve, L5 to S2	• Ilium (posterior gluteal line) • Sacrum and coccyx (posterior surfaces)	• Femur (gluteal tuberosity) • Iliotibial band
Gluteus medius • Superior gluteal nerve, L4 to S1	• Ilium (outer surface, between posterior and anterior gluteal lines)	• Femur (lateral surface of greater trochanter)
Gluteus minimus • Superior gluteal nerve, L4 to S1	• Ilium (outer surface, between anterior and inferior gluteal lines)	• Femur (anterior surface of greater trochanter)

Muscle and innervation	Origin	Insertion
Muscles of the lower extremities (continued)		
Muscles that move the femur (continued)		
Gracilis • Obturator nerve, L2 to L3	• Symphysis pubis • Pubic arch	• Tibia (medial surface, just below condyle)
Iliopsoas • Femoral and second to fourth lumbar nerves	• Psoas major: vertebrae (transverse processes and bodies of last thoracic and all lumbar) • Iliacus: iliac crest and fossa	• Femur (lesser trochanter)
Obturatorius externus • Obturator nerve, L3 to L4	• Obturator membrane (outer surface) • Obturator foramen (bony margins)	• Femur (trochanteric fossa)
Obturatorius internus • Nerve to obturatorius internus, L5 to S2	• Obturator membrane (inner surface) • Obturator foramen (bony margins)	• Femur (trochanteric fossa)
Pectineus • Femoral, obturator, or accessory obturator nerves, L2 to L4	• Pubis (superior ramus)	• Femur (posterior surface, just below lesser trochanter)
Piriformis • Sacral plexus, S1 and S2	• Sacrum (anterior surface)	• Femur (superior border of greater trochanter)
Quadratus femoris • Nerve to quadratus femoris, L4 to S1	• Ischial tuberosity	• Femur (shaft, just below greater trochanter)
Tensor fasciae latae • Superior gluteal nerve, L4 to S1	• Iliac crest (anterior portion) • Anterior superior iliac spine	• Fascia lata (iliotibial band)

Muscle and innervation	Origin	Insertion
Muscles of the lower extremities (continued)		

Anterior compartment

Quadriceps femoris • Femoral nerve, L2 to L4	• Rectus femoris: ilium (anterior inferior iliac spine) • Vastus intermedius: femur (anterior surface of shaft) • Vastus lateralis: femur (linea aspera, greater trochanter) • Vastus medialis: femur (linea aspera)	• Tibia (via patella and patellar ligament)
Sartorius • Femoral nerve, L2 to L3	• Anterior superior iliac spine	• Tibia (proximal medial surface, below tuberosity)

Hamstring group

Biceps femoris • Tibial portion of the sciatic nerve, S1 to S3 • Peroneal portion of sciatic nerve, L2 to L5	• Long head: ischial tuberosity • Short head: linea aspera	• Fibula (lateral surface of head) • Tibia (lateral condyle)
Semimembranosus • Tibial portion of the sciatic nerve, L5 to S2	• Ischial tuberosity	• Tibia (medial surface of proximal end)
Semitendinosus • Tibial portion of the sciatic nerve, L5 to S2	• Ischial tuberosity	• Tibia (medial surface of proximal end)

Muscles that move the foot and toes

Anterior compartment

Extensor digitorum longus • Deep peroneal nerve, L4 to S1	• Tibia (lateral condyle) • Fibula (proximal three-fourths of anterior surface) • Interosseous membrane	• Second through fifth toes (dorsal surface of phalanx)
Extensor hallucis longus • Deep peroneal nerve, L4 to S1	• Fibula (anterior surface of middle portion) • Interosseous membrane	• Great toe (dorsal surface of distal phalanx)
Peroneus tertius • Deep peroneal nerve, L4 to S1	• Fibula (distal one-third of anterior surface) • Interosseous membrane	• Fifth metatarsal (dorsal surface)

Muscle and innervation	Origin	Insertion
Muscles that move the foot		

Anterior compartment *(continued)*

| Tibialis anterior
• Deep peroneal nerve (cuneiform), L4 to S1 | • Tibia (lateral condyle, proximal two-thirds of shaft)
• Interosseous membrane | • Tarsal (first cuneiform)
• Metatarsal (first) |

Lateral compartment

| Peroneus brevis
• Superficial peroneal nerve, L4 to S1 | • Fibula (distal two-thirds) | • Fifth metatarsal (lateral side) |
| Peroneus longus
• Superficial peroneal nerve, L4 to S1 | • Fibula (head and upper two-thirds of shaft) | • First metatarsal
• First cuneiform |

Posterior compartment

Flexor digitorum longus • Tibial nerve, L5 to S1	• Tibia (posterior surface)	• Second through fifth toes (distal phalanges)
Flexor hallucis longus • Tibial nerve, L5 to S2	• Fibula (lower two-thirds)	• Great toe (distal phalanx)
Gastrocnemius • Tibial nerve, S1 to S2	• Femur (medial and lateral condyles)	• Calcaneus (via Achilles tendon)
Plantaris • Tibial nerve, L4 to S1	• Femur (lower surface, above lateral condyle)	• Calcaneus (via Achilles tendon)
Popliteus • Tibial nerve, L4 to S1	• Femur (lateral condyle)	• Tibia (proximal portion)
Soleus • Tibial nerve, S1 to S2	• Fibula (posterior surface of proximal one-third) • Tibia (middle one-third)	• Calcaneus (via Achilles tendon)
Tibialis posterior • Tibial nerve, L5 to S1	• Tibia (posterior surface) • Fibula (posterior surface) • Interosseous membrane (posterior surface	• Navicular bone • All three cuneiforms • Cuboid bone • Second through fourth metatarsals

Muscle and innervation	Origin	Insertion
Muscles that move the foot and toes (continued)		
Dorsal muscle		
Extensor digitorum brevis • Deep peroneal nerve, L5 to S1	• Calcaneus (lateral surface)	• Tendon of extensor digitorum longus
Plantar muscles		
Abductor digiti minimi pedis • Lateral plantar nerve, S2 to S3	• Calcaneus • Plantar aponeurosis	• Fifth toe (proximal phalanx)
Abductor hallucis • Medial plantar nerve, L5 to S1	• Calcaneus	• Great toe (proximal phalanx), with tendon of flexor hallucis brevis
Adductor hallucis • Lateral plantar nerve, S2 to S3	• Oblique head: second, third, and fourth metatarsals • Transverse head: ligaments of metatarsophalangeal joints	• Great toe (proximal phalanx)
Flexor digiti minimi brevis pedis • Lateral plantar nerve, S2 to S3	• Fifth metatarsal	• Fifth toe (proximal phalanx)
Flexor digitorum brevis • Medial plantar nerve, L5 to S1	• Calcaneus • Plantar aponeurosis	• Second through fifth toes (middle phalanges)
Flexor hallucis brevis • Medial plantar nerve, L5 to S1	• Cuboid bone • Lateral cuneiform	• Great toe (proximal phalanx)
Interossei dorsales pedis • Lateral plantar nerve, S2 to S3	• Adjacent metatarsal (bases) • Second toe (both sides) • Third and fourth toes (lateral side)	• Proximal phalanges of second, third, and fourth toes
Interossei plantares • Lateral plantar nerve, S2 to S3	• Third through fifth metatarsals	• Same toe (proximal phalanx)
Lumbricales pedis • First lumbrical by the medial plantar nerve, L5 to S1, and second through fourth lumbricals by the lateral plantar nerve, S2 to S3	• From tendons of flexor digitorum longus	• Into tendons of extensor digitorum longus
Quadratus plantae • Lateral plantar nerve, S2 to S3	• Calcaneus	• Into tendons of flexor digitorum longus

Appendix B: Understanding the Americans with Disabilities Act

The Americans with Disabilities Act (ADA) was written to eliminate discrimination against individuals with disabilities and to ensure that there are clear avenues of legal redress when such discrimination occurs. Enacted on July 26, 1990, the ADA gives civil rights protection to persons with disabilities and guarantees them equal access to employment, public services, public accommodations, and telecommunications.

The ADA defines *disability* as "A physical or mental impairment that substantially limits one or more of the major life activities of such individual; a record of such an impairment; or being regarded as having such an impairment" even if the impairment doesn't actually exist. The illegal use of drugs and sexual preference aren't considered disabilities.

The ADA is divided into five titles: employment, public services, public accommodations, telecommunications, and miscellaneous provisions.

Title I: Employment

The ADA requires that all businesses with 15 employees or more provide accommodations to protect the rights of disabled individuals in their employ. Public entities are required to do the same, regardless of size.

Businesses may not discriminate in hiring based on a person's disability. They can't ask if a person has a disability but may ask about his ability to perform certain job-related skills. A job offer may be contingent on passing a medical examination, but only if it's required of all other prospective employees.

Businesses must provide reasonable accommodations to allow disabled employees to perform their jobs fully and enjoy the benefits of their employment as long as it doesn't cause undue hardship to the business. Undue hardship may include such issues as excessive costs of remodeling or a significant change in the business's ability to function as a result of the new accommodations. Examples of reasonable accommodations include making a facility readily accessible to an employee, restructuring a job, modifying work schedules, modifying equipment to allow the person to complete the job successfully, and providing qualified readers, interpreters, or other aides and services to ensure effective communication.

Title II: Public services

Public services include any programs or services offered through state and local governments, such as public welfare agencies, a city's performing arts center, and public transportation. These services or programs must be accessible to all people, including those with disabilities. If the service isn't accessible and accommodations to that service aren't possible, other options must be available to provide equal service. An example of this would be providing paratransit services to individuals with disabilities as an alternative to other available public transportation provided by a public entity. As in Title I, if the required accommodations can be shown to cause undue financial or administrative hardship on the public entity, the entity will only be required to make those accommodations that don't cause a burden. However, the ADA requires that all new construction and all newly ordered buses and rail cars be made handicap-accessible.

Title III: Public accommodations

Public accommodations include private entities, such as doctors' offices, hospitals, restaurants, grocery stores, hotels, stores, business offices, libraries, schools, and day care centers. (Private clubs and religious buildings or organizations are excluded from the act.) The ADA requires that private entities make accommodations to allow all persons to enjoy their services. Services can't be denied to a person because they have a disability or because they're associated with someone who has a disability. If a service finds that the required changes cause excessive financial burden or that the area in question can't be made accessible, it may provide the service in a different area. The service provided, however, must be equal to the service that is offered to others.

Under the ADA, physical therapists are required to treat any patient as long as it's within their area of expertise. Therapists may not refer a patient to another facility or refuse to treat him simply because they don't feel comfortable treating that patient. For example, a patient with human immunodeficiency virus (HIV) infection who comes to an orthopedic physical therapy clinic for an orthopedic problem can't be referred elsewhere simply because the therapist

doesn't feel "equipped" to deal with an HIV-positive patient. Because no special equipment is needed to deal with this patient's orthopedic problem, it would be in violation of the ADA to refuse such treatment. If a referral is made, it must be based on the treatment the person is requesting.

Title IV: Telecommunications

The telecommunications section of the ADA covers telecommunications services and televised public service announcements. The ADA requires companies that offer telephone services to the general public to also offer an efficient communication service for hearing- or speech-impaired individuals. Telecommunications relay services enable a hearing- or speech-impaired individual using a telecommunications device for the deaf (TDD) or similar device to communicate with an unimpaired individual through the use of a relay operator. The service should operate for 24 hours every day, with confidential communication and rates equivalent to voice-based communication services.

The ADA also requires any public service announcement funded by the federal government to include closed-captioning for hearing-impaired individuals.

Title V: Miscellaneous provisions

Title V comprises various additional issues, including protection from discrimination against or intimidation of a person exercising their rights under the ADA, regulations set by the Architectural and Transportation Barriers Compliance Board, activities of Congress, technical assistance to individuals or businesses to help them understand the requirements of the ADA, and attorneys' fees.

Resources

Many resources are available for individuals and businesses inquiring about the ADA. There are 10 federally funded ADA Regional Business and Disability Technical Assistance Centers located throughout the United States to help educate and assist those interested in the ADA and the accommodations required.

The Department of Justice also offers technical assistance on standards for accessibility and other ADA provisions through their ADA Information Line for documents and questions: (800) 514-0301 (voice) or (800) 514-0383 (TDD).

The federal government also offers tax incentives to help with the cost of modifications to meet the requirements of the ADA and decrease the financial strain put on businesses and services.

Physical therapists can act as advocates for patients, educating them on the requirements of the ADA and their rights to all programs and services. If a patient voices a concern about the inaccessibility of a service,

review with them the possible modifications the service can make and encourage them to speak to the management of the service. Modifications can be as simple as removing objects in hallways to allow a wheelchair to pass, requesting a communication aid, or lowering a paper towel holder in a bathroom. Other possible modifications can include widening doorways, adding a temporary or permanent ramp or painting lines to create an accessible parking space. If such changes don't occur, the next step would be to direct the patient to a mediation service to help him deal with this discrimination. If all else fails, the patient may file a complaint with the Department of Justice, at this address:

> Disability Rights Section
> Civil Rights Division
> Department of Justice
> P.O. Box 66738
> Washington, DC 20035-6728

The ADA is another way to encourage equal rights for all Americans. The Justice Department is available to enforce the ADA in any justified complaint by encouraging voluntary compliance or taking legal action, if necessary. Any person who feels they have been discriminated against because of their disability or an association with a person who has a disability should feel free to come forward and press their complaints.

Appendix C:
English–Spanish words and phrases

Pronouns

Pronouns in Spanish are either masculine or feminine. The *you* pronoun has two forms: familiar and formal.

Singular forms

I	yo
you	tú (familiar)
you	usted (formal); abbreviated Vd. or Ud.
he	él
she	ella

Plural forms

we	nosotros (masculine)
we	nosotras (feminine)
you	vosotros (familiar, masculine)
you	vosotras (familiar, feminine)
you	ustedes (formal); abbreviated Vds. or Uds.
they	ellos (masculine)
they	ellas (feminine)

Greetings and introductions

Hello.	¡Hola!
My name is ___.	Me llamo_____.
What is your name?	¿Cómo se llama Ud.?
It's nice to meet you.	Mucho gusto en conocerle.
How are you?	¿Cómo está Ud.?
please	por favor
thank you	gracias
yes	sí
no	no
sometimes	a veces
never	nunca
always	siempre
signature	firma
good-bye	hasta luego *or* adios

Cardinal numbers

1	uno
2	dos
3	tres
4	cuatro
5	cinco
6	seis
7	siete
8	ocho
9	nueve
10	diez
11	once
12	doce
13	trece
14	catorce
15	quince
16	diez y seis *or* dieciséis
17	diez y siete *or* diecisiete
18	diez y ocho *or* dieciocho
19	diez y nueve *or* diecinueve
20	veinte

Anatomic terms

abdomen	abdomen *or* vientre
ankle	tobillo
arm	brazo
back	espalda
buttocks	nalgas
calf	pantorrilla
chest	pecho
ear	oreja
elbow	codo
eye	ojo
face	cara
finger	dedo de la mano
foot	pie
groin	ingle
hair	cabello *or* pelo

hand	mano
head	cabeza
heel	talón
hip	cadera
knee	rodilla
leg	pierna
lip	labio
mouth	boca
neck	cuello
nose	nariz
shin	espinilla de la pierna
shoulder	hombro
thigh	muslo
throat	garganta
toe	dedo del pie
tongue	lengua
wrist	muñeca

General therapies and treatments

Instructions

Instrucciones

Bend over backward.	Inclínese Ud. hacia atrás.
Bend over forward.	Inclínese Ud. hacia adelante.
Don't talk.	No hable Ud.
Lean backward.	Recuéstese Ud.
Lean forward.	Inclínese Ud. hacia adelante.
Lie down.	Acuéstese Ud.
Lie on your back.	Acuéstese Ud. boca arriba.
Lie on your side.	Acuéstese Ud. de lado.
Lie on your left side.	Acuéstese Ud. lado izquierdo.
Lie on your right side.	Acuéstese Ud. lado derecho.
Lie on your stomach.	Acuéstese Ud. boca abajo.
Roll over.	Dé Ud. una vuelta.
Sit down.	Siéntese Ud.
Sit up.	Enderécese Ud.
Stand up.	Póngase Ud. de pie.
Turn to the side.	Voltéese Ud. hacia un lado.
I'm going to take your vital signs.	Voy a tomarle a Ud. los signos vitales.

I'm going to take your blood pressure.	Voy a tomarle a Ud. la presión sanguínea.
I'm going to take your pulse.	Voy a tomarle a Ud. el pulso.
I'm going to take your respirations.	Voy a tomarle a Ud. la respiración.
I'm going to take your temperature.	Voy a tomarle a Ud. la temperatura.
Are you comfortable?	¿Está Ud. confortable?

Respiratory system / El sistema respiratorio

Do you have chest pain?	¿Tiene Ud. dolor de tórax (pecho)?
— Is it constant?	— ¿Es constante?
— Is it intermittent?	— ¿Es intermitente?
— Where is it located?	— ¿Dónde se localiza el dolor?
Do you have shortness of breath?	¿Sufre Ud. de falta de respiración?
— Is it constant?	— ¿Es constante?
— Is it intermittent?	— ¿Es intermitente?
Does position, medication, or relaxation relieve it?	— ¿Qué postura, medicamento, o descanso la alivia?

Cardiovascular system / El sistema cardiovascular

Do you exercise routinely?	¿Hace Ud. ejercicio rutinariamente?
— Which exercises do you perform?	— ¿Qué tipo de ejercicio hace?
— How often do you exercise?	— ¿Con qué frecuencia hace ejercicio?
— How intensely do you exercise?	— ¿Con qué intensidad hace el ejercicio?
— How long do you spend exercising?	— ¿Por cuánto tiempo hace Ud. ejercicio?

Miscellaneous / Misceláneo

Let me show you how to do it.	Permítame enseñarle como hacerlo.
Let's practice together.	Vamos a ensayar junto(a)s.
I want you to do it yourself.	Quiero que Ud. lo haga por sí solo(a).
I will watch to make sure you can do it correctly.	Le observaré para estar seguro(a) que Ud. lo puede hacer por sí solo(a).

Appendix D: Common abbreviations and acronyms

This list identifies abbreviations that physical therapists commonly use or see in documentation in medical charts.

≈	approximately
≅	approximately equal to
c̄	with
p̄	after, following
s̄	without
<	less than
>	greater than
ā	before
ABD	abduction
ABG	arterial blood gas
ADD	adduction
ADL	activities of daily living
AFIB	atrial fibrillation
AFO	ankle-foot orthosis
AGA	appropriate to gestational age
AMA	against medical advice
amb	ambulation
ARDS	acute respiratory distress syndrome; adult respiratory distress syndrome
ARF	acute renal failure; acute respiratory failure; acute rheumatic fever
AROM	active range of motion
ASA	acetylsalicylic acid (aspirin)
ASD	atrial septal defect
AV	arteriovenous; atrioventricular
AVM	arteriovenous malformation; atrioventricular malformation
BBB	bundle-branch block
BID, b.i.d.	twice a day
BMR	basal metabolic rate

BP	blood pressure
BPM	beats per minute
BSA	body surface area
BUN	blood urea nitrogen
C	Celsius; centigrade; certified; cervical
Ca	calcium
CABG	coronary artery bypass grafting
CAD	coronary artery disease
CAPD	continuous ambulatory peritoneal dialysis
CBC	complete blood count
CC	Caucasian child; chief complaint; common cold; creatinine clearance; critical care; critical condition
CF	cardiac failure; cystic fibrosis
CG	contact guard
CHB	complete heart block
CHD	childhood disease; congenital heart disease; congenital hip disease
CK	creatine kinase
CK-MB	MB isoenzyme of creatine kinase
CMV	continuous mandatory ventilation; cytomegalovirus
CNS	central nervous system
CO	carbon monoxide cardiac output
CO_2	carbon dioxide
COLD	chronic obstructive lung disease
cont.	continue

COPD	chronic obstructive pulmonary disease
CPAP	continuous positive airway pressure
cpm	counts per minute; cycles per minute
CS	close supervision
CSF	cerebrospinal fluid
CT	clotting time; coated tablet; compressed tablet; computed tomography; corneal transplant
CV	cardiovascular; central venous
CVA	cerebrovascular accident; costovertebral angle
CVP	central venous pressure
Cx	cancel crutch
D	dependent
D/C	discharge; discontinue
dB	decibel
DD	differential diagnosis; discharge diagnosis; dry dressing
DF	dorsiflexion
DIC	disseminated intravascular coagulation
DJD	degenerative joint disease
DKA	diabetic ketoacidosis
DNR	do not resuscitate
DOA	date of admission; dead on arrival
DOMS	delayed onset muscle soreness
DS	distant supervision; double-strength
DTR	deep tendon reflex
DVT	deep vein thrombosis
ECG	electrocardiogram
ECHO	echocardiography
ECT	electroconvulsive therapy
EEG	electroencephalogram
EENT	eyes; ears; nose; throat
EF	ejection fraction

EMG	electromyography
ERCP	endoscopic retrograde cholangiopancreatography
ERV	expiratory reserve volume
ES, e stim	electrical stimulation
ESR	erythrocyte sedimentation rate
eval.	evaluation; evaluate
ext.	extension
FEF	forced expiratory flow
FEV	forced expiratory volume
flex.	flexion
FRC	functional residual capacity
FUO	fever of undetermined origin
FVC	forced vital capacity
g, gm, GM	gram
gr	grain
GT	gait training
gtt	drops
h.s.	at bedtime
Hb	hemoglobin
Hct	hematocrit
HDL	high-density lipoprotein
HDN	hemolytic disease of the newborn
HEP	home exercise program
HF	heart failure
HHA	household activities; home health aide
HHNS	hyperosmolar hyperglycemic nonketonic syndrome
HS	half-strength; hour of sleep; house surgeon
Hz	hertz
I & D	incision and drainage
I	independent
I.V.	intravenous
IABP	intra-aortic balloon pump
IADL	instrumental activities of daily living

IC	inspiratory capacity
ICD	implantable cardioverter-defibrillator
ICF	intracellular fluid
ICP	intracranial pressure
ID	identification; initial dose; inside diameter; intradermal
IMV	intermittent mandatory ventilation
IPPB	intermittent positive-pressure breathing
IRV	inspiratory reserve volume
IU	International Unit
IVP	intravenous pyelography
IVPB	intravenous piggyback
J	joule
JVD	jugular venous distention
KAFO	knee-ankle-foot orthosis
kg	kilogram
KUB	kidney-ureter-bladder
KVO	keep vein open
L	left; liter; lumbar
LA	left atrium; long-acting
LBB	left bundle branch
LDL	low-density lipoprotein
LE	lower extremity
LLQ	left lower quadrant
LOC	level of consciousness
LR	lactated Ringer's solution
LSB	left scapular border; left sternal border
LTC	long-term care
LUQ	left upper quadrant
LV	left ventricle
m	meter
m²	square meter
MAFO	molded ankle-foot orthosis
MAO	maximal acid output; monoamine oxidase
max. A	maximum assistance

mcg, μg	microgram
MD	manic depressive; medical doctor; muscular dystrophy
mEq	milliequivalent
mg	milligram
MHz	megahertz
min. A	minimal assistance
μl	microliter
mm³	cubic millimeter
MMEF	maximal midexpiratory flow
mmol	millimole
MMT	manual muscle test
mod. A	moderate assistance
mod. I	modified independence
MS	mitral sounds; mitral stenosis; morphine sulfate; multiple sclerosis; musculoskeletal
MUGA	multiple-gated acquisition (scanning)
MVV	maximal voluntary ventilation
N/A	not applicable
N/R	not remarkable
Na	sodium
NaCl	sodium chloride
NCV	nerve conduction velocity
NG	nasogastric
NKA	no known allergies
NPO	nothing by mouth
NS, NSS	normal saline solution (0.9% sodium chloride solution)
NSAID	nonsteroidal anti-inflammatory drug
O_2 sat.	oxygen saturation
OTC	over-the-counter
P.O.	by mouth; postoperative
p.r.n.	as needed
PAC	premature atrial contraction
$Paco_2$	partial pressure of arterial carbon dioxide

Pao$_2$	partial pressure of arterial oxygen
PAT	paroxysmal atrial tachycardia
PCA	patient-controlled analgesia
PE	pelvic examination; physical examination; pulmonary embolism; pleural effusion
PEEP	positive end-expiratory pressure
PEFR	peak expiratory flow rate
per	by; through
PF	plantar flexion
PMI	point of maximum impulse
PND	paroxysmal nocturnal dyspnea; postnasal drip
PP	partial pressure; peripheral pulses; postpartum; postprandial; presenting problem
PROM	passive range of motion
PT	physical therapy; physical therapist; prothrombin time
pt.	patient
PTCA	percutaneous transluminal coronary angioplasty
PTT	partial thromboplastin time
PVC	premature ventricular contraction; polyvinylchloride
q	every
q. a.m.	every morning
q.d.	every day
q.h.	every hour
q.id.	four times daily
q.n.	every night
R	right
RA	renal artery; rheumatoid arthritis; right arm; right atrium
RBB	right bundle branch
RBC	red blood cell
RDA	recommended daily allowance
RLQ	right lower quadrant
ROM	range of motion
RPE	rating of perceived exertion
RR	respiratory rate
RUQ	right upper quadrant
RV	residual volume; right ventricle
Rx	treat; treatment
S	supervision
S.C., SQ	subcutaneous
SA	sinoatrial
SIMV	synchronized intermittent mandatory ventilation
SL, sl.	sublingual
SOB	shortness of breath
SPT	stand pivot transfer
stat	immediately
STD	sexually transmitted disease
STS	stand turn sit transfer
TC	telephone call
TENS	transcutaneous electrical nerve stimulation
TIA	transient ischemic attack
TID, t.i.d.	three times a day
TLC	total lung capacity
TMJ	temporomandibular joint
tol.	tolerate
TPN	total parenteral nutrition
TSH	thyroid-stimulating hormone
tx	transfer
UE	upper extremity
UV	ultraviolet
VAD	vascular access device; ventricular assist device
VO	verbal order
VT	tidal volume
W/C	wheelchair
WBC	white blood cell
↔	to and from
↑	up, increase
↓	down, decrease

Selected references

American College of Sports Medicine. *ACSM's Guidelines for Exercise Testing and Prescription,* 5th ed. Philadelphia: Lippincott Williams & Wilkins, 1995.

Blackburn, J.R., and Morrissey, M.C., "The Relationship Between Open and Closed Kinetic Chain Strength of the Lower Limb and Jumping Performance," *Journal of Orthopedic & Sports Physical Therapy* 27(6): 430-35, June 1998.

Campbell, S.K. *Physical Therapy for Children.* Philadelphia: W.B. Saunders Co., 1994.

ECG Cards, 3rd ed. Springhouse, Pa.: Springhouse Corp., 2000.

Fauci, A.S., et al., eds. *Harrison's Principles of Internal Medicine,* 14th ed. New York: McGraw-Hill Book Co., 1998.

Guide to Physical Therapy Practice. Alexandria, Va.: American Physical Therapy Association, 1999.

Guidelines for Cardiac Rehabilitation and Secondary Prevention Programs, 3rd ed. Champaign, Ill.: Human Kinetics, 1999.

Illustrated Guide to Diagnostic Tests, 2nd ed. Springhouse, Pa.: Springhouse Corp., 1998.

Jette, A. "Using Health-Related Quality of Life Measures in Physical Therapy Outcomes Research," *Physical Therapy* 73(8):528-37, August 1993.

Kisner, C., and Colby, L.A. *Therapeutic Exercise Foundations and Techniques,* 3rd ed. Philadelphia: F.A. Davis Co., 1996.

Lewis, C.B., and Bottomley, J.M. *Geriatric Physical Therapy: A Clinical Approach.* Stamford, Conn.: Appleton & Lange, 1994.

Lusardi, M.M., and Nielsen, C. *Orthotics and Prosthetics in Rehabilitation.* Newton,

Mass.: Butterworth-Heinemann Medical, Ltd., 1999.

Palmer, M.L., and Epler, M.E. *Fundamentals of Musculoskeletal Assessment Techniques,* 2nd ed. Philadelphia: Lippincott Williams & Wilkins, 1998.

Professional Guide to Diseases, 6th ed. Springhouse, Pa.: Springhouse Corp., 1998.

Professional Guide to Signs and Symptoms, 2nd ed. Springhouse, Pa.: Springhouse Corp., 1997.

Rothstein, J.M., et al. *The Rehabilitation Specialist's Handbook,* 2nd ed. Philadelphia: F.A. Davis Co., 1998.

Schurr, D., and Cook, T. *Prosthetics and Orthotics.* Stamford, Conn.: Appleton & Lange, 1990.

Shumway-Cook, A., et al. "Predicting the Probability for Falls in Community Dwelling Older Adults," *Physical Therapy* 77(8):812-19, August 1997.

Tan, J. *Practical Manual of Physical Medicine and Rehabilitation.* St. Louis: Mosby–Year Book, Inc., 1998.

Tierney, L.M., et al. *Current Medical Diagnosis and Treatment,* 38th ed. Stamford, Conn.: Appleton & Lange, 1999.

Wenger, N.K., et al. *Cardiac Rehabilitation. Clinical Practice Guideline No. 17.* Rockville, Md.: U.S. Department of Health and Human Services, Public Health Service, Agency for Health Care Policy and Research, and the National Heart, Lung, and Blood Institute. AHCPR Publication No. 96-0672, October 1995.

Index

t refers to a table; i refers to an illustration.

t refers to a table; i refers to an illustration.

t refers to a table; i refers to an illustration.